Springer Series on Advanced Practice Nursing

Terry T. Fulmer, PhD, RN, FAAN, Series Editor
New York University School of Nursing

Advisory Board: Susan J. Kelley, RN, PhD, FAAN; Ann L. Horgas, RN, PhD; Dorothy D. Rentschler, PhD, MA, BSN, RN; Dorothy A. Jones, EdD, RNC, ANP, FAAN; Judith Haber, PhD, APRN, BC, FAAN

2003   **Nurse Practitioners: Evolution of Advanced Practice, 4th Edition**
Mathy Doval Mezey, EdD, RN, FAAN, Diane O. McGivern, RN, PhD, FAAN, Eileen M. Sullivan-Marx, PhD, CRNP, FAAN, Editors, and Sherry A. Greenberg, MSN, RN, BC, Managing Editor

2000   **Outcome Assessment in Advanced Practice Nursing**
Ruth M. Kleinpell, PhD, RN, ACNP, CCRN

1999   **Advanced Practice Nursing: A Guide to Professional Development, 2nd Edition**
Mariah Snyder, PhD, RN, FAAN, and Michaelene P. Mirr, PhD, RN, CS

1998   **Practice Issues for the Acute Care Nurse Practitioner**
Ruth M. Kleinpell, PhD, RN, CCRN, and Mariann Piano, PhD, RN

1998   **Nurses, Nurse Practitioners: Evolution to Advanced Practice, 3rd Edition**
Mathy D. Mezey, RN, EdD, FAAN, and Diane O. McGivern, RN, PhD, FAAN

1997   **Developing a Private Practice in Psychiatric Mental-Health Nursing**
Susanne Fine, PhD, RN, CA

1997   **The Acute Care Nurse Practitioner**
Barbara J. Daly, PhD, RN, FAAN

1995   **Advanced Practice Nursing: A Guide to Professional Development**
Mariah Snyder, PhD, RN, FAAN, and Michaelene P. Mirr, PhD, RN, CS

1994   **Nurse–Physician Collaboration: Care of Adults and the Elderly**
Eugenia L. Siegler, MD, and Fay W. Whitney, PhD, RN, FAAN

1993   **Nurses, Nurse Practitioners: Evolution to Advanced Practice, 2nd Edition**
Mathy D. Mezey, RN, EdD, FAAN, and Diane O. McGivern, RN, PhD, FAAN

Mathy Doval Mezey, EdD, RN, FAAN, received her undergraduate and graduate education at Columbia University. She taught at Lehman College of the City University of New York and at the University of Pennsylvania School of Nursing where she directed the geriatric nurse practitioner program and the Robert Wood Johnson Foundation Teaching Nursing Home Program. Since 1991 she has been the Independence Foundation Professor and Director of the John A. Hartford Foundation Institute for the Advancement of Geriatric Nursing at New York University. Dr. Mezey has authored 5 books and has over 60 publications that focus on the preparation of advanced practice nurses to care for older adults, nursing practice with older adults and bioethical issues that affect decisions at the end of life. She is Editor for the Springer Series in Geriatric Nursing and of the Springer publication *The Encyclopedia of Elder Care.*

Diane O'Neill McGivern, RN, PhD, FAAN received her Bachelor of Science Degree in Nursing from St. John's College in Cleveland, Ohio and her MA and PhD from New York University. She has taught at Lehman College, the University of Pennsylvania, and New York University. Dr. McGivern has been widely honored within nursing and the health care professions. She was a Robert Wood Johnson Health Policy Fellow, and is a member of American Academy of Nursing and on the board of the Nurses' Educational Fund. She has written widely on professional practice preparation, particularly advanced practice nursing. She is Editor for the Springer Series on Teaching of Nursing. Dr. McGivern was elected by the New York State Legislature in 1991 to serve on the Board of Regents, the policymaking body for education in the state. She has served as Vice-Chancellor and currently chairs the Higher Education and Professions Committee.

Eileen M. Sullivan-Marx, PhD, CRNP, FAAN, received her Bachelor of Science in nursing from the University of Pennsylvania, a Master of Science degree from the University of Rochester School of Nursing, and her doctorate from the University of Pennsylvania. She is an Associate Professor at the University of Pennsylvania School of Nursing and Associate Dean for Practice and Community Affairs. With over 30 publications and numerous national presentations, Dr. Sullivan-Marx's research focuses on outcomes of care for vulnerable older adults and includes demonstration of the effectiveness of nurse-managed programs, restraint reduction in nursing homes, and policy issues on access and payment for health care services. From 1993 to 2002, she represented nursing on the American Medical Association's Relative Value Update Committee that sets work values for the Medicare Fee Schedule. Dr. Sullivan-Marx has won several practice and research awards including the Springer Publishing Company Research Award in 1998.

Sherry A. Greenberg, MSN, RN, BC, received her Bachelor of Science in Nursing and Master of Science in Nursing from the University of Pennsylvania School of Nursing. She has worked as a gerontological nurse practitioner in ambulatory, acute and institutional long-term care settings. From 1997 to 2001, Ms. Greenberg coordinated the Advanced Practice Nursing Program in Geriatrics at New York University. Currently she practices in New Jersey in the outpatient Geriatric Assessment Program at Overlook Hospital.

Nurse Practitioners
Evolution of Advanced Practice
Fourth Edition

Mathy D. Mezey, EdD, RN, FAAN
Diane O. McGivern, RN, PhD, FAAN
Eileen M. Sullivan-Marx, PhD, CRNP, FAAN
Editors

Sherry A. Greenberg, MSN, RN, BC
Managing Editor

 Springer Publishing Company

Springer Publishing Company, Inc.
536 Broadway
New York, NY 10012-3955

Acquisitions Editor: Ruth Chasek
Production Editor: Pamela Lankas
Cover design by Joanne Honigman

03 04 05 06 07 / 5 4 3 2 1

Library of Congress Cataloging-in-Publication Data

Nurse practitioners : evolution of advanced practice / Mathy D. Mezey, Diane O.
    McGivern, Eileen M. Sullivan-Marx, editors. — 4th ed.
        p. ; cm. — (Springer series on advanced practice nursing)
    Rev. ed. of: Nurses, nurse practitioners. c1999.
    Includes bibliographical references and index.
    ISBN 0-8261-7772-7
        1. Nurse practitioners. 2. Primary care (Medicine) I. Mezey, Mathy Doval.
    II. McGivern, Diane O'Neill. III. Sullivan-Marx, Eileen. IV. Nurses, nurse
    practitioners. V. Series.
        [DNLM: 1. Nurse Practitioners. 2. Primary Health Care. WY 128 N9735 2003]
    RT82.8.N884 2003
    610.73'06'92—dc22

                                                                    2003057354

Printed in the United States of America by Maple-Vail Book Manufacturing Group.

Dedicated to

Barbara Bates

The history and evolution of the advanced practice nursing movement has many heroines and heroes. Early on, those of us who were learning advanced practice skills and teaching students the new curricular content of physical assessment and other primary care skills were indebted to Barbara Bates for her book, *A Guide to Physical Examination and History Taking*. Barbara Bates, MD worked to improve public access to health care by encouraging greater collaboration between physicians and nurses and expanded practice opportunities for nurses. She and Joan Lynaugh collaborated to inform and encourage faculty, new advanced practice nurses, and physicians to provide the appropriate level of care to patients and improve outcomes. Dr. Bates inspired collaboration, modeled collegiality, and helped to create the dialogue that encouraged the evolution of the nurse practitioner movement.

CONTENTS

Foreword by Loretta C. Ford xi
Preface xiii
Acknowledgments xv
Contributors xvii

PART I Perspectives: History, Education, Philosophy, and Research   1

1 Advanced Practice Nursing: Preparation and Clinical Practice   3
   Diane O. McGivern, Eileen M. Sullivan-Marx,
   and Mathy D. Mezey

2 Philosophical and Historical Bases of Advanced Practice   37
   Nursing Roles
   Ellen D. Baer

   Commentary: Philosophical and Historical Bases   54
   of Advanced Practice Nursing Roles
   Julie Fairman

3 Primary Care as an Academic Discipline   65
   Claire M. Fagin

4 Research in Support of Nurse Practitioners   84
   Frances Hughes, Sean Clarke, Deborah A. Sampson,
   Julie Fairman, and Eileen M. Sullivan-Marx

5 Long-Term Outcomes of Advanced Practice Nursing   108
   Harriet J. Kitzman and Susan Groth

PART II The Practice Arena: Many Roles, Many Settings   133

6 Advanced Practice Nurses in Acute-Care Services   135
   Deborah E. Becker and Therese S. Richmond

7   Advanced Practice Nurses in Managed Care   150
    Patricia M. Barber and Marina Burke

8   Nurse Practitioners in the School-Based Health   166
    Care Environment
    Judith B. Igoe

9   Meeting the Needs of Older Adults for Primary Health Care   192
    Diane Stillman, Neville E. Strumpf, and Geraldine Paier

10 Advanced Practice Psychiatric–Mental Health Nursing   215
    Madeline A. Naegle

11 Advanced Practice in Holistic Nursing   233
    Carla Mariano

12 Nurse-Midwifery and Primary Health Care for Women   254
    Joyce E. Thompson

13 Nurse Anesthetists: Evolution From Critical Care   269
    Practitioners to Anesthesia Providers
    William P. Fehder

14 Roles of Nurse Practitioners in the U.S. Department   284
    of Veterans Affairs
    Karen R. Robinson and Robert Petzel

    PART III Voices From the Field   303

15 The Voice of Experience: The Nuts and Bolts   305
    of Advanced Practice for Nurse Practitioners
    Joseph P. Colagreco and Carl A. Kirton

16 Marginalized Patients, Family Nurse Practitioners,   321
    and Nurse-Managed Health Centers:
    Caring for Residents in Public-Housing-Based
    Nursing Centers
    Susan M. Beidler and Donna Torrisi

17 Primary Care in the Home: The Nurse Practitioners' Role   333
    JoAnn Hunt Stracuzzi and Lynn T. Rinke

18 Surgical Intensive Care Unit Nurse Practitioner   347
    Sabrina D. Jarvis

19 Physician–Nurse Practitioner Relationships   355
    William Kavesh

20 Pediatric Nurse Practitioner and Pediatrician: 367
        Collaborative Practice
          Carol Boland and Susan Leib

21 Adolescent Family Practice   376
          Ann L. O'Sullivan

        PART IV Payment, Policy, and Politics   **389**

22 Systems of Payment for Advanced Practice Nurses   391
          Eileen M. Sullivan-Marx and David Keepnews

23 Licensure, Certification, and Credentialing   415
          Frances K. Porcher

24 Workforce Policy Perspectives on Advance Practice Nursing 431
          Linda H. Aiken

25 Academic Nursing Practice: Implications for Policy   443
          Lois K. Evans, Melinda Jenkins, and Karen Buhler-Wilkerson

Index   471

FOREWORD

Nothing could be more propitious to herald the 21st century than this fourth edition of *Nurse Practitioners: Evolution of Advanced Practice*. Like earlier editions, it is a signature piece. It expands on the third edition with reflective commentaries, descriptions of innovative advanced practices, and analyses of current issues in research, education, and legislation. As such, it chronicles the depth and breadth of advanced practice nursing (APN) historically, clinically, professionally, organizationally, legally, and politically since the advent of the third edition. In fact, each edition adds another building block to the professional progress of advanced practice nursing.

This edition is organized into four parts, each of which is introduced by one of the editors. The introductions guide the reader to the major components in the parts and offer challenging commentaries on the environments, the practitioners, and the issues in advanced practice nursing. Part I addresses the philosophical and historical aspects of APN with the conceptual academic and long-term outcome research bases for practice at the advanced level. These lead into the second and third parts, which orient the reader to various views and voices of specialty practices and the many functional issues of APN. In Part IV, the issues of payment, policy, and politics are thoughtfully analyzed and discussed. With their assistance and insights, the editors have made this comprehensive and informative fourth edition a vital descriptive link in the illustrious, if tortuous, history of APN. Further, chapter authors have addressed the broad concept of advanced practice nursing including a range of practitioners and practice settings. These contributors have aptly captured the ferment, fervor, and facts on advanced practice nurses that have brought the health professions, the public, and the policymakers to higher levels of understanding and support. Further explored in this publication are problems that exist in the control of practice, deficits in authorization and reimbursement for expansions in the scope of practice, and recognition and reward of advanced practice nurses.

Students and faculty, practitioners, policy makers, researchers, nurse generalists, and employers of advanced practice nurses will find valuable information, insights, and perhaps even inspiration in the long, challenging evolution of advanced practice nursing from an expanded role concept to the role of full-fledged professional. No longer are nurse practitioners and other advanced practice nurses just expanding a role; they are now a vital professional nursing force ready to do battle in the public interest. They are a force prepared, poised, and positioned to enter the 21st century as expert clinicians, innovative leaders, and wise statespersons.

LORETTA C. FORD, RN, EdD, PNP, FAAN, FAANP
Cofounder, with Pediatrician Henry Silver,
of the Pediatric Nurse Practitioner Role (1965)
Professor and Dean Emeritus
University of Rochester
School of Nursing
Rochester, New York

PREFACE

"Everyday our numbers grow and these will speak for us."
—Frederick Douglass.

With the onset of the nurse practitioner movement, the first edition of this book, originally titled *Nurses, Nurse Practitioners,* was a sentinel that heralded the arrival of nurse practitioners in society. Each subsequent edition echoed continued exhilaration as society, nurses, nurse practitioners, and advanced practice nurses bridged gaps in health care for children, women, and men of all ages. Today, with over 100,000 advanced practice nurses well established in practice, we are pleased to bring you an unprecedented fourth edition, entitled *Nurse Practitioners: Evolution of Advanced Practice.*

In this new edition we continue to chronicle the rich developments in advanced practice nursing and the accomplishments of both the new and more mature generations of nurse practitioners, clinical nurse specialists, nurse-midwives, and nurse anesthetists. This book is intended to present a vibrant celebration of accomplishments, a testimony to founders, a proclamation of a new generation of bright and committed leaders, and a compendium of knowledge, in one volume, that will be extremely valuable to students considering generalist and advanced practice, students and faculty in advanced practice programs, new advanced practice graduates, employers and other providers, and policymakers. The authentic voices of clinicians, clinical leaders, academicians, and researchers provide a broad and balanced picture of this important part of professional nursing.

We know you will find each chapter informative and, in some cases, inspirational. New chapters on the nuts and bolts of practice, outcomes research, certified registered nurse anesthetists, acute care nurse practitioners, Veterans Affairs, the nurse workforce, holistic care, and home care have been added. Significant updates in research supporting nurse practitioners, payment structures, managed care, politics, and historical background from well-known sages and exciting new leaders in the field bring fresh views on the complexity of issues facing advanced practice nurses today.

We celebrate with you in the richness of this new edition that chronicles the unfolding and unending horizon for nurses and nurse practitioners.

MATHY D. MEZEY
DIANE O. MCGIVERN
EILEEN M. SULLIVAN-MARX

ACKNOWLEDGMENTS

We wish to acknowledge our gratitude to the following people: Sherry Greenberg, whose valuable support and excellent organization kept this project on track and ensured that authors and editors completed their work in a timely way. Ruth Chasek, for her quiet persistence and helpful suggestions. Pamela Lankas, for her exquisite attention to detail. Ursula Springer, whose dedication to nursing and the quality of nursing literature inspires new generations of authors and editors. Our authors, for their wonderfully wise and well-informed chapters that describe and encourage advanced practice.

CONTRIBUTORS

Linda H. Aiken, PhD, FAAN, FRCN, RN
Claire M. Fagin Leadership
  Professor in Nursing
Professor of Sociology, and Director
  of the Center for Health
  Outcomes and Policy Research
University of Pennsylvania
  School of Nursing
Philadelphia, Pennsylvania

Ellen D. Baer, PhD, RN, FAAN
Wallace Gilroy Professor of Nursing
University of Miami
Miami, Florida

Professor Emerita of Nursing
University of Pennsylvania
  School of Nursing
Philadelphia, Pennsylvania

Patricia M. Barber, RN, MPA
Healthcare Consultant
Portland, Maine
Assistant Director
Marketing and Communications
  Occupational Health Associates
  of Maine PA

Deborah E. Becker, MSN, CRNP, BC
Associate Director
Adult Acute Care Nurse
  Practitioner Program
University of Pennsylvania
  School of Nursing
Philadelphia, Pennsylvania

Susan M. Beidler, PhD, MBe, MSN, BC
Assistant Professor
Florida Atlantic University
Christine E. Lynn College of Nursing
Boca Raton, Florida

Carol Boland, MSN, APRN
Pediatric Nurse Practitioner
Ridgefield Pediatric Associates
Ridgefield, Connecticut

Karen Buhler-Wilkerson, PhD, RN, FAAN
Professor of Community Nursing
University of Pennsylvania
  School of Nursing
Philadelphia, Pennsylvania

Marina Burke, MSN, BA, RN, ANP
Nurse Practitioner
The Visiting Doctors Program
The Mount Sinai Medical Center
New York, New York

Sean Clarke, PhD, RN, CRNP, CS
Assistant Professor and Associate
  Director of the Center for Health
  Outcomes and Policy Research
University of Pennsylvania
  School of Nursing
Philadelphia, Pennsylvania

Joseph P. Colagreco, MS, APRN,
   BC, NP-C
Clinical Assistant Professor of Nursing
Division of Nursing
The Steinhardt School of Education
New York University
New York, New York

Deborah Cross, MPH, CRNP
Lecturer and Clinical Coordinator
Adult Health and Gerontology
   Nurse Practitioner Program
University of Pennsylvania
   School of Nursing
Philadelphia, Pennsylvania

Lois K. Evans, DNSc, RN, FAAN
Viola MacInnes/Independence
   Professor
University of Pennsylvania
   School of Nursing
Philadelphia, Pennsylvania

Claire M. Fagin, PhD, RN, FAAN
Program Director: Building Academic
   Geriatric Nursing Capacity
A John A. Hartford Foundation
   Initiative
American Academy of Nursing
Washington, D.C.

Dean Emerita and Professor Emerita
University of Pennsylvania
   School of Nursing
Philadelphia, Pennsylvania

Julie Fairman, PhD, RN, FAAN
Associate Professor
Associated Scholar
Center for the Study of the History
   of Nursing
University of Pennsylvania
   School of Nursing
Philadelphia, Pennsylvania

William P. Fehder, PhD, CRNA
Associate Professor of Nursing
Drexel University College of
   Nursing and Health Professions
Philadelphia, Pennsylvania

Susan Groth, MSN, RNC, WHNP
Senior Associate
University of Rochester
   School of Nursing
Rochester, New York

Frances Hughes, MA, RN, FCON
   (Aoteroa), FANZCMHN
International Health Care Harkness
   Fellow (Col RNZNC)
Chief Advisor Nursing
Ministry of Health
Wellington, New Zealand

Judith B. Igoe, MS, RN, FAAN
Associate Professor and Director
Office of School Health
School of Nursing
University of Colorado Health
   Science Center
Denver, Colorado

Sabrina D. Jarvis, ACNP, FNP,
   MS, CCRN
Surgical Intensive Care Unit Nurse
   Practitioner
Veteran's Affairs Salt Lake City
   Health Care System
Orem, Utah

Melinda Jenkins, PhD, APRN
Assistant Professor of Primary Care
University of Pennsylvania
   School of Nursing
Philadelphia, Pennsylvania

William Kavesh, MD, MPH
Director of Geriatric Primary Care
Philadelphia Veterans Affairs
  Medical Center
Philadelphia, Pennsylvania

Clinical Assistant Professor
  of Medicine
University of Pennsylvania
  School of Medicine
Fellow of the Institute on Aging
University of Pennsylvania
  Health System

**David Keepnews, PhD, JD, RN,
  FAAN**
Assistant Professor
Department of Biobehavioral
  Nursing and Health Systems
University of Washington
  School of Nursing
Seattle, Washington

Adjunct Assistant Professor
University of Washington
  School of Law
Seattle, Washington

Carl A. Kirton, MA, RN, APRN, BC
Nurse Practitioner and
  Nurse Manager
Infectious Disease Clinic
Mt. Sinai Medical Center
New York, New York

Adjunct Clinical Associate Professor
Division of Nursing
The Steinhardt School of Education
New York University
New York, New York

Harriet J. Kitzman, PhD, RN
Professor of Nursing
University of Rochester
  School of Nursing
Rochester, New York

Professor of Pediatrics
School of Medicine and Dentistry
University of Rochester
Rochester, New York

Susan Leib, MD
Pediatrician
Ridgefield Pediatric Associates
Ridgefield, Connecticut

Carla Mariano, EdD, RN, HNC
Associate Professor and Coordinator
Advanced Practice Holistic
  Nursing Program
Division of Nursing
The Steinhardt School of Education
New York University
New York, New York

**Madeline A. Naegle, PhD, RN,
  APRN-BC, FAAN**
Associate Professor of Nursing and
  Coordinator
Advanced Practice Psychiatric-
  Mental Health Nursing
Division of Nursing
The Steinhardt School of Education
New York University
New York, New York

**Ann L. O'Sullivan, PhD, CRNP,
  FAAN**
Professor of Primary Care Nursing
University of Pennsylvania
  School of Nursing
Philadelphia, Pennsylvania

Pediatric Nurse Practitioner
The Children's Hospital
  of Philadelphia
Philadelphia, Pennsylvania

Geraldine S. Paier, PhD, RN
Gerontologic Nurse Consultation
  Service
University of Pennsylvania
  School of Nursing
Philadelphia, Pennsylvania

Robert Petzel, MD
Network Director
Health Care Veterans Integrated
  Service Network (VISN 23)
Member of the Department
  of Medicine
University of Minnesota
Minneapolis, Minnesota

**Frances K. Porcher, EdD, RN,
  CPNP**
Assistant Professor
Pediatric Nurse Practitioner
  Program Coordinator
Medical University of South Carolina
Charleston, South Carolina

**Therese S. Richmond, PhD, CRNP,
  FAAN**
Associate Professor of Trauma and
  Critical Care Nursing
Director, Adult Acute Care Nurse
  Practitioner Program
University of Pennsylvania
  School of Nursing
Philadelphia, Pennsylvania

Lynn T. Rinke, MS, RN
Executive Vice President
Chief Operating Officer
The Visiting Nurse Association
  of Greater Philadelphia
Philadelphia, Pennsylvania

Karen R. Robinson, PhD, RN, FAAN
Associate Director for Clinical
  Operations
Department of Veterans Affairs
  Medical Center
Fargo, North Dakota

Adjunct Assistant Professor
University of Minnesota
  School of Nursing
Minneapolis, Minnesota

**Deborah A. Sampson, MSN, RN,
  CRNP**
Doctoral Candidate
University of Pennsylvania
  School of Nursing
Philadelphia, Pennsylvania

Diane Stillman, MSN, RN, CS
Consultant
University of Pennsylvania
  School of Nursing
Philadelphia, Pennsylvania

**JoAnn Hunt Stracuzzi, MSN, RN,
  CRNP**
Adult Nurse Practitioner
VNA House Calls
VNA of Greater Philadelphia
Philadelphia, Pennsylvania

**Neville E. Strumpf, PhD, RN, C,
  FAAN**
Edith Clemmer Steinbright Professor
  in Gerontology
Director, Hartford Center of
  Geriatric Nursing Excellence
University of Pennsylvania
  School of Nursing
Philadelphia, Pennsylvania

Joyce E. Thompson, RN, CNM,
  DrPH, FAAN, FACNM
Bernardine M. Lacey Professor of
  Community Health Nursing
Western Michigan University
  Bronson School of Nursing
Kalamazoo, Michigan

Donna Torrisi, MSN, CRNP
Robert Wood Johnson Executive
  Nurse Fellow
Director, Family Practice and
  Counseling Network
Abbottsford Family Practice
  and Counseling
Philadelphia, Pennsylvania

PERSPECTIVES: HISTORY, EDUCATION, PHILOSOPHY, AND RESEARCH

Part I provides a context for understanding the history, evolution, and current and future states of advanced practice nursing. The chapters in Part I also are a frame of reference for understanding and analyzing Parts II–IV, which describe individual practitioners' experiences, development of advanced practice specialties by academic and clinical innovators, and the important determinants of policy and politics.

Of the three chapters in Part I that appeared in the third edition, two are now accompanied by contemporary commentary. The inclusion of these two chapters, by Baer and Fagin, highlights the timelessness and correctness of their arguments. Baer's chapter contains a commentary by Fairman, who emphasizes Baer's perspective on nurse practitioners' autonomy and authority based on educational preparation, legislation, and consumer recognition. Fairman endorses this argument by adding a fourth dimension, the nurse's relationship to the patient. Fagin, in her introduction to her own original chapter, reconfirms that primary care is a distinct and traditional nursing service. Primary care and advanced practice are grounded in nursing, and she therefore questions the attitude of some nurse practitioners who disassociate themselves from identification with nursing.

The enormous potential of advanced practice nursing, as reflected in the chapters in Parts II and III, is validated by the extensive research reviewed and discussed by Hughes and colleagues and the long-term outcomes research presented by Kitzman and Groth. Both chapters underscore the evolution of research on advanced practice, evolution consistent with the maturational development of the role. Early research was a "self-conscious" proof of worth; now we are moving on to research that focuses on the unique nature of advanced practice and the outcomes of that highly nuanced model. The long-term outcomes research in Kitzman and Groth's chapter is, in a sense, the response to some of the questions posed at the end of the previous chapter (Hughes et al.) regarding what research is needed to move advanced practice nursing forward.

Finally, the editors who coauthored the first chapter hope that the information presented there raises questions, ideas, and discussion about the directions taken in education and practice and what issues should occupy our attention in the near future.

Chapter 1

ADVANCED PRACTICE NURSING: PREPARATION AND CLINICAL PRACTICE

Diane O. McGivern, Eileen M. Sullivan-Marx, and Mathy D. Mezey

In the almost 40 years of nurse practitioner role development, an extraordinary range of specialty roles and practice settings have flourished (Ford, 1997), studies of effectiveness have been published, and innovative models of practice implemented and evaluated. New roles, settings, and arrangements continue to develop. Language and terminology continue to evolve to encompass nurse practitioners, clinical nurse specialists, nurse anesthetists, and nurse-midwives under the umbrella of advanced practice nursing. This chapter traces the evolution of advanced practice nursing preparation and clinical practice, touching on the history and definition, workforce realities and projections, factors shaping practice and education and the link between the two, and projections for the future.

HISTORY AND DEFINITION

The development of the first nurse practitioner program in 1965 by Loretta Ford and Henry Silver was a seminal event in that it was based on a "nursing model focused on the promotion of health in daily living, growth and development for children in families as well as the prevention of disease and disability" (Ford, 1982, 1986). Ford noted that societal needs and nursing's potential led to the development of nurse practitioners; the primary care physician shortage, which is described as a major contributing factor to the expansion of nurse practitioners in other parts of the country (see Fairman's commentary in chapter 2 of this edition; Elder & Bullough, 1990; McGivern, 1986) is defined by Ford and others as the *opportunity*, not the reason, for the new role (Ford, 1982; Lewis & Lewis, 2002).

Other programs expanded this effort, including the home-care demonstration project at the University of Kansas Medical Center developed by Lewis in 1969 (Lewis & Lewis, 2002), the integration of primary care skills into the baccalaureate nursing curriculum of City University's Lehman College in the 1970s (McGivern, Mezey, & Baer, 1976), and the "Primex" research and demonstration project described by Linn and Lewis in the 1970s (Lewis & Lewis, 2002; Linn & Lewis, 1976).

Resistance to the nurse practitioner role initially came from the academic nursing community, the medical profession, and some federal agencies, but the idea was born at a time of general concern on the part of consumers about accessible, affordable, and humane care. Bolstered by the supportive health care environment of the 1960s and 1970s, nurse practitioners created a role that served populations in many settings and became more fully integrated into baccalaureate and master's nursing programs. An extensive number of studies confirmed the quality, cost effectiveness, productivity, clinical decision-making skills, and job satisfaction of nurse practitioners, making this the most evaluated role in any discipline (see chapters 4 and 5; Brown & Grimes, 1993, 1995; Horrocks, Anderson, & Salisbury, 2002; Rudy et al., 1998; U.S. Congress, Office of Technology Assessment, 1986).

Organizational recognition of the nurse practitioner role was reflected in the rapid establishment of a number of important affiliations: the American Nurses Association Council on Primary Health Care Nurse Practitioners in 1977, the National Organization of Nurse Practitioner Faculties in 1980, The New York State Coalition of Nurse Practitioners in 1981, the National Council of Gerontological Nurse Practitioners in 1983, the National Association of Neonatal Practitioners in 1984, and, in 1985, The National Alliance of Nurse Practitioners and The American Academy of Nurse Practitioners (Lewis & Lewis, 2002).

The evolution of preparatory programs for nurse practitioners, from physician- and nurse-taught certificate programs to well-integrated content in baccalaureate and master's degree programs, was relatively rapid and consistent across the country (McGivern, 1986). The rapid development of expert clinicians produced two models of specialization in nursing: the consultative nursing model of clinical nurse specialists and the collaborative model of practitioners, midwives, and anesthetists (Bullough, 1992). These models shared a commitment to research and utilization of knowledge from other disciplines but differed for several decades in their emphasis on nursing theory, medical content, direct service activities, and practice settings.

Driven by assertions that the curricular content for clinical nurse specialist (CNS) and nurse practitioner (NP) programs have become more congruent, that the practice setting distinctions have blurred, and that there is value-added when the history of evaluation and success of reimbursement for nurse practitioners is added to the mix, more and more programs decided to prepare advanced practice nurses for a "blended" role, making the graduates eligible to take both the CNS and NP certification examinations (Cukr, Jones, Wilberger, Smith, & Stopper, 1998; McCabe & Grover, 1999). However, consensus has not been reached, and clinical nurse specialists as distinct practitioners are again seen as necessary in order to supply the expertise leached from hospitals through downsizing, re-engineering, and retirement of senior, skilled nurses.

The National Council of State Boards of Nursing (NCSBN, 1992) defines advanced practice nursing as

> the advanced practice of nursing by nurse practitioners, nurse anesthetists, nurse-midwives, and clinical nurse specialists, based on the following: knowledge and skills required in basic nursing education; licensure as a registered nurse; graduate degree and experience in the designated area of practice which includes advanced nursing theory; substantial knowledge of physical and psychosocial assessment; appropriate interventions and management of health care status. The skills and abilities essential for the advanced practice role within an identified specialty area include: providing patient/client and community education; promoting stress prevention and management; encouraging self-help; subscribing to caring; advocacy; accountability; accessibility; and collaboration with other health and community professionals.

The Council also noted that "each individual who practices nursing at an advanced level does so with substantial autonomy and independence resulting in a high level of accountability" (NCSBN, p. 4).

WORKFORCE REALITIES AND PROJECTIONS

The sustained decline in basic nursing program enrollments, projected shortages of generalist and advanced practice nurses, and the declining numbers of nurse faculty are current and fundamental workforce issues (Janofsky, 2002; O'Grady, 2002; U.S. Dept. of Health and Human Services [DHHS], 2002). The projected long-term shortages of baccalaureate-prepared professional nurses, the pool of potential master's-prepared advanced practice nurses, and the impact of declining numbers of nursing faculty negate the old models of workforce projection and the usual cycling of surplus and shortage and pose new sets of variables.

The expansion of master's programs and enrollments in the mid-1990s was fueled by the loss of nurse-generalist positions in tertiary care settings, the expansion of community-based more autonomous practices, new reimbursement opportunities, and colleges' and universities' programmatic efforts to expand enrollments. The decrease in the number of nurse-generalists in hospitals and their replacement by less well prepared, and in some cases unlicensed, personnel has recreated the scenario that first produced the need for specialized nurses in the mid-1950s. Expert clinicians once again are providing the modeling and direction for less well-prepared workers who are caring for more acute and complex patients and providing direct care and consultation related to increasingly sophisticated technology-based diagnosis and treatment.

Community-based health care agencies, such as home and institutional long-term care, have increasingly expanded and attracted advanced practice nurses from acute care settings. These agencies seemed to be the platform for expansion of nurse practitioner roles. However, evolution of the advanced practice role in many geographic areas has been negatively impacted by federal and state attempts to limit payments, services, and client eligibility.

The well-publicized unpredictability of the health care system depressed baccalaureate enrollments and stimulated academic programs to expand master's programs, particularly nurse practitioner programs, in order to increase overall enrollments and capture new recruits with degrees in other fields. More recently, popular media and targeted advertising campaigns highlighting the "new" nursing shortage and explaining contemporary nursing roles along with a loss of jobs in other sectors are stimulating enrollments. Recent research by Needleman, Buerhaus, Mattke, Stewart, and Zelevinsky (2001) and Aiken, Clarke, Sloane, Sochalski, and Silber (2002) demonstrates a direct relationship between nurse staffing and patient outcomes, but the impact that will have on the public, the hospital industry, and future selection of nursing as an academic and career choice remains to be seen.

Changes in accreditation, regulation, and state laws affecting other health professions—specifically medicine, by limiting residents availability to 80 hours a week and mandating 10 hours between shifts—will have an impact on nurse practitioner and physician assistant utilization (Abelson, 2002; Altman & Grady, 2002; "Sleep-deprived," 2002). These changes and the decline in applications to all health professions programs raise questions about the continued evolution of practices, interdisciplinary practice potential, and the overall balance of generalist primary care practice and specialty and subspecialty practice.

Predictions regarding local and national supply and demand for advanced practice nurses are also difficult to discuss with precision. Although advanced practice nurses are seen as particularly well prepared for the rapidly evolving health care environment, expansion of the advanced practice nursing role is constrained by the relatively limited number of nurses appropriately prepared and credentialed in advanced practice. As of 2000, there were 196,279 advanced practice nurses, including 88,186 nurse practitioners, 54,374 clinical nurse specialists, 29,844 nurse anesthetists, and 9,232 nurse-midwives. These practitioners are not necessarily prepared in master's-level advanced practice programs (U.S. DHHS, 2002).

The immediate response of many academic institutions to the need for and interest in advanced practice nursing is reflected in the increased numbers of institutions offering such programs at the master's level. As of 2002 there were 325 colleges and universities offering master's nurse practitioner nursing programs, in contrast to 274 in 1998. Programs, in order of prevalence of specialty practice preparation, include family nurse practitioners, adult primary care, adult acute care/critical care, pediatrics, gerontological/geriatrics, women's health care, psychiatric/mental health, and neonatal. This rank order has not changed since 1998. Nurse practitioner students are 52.3% of all master's students and 61.6% of graduates (Berlin, Stennett, & Bednash, 2002).

Advanced practice nursing, defined by master's degree preparation and certification, is necessarily dependent on sufficient numbers of nurses with the requisite baccalaureate preparation. The current configuration of nursing education programs and numbers of graduates is incongruent with health workforce needs, although the distribution of graduates has changed significantly between 1992 and 1999. The number of associate degree graduates is declining at a faster rate than the number of baccalaureate graduates. As of 1999, baccalaureate graduates constituted 44% of all graduates, up from the 1992 level of 27%; associate degree graduates were at 52%, down from 64%. Unfortunately, baccalaureate graduations have declined overall between 1997 and 2001 from 24,423 to 19,035 (Berlin et al., 2002; U.S. DHHS, 2002).

Enrollments are also affected by the limited clinical placements for students in advanced practice nursing programs and competition with the better-paying service sector for clinician-faculty, which increases part-time faculty and thereby creates significant difficulties in coordination for full-time faculty and administrators. The number of students who graduate annually is further limited by the inability of most students to attend advanced practice programs on a full-time basis. Academic programs accommodate to these pressures and their own budgetary constraints in a variety of ways, including limiting enrollments, requiring students to contract for their own clinical practica placements, and reducing faculty field supervision.

The general uncertainty about the economics of the health care system reduces the impetus for students, academic institutions, and clinical service providers to aggressively plan for the advanced practice model in other than incremental steps. Students are predominantly part time (Berlin et al., 2002), and in many regions where continued threats of downsizing and reorganizing of health care institutions create uncertainty, students are preparing for advanced practice while staying in current practice roles in their employing agencies and institutions without specific plans to move into new practice opportunities.

Added to the decline in the overall number of new entrants and graduate from nursing programs is the increasing gap in diversity. The current nursing supply does not reflect the increasing diversity in the general population. Eighty percent of nurses are identified as White, non-Hispanic, in contrast to 71% in the general population; Black, 4.9% versus 12.2%; and 2.0% Hispanic, in contrast to the fast-growing representation in the general population of 11.4%. Emphasis on recruitment of these underrepresented groups is necessary to create a profession sensitive to cultural differences and as an opportunity to enhance enrollments and graduations.

Enrollments are also influenced by the limited number of available and appropriate clinical placements, competition with the better-paying service sector for expert clinician-faculty, limited institutional budgets that fail to support a sufficient number of full-time faculty, and limited candidates for faculty positions. Annual graduations are depressed by the large cadre of part-time students who take three to five years to complete their program (Berlin et al., 2002).

Demand is subject to a variety of factors. Despite hospital downsizing, there is increased hospital employment of nurses; expansion is occurring in areas traditionally requiring baccalaureate and higher degrees, including community health and managed care/case management. The future physician availability for primary care is unclear in light of the 6-year decline in applications to U.S. medical schools. The 33,501 applications filed in 2002 represent a 29% decline from 47,000 applications made in the peak year 1996 (Mangan, 2002).

Demand is also influenced by perceptions about standardization of preparation and credentialing. Institutional and organizational employers, insurers, and consumers want assurances that support credibility for practice and reimbursement claims (see chapter 7). While consistency in preparation and credentialing in master's programs is enhanced through criteria established by the American Association of Colleges of Nursing (AACN), the National Organization of Nurse Practitioner Faculties (NONPF), the American College of Nurse Midwives, other specialty organizations, and the American Nurse Credentialing Center, there is strong sentiment for even more standardization, consistency, and transparency to be made available through professional and governmental agencies (NONPF & AACN, 2002; U.S. DHHS, 2002).

The recently introduced federal legislation, the Nurse Reinvestment Act, provides for scholarships; nurse information and recruitment programs aimed at elementary, middle, and secondary school students; and special emphasis on training in long-term care of the elderly. While appropriations for this federal legislation have not yet been established, states are launching their own initiatives. In Florida for example, $4,000 scholarships are being offered to encourage enrollment.

Finally, supply of and demand for advanced practice nurses will continue to be strongly influenced by the geographic differences in health care systems reorganization, the continued impact of managed care on access and availability of health services, and regional bias toward mid-level providers (Kovner & Rosenfeld, 1997).

FACTORS SHAPING THE PRACTICE ENVIRONMENT

Practice and education are being influenced by cross-cutting trends and influences that are having widespread and multiplying effects on higher education and clinical practice. Specifically, clinical practice is being affected by the health care system economy, the resulting pressures on providers to enhance efficiency and effectiveness, diversity and disparity among populations, and the corporatization of health care.

Health Care Environment and Economy

The current economic decline in the United States and globally, the loss of trust in large national and multinational business firms, and post-Cold War instability in international relations have produced subtle and not-so-subtle changes in the general economy and social commitment to broader health and welfare programs (Lang, 2002). The general economic decline and the continued press for health care cost containment will continue to have a significant impact on the environment in which health care professionals practice. The cost-containment strategies of managed care and its permutations continue to shape the overall care environment. The cost debate will increasingly incorporate the quality dimension, although at some point of declining payment, there is a question of how quality can be preserved. In a number of instances, that question has already been raised.

The influence of managed care on professional practice has been perceived to be both positive and negative. One state survey indicated that the managed care environment influenced professional practice by encouraging exploration of new approaches to cost-effective quality care, expansion of nurse practitioners' primary care role, and more effective collaboration with patients and clients, thereby promoting personal health care responsibility (Harrison, 1999) Others have seen managed care as stifling the expansion of advanced practice nurses.

The cost, quality, and health care system debate is stymied by the ambivalence of the American public on the appropriate role of government in solving the dilemma of access, cost, and level of consumers' contributions. Although most Americans feel there should be more rationality to the health care system, most also believe the government is incapable of effectively and efficiently managing a system that provides care to all, whether the solutions include tax credits, expansion of Medicaid, Child Health Plus, or mandatory employer-based systems for part-time, temporary, new, and former employees (Hendrix, 2002; "Paralysis," 2002). This national ambiguity will delay any but the most incremental system change.

Pressure on Providers to Enhance Efficiency and Effectiveness

The complex scenario created by declining reimbursement, increasing regulatory pressures, and the drive for quality and cost containment has prompted several responses by organized nursing and advanced practice nurses, including a commitment to evidence-based practice and quality improvement, strategies believed to be both fiscally and clinically sound (Agency for Healthcare Research and Quality [AHRQ], 2002b; DeBourgh, 2002; Starr, 2002). This is a positive response to the pressures of cost control and quality outcomes and is the opportunity for advanced practice nurses to play a role in both efforts.

Advanced practice nurses need to measure and report practice outcomes related to patients as well as the benchmarks identified by regulatory agencies and consumer groups. Evidence-based practice may have several important outcomes beyond clinical effectiveness and cost containment. First, evidence-based practice may bring physicians and nurses closer to shared goals and processes of patient care. Second, payers and providers may be reassured by reductions in practice variability and improved care outcomes. Finally, evidence-based practice may improve patients' adherence to therapeutic regimens, thereby also improving care and decreasing cost (Keckly, 2002).

Financial and Professional Recognition

Recognition of advanced practice nursing's central role in health care is directly linked to compensation, credentialing, and prescriptive, admitting, and other privileges and remains high on nursing's legislative and policy agenda. The focus on financial and professional recognition is the topic of several chapters in this book. In addition to public recognition of the expert authority of nurses, the most immediate recognition of a professional group's authority to practice is payment; barrier to payment is a code for the other recognition issues, including education, gender, status, and competition with other providers (see chapters 2, 7, and 22).

Although content on reimbursement and the structure of the health care finance system is commonly included in advanced practice programs, nurses are still not knowledgeable about the sources of revenue that support their practice sites. While advanced practice nurses are generally unaware of sources of payment, probably because they are largely salaried, professional associations and lobbyists have generated support for third-party payment for advanced practice nursing services from Medicaid, Medicare, and some managed care organizations. Improved access to managed care panels and elimination of the supervision requirements in many state practice laws are necessary to facilitate access to advanced practice services.

Other important sources of professional recognition, including credentialing, compensation, and prescribing and admitting privileges, are covered in other chapters in this book, including 7, 15, and 22.

Health Disparities

While there is volatility in the health care environment, there has been a consistency over time in the themes of both public rhetoric and legislation, including concern about the continued rise in health care costs, the number of uninsured and underinsured, incremental expansion of coverage, anticipation of expanding needs of certain populations such as the elderly, and the impact of technology on care and cost.

The widening gulf between the health care "haves and have nots" will continue to create a dilemma for practitioners and potential clients. The effects of both public and private sector pressure to reduce the amount spent on care, health maintenance organization panels limited acceptance of nurse practitioners, and the pressure to reduce eligibility, benefits, and access raise significant issues of safety and quality of care in all health care settings (American Nurses Association [ANA], 2002a, 2002b). The nation is moving toward a distinctly tiered system in which many will have limited options and many will have neither insurance coverage nor the capacity to pay. Specifically, it is anticipated that there will be three groups; a well-educated, well-financed group that will have options and a voice in decisions; a mid-level group that will have limited choices and limited eligibility; and a third group that will have intermittent or no coverage. These increasing disparities in access to care (Lieberman, 2002), prescription drugs (Safran, 2002), and safe and effective services (ANA, 2002a, 2002b) confront patients and advanced practice nurses alike.

The rise in the number of uninsured from 38.7 million in 2000 to 45.6 million in 2002 to a projected 54 million by 2007 (Shiels, 1999) is associated with changes from long-term employment and employment-based coverage to employment in smaller organizations without benefits, the inability to assume costs of co-payments and deductibles, and the increased cost of insurance purchased in the private market. The new economic environment will lead to an increase in premiums that will reflect the increased use of prescription drugs and expanded use of services secondary to demands for broader choices in managed care plans (Ginsberg, 2002; Lieberman, 2002).

For the uninsured, the problems of access are twice as difficult as those for people who are covered by private insurers or Medicaid and three times greater than those covered by Medicare (Cunningham & Kemper, 1998). Disparities in access and treatment have several consequences, including over 18,000 deaths annually because diagnosis or appropriate care is delayed or there is no access to preventive care (Institute of Medicine, 2002). For low-income rural and urban groups, children, African-American and Hispanic populations, family income and lack of insurance prevent development of a relationship with a primary care provider, further contributing to health disparities (Blankfield et al., 2002; Merzel & Moon-Howard, 2002). Unless systemic changes are effected, these inequities will increase in concert with the projected expansion of minority populations from 2000 to 2030, during which time the African-American population will increase from 12 % to 13%, Hispanics from 13% to 19%, and Asians from 4% to 7% (Betancourt, Green, & Carillo, 2002; Hargraves, 2002; Louie, 2001).

Increasingly, advanced practice nurses will struggle with defining their professional responses to the plight of the uninsured and underinsured as employing institutions, organizations, and group practices lack the flexibility of cross subsidy to accommodate free or discounted pricing (Hendrix, 2002). Services of advanced practice nurses that could meet the needs of these populations will not be available without changes in the reimbursement system; fewer barriers to practice, including technologic links to physicians, who are not well-distributed geographically (Aiken & Salmon, 1994); greater access to capital; and greater access to consultation. Nursing has traditionally focused on the disparities among groups, and nurse researchers are examining the health-related problems of vulnerable populations, prompted by the legal, political, and economic events of the second half of the 20th century, including the dismantling of federal agencies and programs during the Reagan years and the futile attempt to develop health care reform in the Clinton administration (Downs, 1986; Flaskerud et al., 2002). Researchers have identified priorities for groups that must be addressed to meet the goals of Healthy People 2010 (Burnes-Bolton, 2001; delaCruz, McBride, Compas, Calixto, & VanDerveer, 2002; Louie, 2001; Parker, Haldane, Kelfner, Strickland, & Tom-Orme, 2002; Portillao et al., 2001).

Remedies to the gaps in health care undertaken by advanced practice nurses include lobbying for incremental increases in coverage to include services by advanced practice nurses; collection of data by health plans to document care for racial and ethnic minority groups (Nerenz, 2002); utilizing the quality improvement process and participating in research that establishes relationships among nursing care and patient outcomes, including examination of Nursing Sensitive Quality Indicators (ANA, 2002a; 2002b); and recruitment of potential advanced practice students from health professional shortage areas and educating them in their home communities (Kippenbrock, Stacy, Tester, & Richy, 2002). Advanced practice nurses should also take leadership roles in advancing organizational, systemic, and clinical cultural competence (Betancourt et al., 2002).

Corporatization of Health Care

In tandem with the overall business flavor of health care is the intensifying corporate character of professional practice that encourages fiscal over clinical decisions, nonprofessional/business control of licensed professionals' practice, and employee status for an increasing number of health professionals. The services of managed care companies blur the distinction between professional judgment and utilization review. This decline in the distinction among insuring, financing, and clinical decisions continues to influence the access to, eligibility for, and availability of services.

The cost containment, limited reimbursement, and reduced staffing dynamic is not the only indication of the corporatization of health care and professional practice. Other developments are having a profound effect on professional practice, including the push by business corporations to provide everything from physical and occupational therapy services to veterinary medicine services. Management service organizations (MSOs) are attempting to expand into supervision and profit sharing of professional practices. State law governs professional titles, scope of practice and the extent of overlap among professions' services, and the formation of professional partnerships and professional service corporations, but states are struggling to keep up with these incursions into the professional practice arena (University of the State of New York [USNY], 2000).

FACTORS SHAPING PROFESSIONAL EDUCATION

Nursing education is influenced directly by all the factors that shape higher education generally, including funding, philosophy and mission of higher education, the movement toward internationalization of education and institutional priorities for international outreach, and the factors that drive professional educational preparation.

DIRECTIONS IN HIGHER EDUCATION

In response to the general economy and states' fiscal response to the recession, institutions of higher education, both public and private, are facing significant budget constraints. Reduction in state tax revenues have led to reduced support for public institutions, while at the same time endowment earnings and donations are down, leading to pressure on private institutions. Reduced funding for colleges and universities has resulted in tuition increases of 6% to 10%, an increasing demand for financial aid and thus students' post-graduation debt, and a shift in selection from small independent colleges to larger public institutions with lower tuition costs (Schemo, 2002; Young, 2002). Approximately 18% of nursing programs are in baccalaureate colleges (Carnegie Classification) and vulnerable to this shift (Berlin et al., 2002).

Institutional budget reallocations are creating gaps in library and information services, depressing advances in technology-based instruction and information retrieval (Smallwood, 2002). Budget constraints have also led to an increasing number of part-time faculty, particularly in field-intensive higher cost programs in fine arts, social sciences, and health sciences including nursing (46.6% part-time faculty). Part-time faculty increased overall by 79% from 1981 to 1999. The Department of Education's Study of Postsecondary Faculty noted that 62% of all instructional faculty are now either part time (49%), full time nontenure track (7%), and full time without tenure (6%) (E. Anderson, 2002; Walsh, 2002).

Other higher education issues include increasing federal and state interest in, and potentially greater regulatory oversight of, institutional outcomes such as retention and graduation rates, graduate pass rates on professional licensing examinations, and improved articulation between community and senior colleges. A 2002 U.S. Department of Education report suggests that colleges be held accountable for institutional effectiveness in retaining and graduating students in a timely manner and report to state and federal governments on these measures (Burd, 2002). Depending on the perspective, this could lead to diminished access for less well prepared and upwardly mobile students, frequently found in nursing programs, as institutions attempt to preserve better outcome measures. Or it could stimulate institutions to provide improved advising, lower faculty-student ratios, increase faculty interest in students, and other strategies known to support academic achievement (Wilson, 2002).

Internationalization

Internationalization is taking several forms in higher education. American institutions are accepting an increasing number of new immigrants, and at the same time are expanding their own presence into other countries. The large number of students born in other countries brings to some institutions an intense demand for English language immersion, remediation services, and other support services. Foreign graduates, including physicians and other health professionals, are applying to schools of nursing assuming their past experiences will facilitate completion of generalist and advanced practice nursing programs.

A second development extends the study abroad concept, which has been an important option in many colleges and universities, by offering programs to nationals in countries seeking English language education and specialized programs. Typically, an American college partners with a local institution that is interested in providing English language education, will recruit students with the cachet of an American university degree, and can thus provide access to specialized programs not available locally. As these programs expand, and as countries other than the United States adopt roles for advanced practice nurses, policy and regulatory issues will arise for nursing program graduates in terms of their eligibility for licensure and certification, practice jurisdictions, and how graduates will fit into the education and practice structures of their country.

Professional Education

Despite the general interest in master's programs to prepare advanced practice nurses, there are significant factors that continue to mitigate against expanding programs and enrollments. These forces include reduced state appropriations and constrained college and university funding, increased competition for federal start-up funds for new programs, the identified costs of students in the clinical setting in a corporate culture that does not necessarily value teaching and research, new competition with medical students and residents for primary care placements and preceptors, shortage of nurse faculty and the competition for clinically expert faculty, and the expanded and prolonged risk management and legal reviews of institutional and agency placement contracts.

While there has been growth in the number of and enrollment in master's programs and the potential for increased utilization of advanced practice nurses across a wide range of settings, operant factors affecting program development make it difficult to predict the future of education of advanced practice nurses in any but the most conservative manner. New program development will be limited by reduction in federal funding and institutional pressure to support high enrollment programs; programs with low enrollments will be collapsed or content integrated into other programs, for example, geriatric content may be included as part of the adult program.

Curriculum

Advanced practice programs strive for a balance between general and specialized content and focus. The argument for more general preparation is linked to cost-effectiveness, available faculty expertise, flexibility, and the graduate's ability to take advantage of a wide range of practice opportunities. Broad areas of preparation also counter the criticism that nursing is mimicking medical specialization. The argument for greater depth and more narrow specialty preparation is that many generalist skills have been incorporated into baccalaureate nursing preparation, the expectations for more autonomous practice and more complex patient care, regardless of setting, requires greater depth of knowledge, and advanced practice nurses work with distinct populations and diseases and/or in defined settings.

Curricular distinctions between nurse practitioner programs and clinical nurse specialists have been discussed with varying degrees of intensity for several decades. Reviews in the early 1990s found that curricular preparation and practice were increasingly similar (Elder & Bullough, 1990; Forbes, Rafson, Spross, & Kozlowski, 1990). The debate muted as the demand for nurse practitioners increased in both inpatient and outpatient settings, the reimbursement system favorably recognized advanced practice nurses, and educational programs were designed to prepare graduates for certification as clinical nurse specialists or nurse practitioners. While the roles that all advanced practice nurses are expected to engage in—provider, consultant, patient educator, and researcher—continue to be addressed in both nurse practitioner and clinical nurse specialist curricula, the debate about the relative importance of each of these roles has resurfaced as hospitals with depleted ranks of experienced senior nurses revive the role of expert consultant/clinical nurse specialist. The role preparation most notably lacking is that of teacher of students in clinical programs. Recruited for their clinical expertise, the clinicians lack the preparation and experience in instruction and evaluation required to assume faculty positions.

Curricular content is increasingly prescribed by specialty organizations, credentialing bodies, state education departments, boards of nursing, and the move toward increased standardization. These prescriptions are prompted by professional interests, third-party payers, consumers, and state agencies requiring more assurances of quality and cost-effectiveness.

Curricular content in advanced practice programs generally includes advanced nursing theory; research and statistics; professional and systems issues; advanced assessment; sciences, including pharmacology and prescriptive authority knowledge and skills, pathophysiology, psychoimmunology, epidemiology, and others, depending on the specialty focus; clinical content; and 400 to 800 hours of precepted clinical experiences congruent with the objectives of the program.

Although the didactic content requirements are generally understood by students, less tangible expectations of the advanced practice programs occasionally catch students unaware even though they are described in program materials and are part of the conversation with faculty. Students who enroll in advanced practice programs often do not appreciate the difference from their current practice in the role expectations or responsibilities of advanced practice until they are far along in the program. Accountability, autonomy, continuous responsibility, and new collaborative relationships with physicians and others are behaviors that some students have not necessarily developed in their generalist nursing practice and ultimately find difficult or impossible to cultivate in their new role. To close the gap in role expectations between basic nursing preparation and advanced nursing practice education, we need to establish an appreciation of advanced practice nursing within the basic curriculum and among generalist nurses.

New specialty program development will be slowed by the budget constraints in the public and private higher education sectors, the limited federal funds available for program start-up or expansion, and the leveling of enrollments in current programs. Although new specialty programs may be delayed, there will be significant content revision and enrichment to meet the demands for cultural competence, greater research skills, more science, enhanced informational and medical technology, and greater levels of expertise at the point of program completion.

Cultural competence is a necessary part of all preparatory programs, even in those here-to-fore homogeneous communities. Cultural competence is viewed as a "strategy to reduce disparities in access to and quality of health care" (Betancourt et al., 2002). In health care it is seen as the ability of systems to provide care to patients with diverse values, beliefs, and behaviors and to tailoring delivery to meet patients' social, cultural, and linguistic needs. From this perspective, cultural competence is viewed as a link between quality improvement and the elimination of racial and ethnic disparities in health care. Academic and clinical service organizations are addressing this through intensive recruitment of members of underrepresented groups and providing content in cross-cultural information and clinical training (Betancourt et al., 2002).

The current spotlight on patient safety and quality improvement initiatives means that advanced practice nurses must have strong preparation in quality measurement and research methodology and the ability to understand the quality of evidence in individual research studies (AHRQ, 2002a, 2002b; Buerhaus & Norman, 2001; McGee, 1996; Steele, 2001). The imperative to strengthen research requirements runs counter to the trend to reduce research course requirements in order to increase clinical content and experiences demanded to reach expectations for greater clinical competence. Despite the attention to evidence-based practice, students and practitioners view research as extraneous to the advanced practice role, relying on preceptors, pharmaceutical, and on-line information (Camiah, 1997; Steele, 2001). Steele (2001) suggested that weakening of research focus is related to an emphasis on clinical faculty and preceptors for practitioner programs and a decline in the number of faculty with a research focus. There will be an imbalance between the public understanding of the evaluation of research findings (Brody, 2002) and nurse practitioners' ability to understand and apply research unless preparatory programs are more effective in their integration and emphasis.

Standardization of preparation and credentialing will create greater pressure on academic programs and students to incorporate and achieve a higher level of skill proficiency by program completion. The pressure to demonstrate greater knowledge and skills is exacerbated by the economic environment of health care delivery, the increasing acuity of both primary and tertiary care, patients' rapid deployment across care settings, and the responsibility of nurses and others to reduce errors (Buerhaus & Norman, 2001). The emphasis on evidence-based practice, national uniform standards, and increased governmental and consumer surveillance add pressure to programs and graduates (Deshefy-Longi, Swartz, & Grey, 2002; Pulchini & Marion, 2000). Structured care approaches (SCAs), including protocols, clinical pathways, decision analysis, and algorithms, are being used to frame "best practices" in order to increase efficiency and reduce costs. Using these approaches, students can organize complex clinical knowledge and make appropriate clinical decisions (O'Neill & Dluhy, 2000).

As with all nursing education, advanced practice curricula need to address the expanded science and technology base for master's programs as well as examine and trend clinical problems and practice patterns (Deshefy-Longi et al., 2002; Donaldson, 2002). Increasingly, genetics is part of the expanded science and technology content essential to include in advanced practice programs. Focus on genetics is important because genetics information, technology, and testing are used in delivery of health care services (G. Anderson, Monsen, Prows, Tinley, & Jenkins, 2000). The AACN through *Essentials of Baccalaureate Education for Professional Nursing Practice,* the National Institute of Nursing Research, and the International Society of Nurses in Genetics through their *Statement on the Scope and Standards of Genetics Clinical Nursing Practice* (G. Anderson et al., 2000) all support genetics as a more visible component of the science core and clinical applications.

The future of advanced practice is dramatically affected by the development of information technology and telecommunications at a speed that outpaces government policy, regulation, or professional oversight. Technology is medical, informational, and assistive—tools for advanced practice nurses, health information consumers, and patients and clients. Telehealth is the practice of health care delivery, diagnosis, consultation, treatment, and transfer of data and education by using interactive audio, visual, and data communications (Jenkins & White, 2001). In the managed care environment, telehealth can increase professional contact, eliminate travel time, and increase the opportunity for collaborative practice and consultation. There is evidence that technology can support effective, efficient nurse-patient interactions and reduce emergency department and unscheduled office visits and repeat hospitalizations as a result of early intervention and symptom management. The curricular integration of technology will have to be enhanced so that nurses can use it effectively and bring applications to patients that will supplement care (Nativio, 2000).

Greater levels of expertise demanded of new graduates require more controlled and technology-based instruction so that all students have the experiences expected of well-prepared clinicians. In order to ensure that all students have equally rigorous and relevant experiences, many professional schools are structuring the inclusion of standardized patient encounters, integrating the case-study approach in clinical and nonclinical courses, and requiring longer hours of clinical practica. The key is balancing technology-based instruction with more traditional instructional methods.

Faculty

The most important aspect of advanced practice preparation is the quality of clinical instruction and supervision. Clinical faculty serving as preceptors and clinical supervisors promote in their students a reflective practice and a heightened awareness of necessary knowledge and skills essential in light of the demand for a greater level of expertise at program completion (DeMarco, Horowitz, & McLeod, 2000; Hayes, 1998). Securing appropriately prepared faculty to teach in advanced practice programs is a major issue in light of the overall long-term faculty shortage, the competition among programs for clinical experts, and the varying degrees of flexibility in academic institutions to combine teaching responsibilities with clinical practice opportunities distinct from student practica supervision.

Once appointed, faculty clinicians present other challenges, including their lack of traditional preparation in teaching, course and curriculum development, and assessment and evaluation; their lack of appreciation for the expectations of the academic culture; and the obligation thus shifted to other faculty. Programs and texts (Thompson, Kershbaumer, & Krisman-Scott, 2001) offered to clinicians address these requirements and underscore the need for additional formal and/or informal programs to prepare clinicians as knowledgeable teachers.

Clinicians bring their network of colleagues and their good working relationships with physicians and others that infuse a practice paradigm into the educational program and improve access to new preceptors and new agencies. Students obviously benefit from working with experts who have, in addition to clinical skills, the skills gained from experience in handling ethical, legal, fiscal, and interpersonal practice issues. Clinical agencies are more cooperative and comfortable dealing with expert clinician faculty, and the preceptors in agencies view these faculty as knowledgeable colleagues. Unfortunately, clinicians often come to the academic setting anticipating less consuming and less stressful work than that of the practice setting. They are unprepared for the diversity of demands and the stress of being responsive to students, patients, clinical agency administrators, and academic colleagues and administrators. Joint appointments create the additional competition between clinical and teaching responsibilities, and the immediacy of clinical demands always dominates.

Nursing faculty are supplemented by other scientists with credentials appropriate to genetics, pharmacology, pathophysiology, and other program requirements; by researchers with a variety of backgrounds; and by experts in legal, ethical, organizational, and fiscal aspects of practice. Physicians continue to serve as faculty in didactic portions of programs and as preceptors in clinical practica. Although the need for medical expertise has decreased considerably with the relative increase in prepared advanced practice faculty, there continue to be advantages to the ongoing physician involvement in preparatory programs. Physicians provide clinical expertise and perspectives and, in the process, become more conversant with advanced practice nursing and confident in the knowledge and skills of students and graduates.

As noted earlier, nontraditional faculties have increased significantly, reflecting full-time master's-prepared nontenure track and part-time faculty status. Master's-prepared clinical faculty are a strength of advanced practice programs, but the imbalance of master's-prepared clinicians to doctorally prepared faculty with research preparation may also contribute to the new advanced practice graduate's lack of research skills. In many institutions, there is also a lack of understanding about the role and standing of master's-prepared clinical faculty, leading to subtle differences in status and value of contribution.

Funding

Despite the need for generalist and advanced practice nurses, federal funding for academic programs; financial aid in the form of scholarships, traineeships, and loan forgiveness; and institutional support in public and private sectors for baccalaureate and higher degree programs is limited.

As practice shifts from structured acute-care settings to ambulatory, home, and community-based settings, the need for better educated, more autonomous practitioners is escalating. Acute-care settings are also changing, with few medical residents in specialty training, the opening of attending physician- and nurse practitioner-managed units, and the overall down-sizing of nursing staff, including the loss of senior clinicians and supervisory staff. But funding for nursing education and clinical training by all levels of government is at odds with anticipated consumer needs and provider skill mix.

Community college programs, supported by county and state governments, prepare graduates for the small but acute inpatient population but are not cost-effective or efficient since graduates eventually seek baccalaureate preparation at additional cost in time and money. Federal funds through Title VIII, The Nurse Education Act, provided only $67.83 million to nursing programs in 1999. During the same year, Medicare support of medical and nursing education was $6.2 billion, with only $166 million or 9.7% directed to nursing and a disproportionate amount of support going to a very small number of geographically concentrated hospital-based diploma programs (AACN, 2002). As noted in chapter 25, schools of nursing are heavily dependent on tuition revenue and lack substantial revenue streams from research and clinical practice that typically support medical education.

The capacity of advanced practice nursing programs could be expanded by redirecting existing levels of funding to appropriate levels of education and preparation of clinicians, including those prepared to teach in academic programs. Thus, funding for advanced practice preparation should be aligned with anticipated need and coordinated by all levels of government. Appropriate government support that makes education more available would address a range of issues, including the need for greater diversity, recruitment of a younger workforce, and enhanced graduate and undergraduate graduation rates through increased full-time study.

Credentialing

Credentialing is a process common to education and practice encompassing a variety of mechanisms that share a set of common goals: to ensure quality, competency, and accountability and to achieve recognition for funding or reimbursement. These goals take on more importance as consumers and payers require assurances of quality and cost-effectiveness. The meaning of each of the current credentialing mechanisms should be widely disseminated to the constituencies requiring the information so that they may select and pay for programs and services knowledgeably.

Credentialing targets individuals, academic institutions, and health care organizations through various mechanisms. (Credentialing of individual practitioners is discussed in chapter 23). Certification is carried out by both governmental and nongovernmental bodies; the process attests that a licensed professional has met certain standards of preparation, experience, and successful testing. In contrast to individual provider certification, some states and professional organizations certify educational programs following review of curricula and practice requirements. Certification in such instances is automatically conferred on graduates who successfully complete the certified program.

Specialty certification still lacks the clarity and consistency of standards because it recognizes both generalist and specialist practice, a range of educational preparation, and other variable criteria, including experience. To be useful to advanced practice nursing, certification should uniformly require advanced practice preparation embedded in master's or post-master's degree programs and represent a uniform level of expertise. Certification should also be continually redefined in keeping with the development of new science and technologies and the natural evolution of scope of practice.

Institutional credentialing includes accreditation of academic institutions and programs and reviews of hospitals and community health care agencies. Accreditation is the process by which nongovernment agencies and organizations review and grant accreditation status to institutions and programs according to stated criteria. Officially designated accrediting bodies—including the Commission on Collegiate Nursing Education (CCNE) and the National League for Nursing Accreditation Commission (NLNAC)—are, in turn, reviewed and recognized by national accrediting bodies and the Department of Education. In health care, the Joint Commission on Accreditation of Healthcare Organizations (JCAHO) and The Community Health Accreditation Program (CHAP) review and accredit hospitals and long-term care facilities and home care agencies, respectively.

The American College of Nurse Midwifery maintains the dual function of specifying curriculum requirements and certification requirements; such credentialing has served to create a standard minimum curriculum that ensures comparability of preparation. In contrast to nurse-midwifery, the lack of comparability in credentialing in most other specialty practice areas fosters unevenness in advanced practice master's programs and different levels of clinical proficiency.

All states have mechanisms for credentialing advanced practice nurses. However, the mechanisms for achieving certification vary by state and include national certification examinations, state boards of nursing and or medicine approval, state examination, completion of academic programs, or some combination. These state variations are confusing to constituent groups and limit practitioner mobility. The interstate compact model proposed in 1997, which requires each state's legislative approval, currently allows generalist nurses cross-jurisdictional authority in 16 states. This model is being proposed for advanced practice nurses (Hardin & Langford, 2001; NCSBN, 2002). Other proposals include a special form of telepractice licensure and "model practice laws" to support national consistency within a profession (University of the State of New York, 2000).

LINKING EDUCATION AND PRACTICE

Formal links between academic programs and clinical practice began in the 1960s (Christman & Grace, 1981; Ford 1981; MacPhail, 1972; Smith, 1965) and centrally involved schools of nursing administrators and faculty in the administration and delivery of nursing services (Christman & Grace, 1981; Ford, 1981). In addition to the dual appointment model, there have been a variety of other affiliation models, such as with nursing homes (Mezey & Lynaugh, 1989; home care programs (see chapter 25) and agencies (see chapter 17), and dedicated units within hospitals.

Although academic programs and health facilities voice a desire to develop alliances that will facilitate recruitment and recognize advantages of sharing faculty and clinical staff expertise, the desired results of these collaborations have been uneven and, in many cases, dependent on the personalities involved. Academic programs and clinical practices have developed a variety of collaborative arrangements tempered by the changing economic and clinical environment. Academic programs have an interest in greater access for students' clinical placements, access to subjects for clinical research, and opportunities to shape clinical care. Clinical practices have the potential benefits of recruiting graduates familiar and skilled in the practice, access to faculty expertise, and the improved quality of care associated with faculty and student participation in patient care. Collaborative efforts are also influenced by the efficiency demands of practitioners, which are affected by the time and attention required by students,

Nursing programs and medical centers' departments of nursing are attempting to integrate the education, research, and clinical practice elements for mutually beneficial reasons. Hospital departments of nursing have lost many of the staff dedicated to staff development, community outreach, and educational liaison work. Hospitals see many opportunities to involve advanced practice nurses in research, evaluation studies, and evidence-based practice, but these activities can cut into clinical time and thus affect productivity. Similarly, advanced practice nurse faculty can enhance nursing departments' efforts to conduct and participate in research because the staff's lack of experience in research can impede involvement in these areas. Successful student affiliations can maximize recruitment efforts and improve staffing ratios. For the clinical and tenure track faculty teaching in advanced practice nursing programs, more direct linkages with hospitals and health care agencies can improve clinical instruction, support more clinical input into curriculum and student practice requirements, and open opportunities for students and faculty to engage in clinically based projects.

While many connections have been forged in the quest to develop clinical practices managed by faculty and students, the reimbursement system and the limited degree to which academic institutions are prepared and able to take financial risk for patient care has depressed advanced practice nursing faculties' practice management ventures. The practices that do exist generate significant information for students with respect to reimbursement, risk management, legal and ethical issues of practice, and the benefits of interprofessional collaboration. The practice projects also demonstrate that collaborative relationships can improve patient care and provide important clinical learning opportunities for faculty, staff, and students (Garrad, Kane, Ratner, & Buchanon, 1991; Mezey & Lynaugh, 1989; Mitty, Bottrell, & Mezey, 1997; Shaughnessey, Kramer, Hittle, & Steiner, 1996; Winslow, 1997).

Effective models of collaboration recognize the scale of the institutions involved, the financial risk aversion of academic institutions, and the unique philosophy and mission. So while collaborations will continue, they will focus on smaller initiatives such as shared appointments, clinical research partnerships, and specific projects and programs.

THE FUTURE OF ADVANCED PRACTICE NURSING

Despite the uncertainty and occasional chaos of the health care system, the future of advanced practice nursing and the profession of nursing is potentially in the most exciting and momentous period in our profession's history. The highly publicized shortage of nurses, higher education's continued endorsement of nursing programs, and standards of practice suggest that nursing can play an even more central role in the evolving health care delivery system.

Nursing's opportunity to make health care accessible, humane, and efficacious depends on assurances that education, clinical training, and standards for individual and institutional credentialing are rigorous and consistent. This is necessary to convey clear information and expectations to consumers and payers. The expansion, more even distribution, and access to and utilization of advanced practice nurses depends on more uniform reimbursement policies and practice privileges that meet consumer and patients' needs consistent with competitive, high-quality and cost-effective care.

In the face of this range of opportunities for advanced practice nursing, what will be the most important areas for the focused attention of educators, practitioners, and policy makers? The following sections briefly discuss five developing areas: new practice opportunities, collaboration and interdisciplinary education and practice, globalization of the advanced practice model, E-health, and disaster preparation.

Practice Opportunities

Institutional and community-based practices will continue to offer new practice options to academically and clinically prepared and credentialed providers. In order to anticipate and produce change, or simply to take advantage of existing opportunities advantageous to their consumers, advanced practice nurses need preparation as experts, socialization as autonomous, accountable, and ethical providers; and grounding in the fiscal, technologic, legal, and political requirements of health care delivery.

Acute and primary care will continue to offer the potential for advanced practice. The continued development of freestanding group practices and the expansion of advanced practice nursing into home care, nursing homes, assisted living facilities, and specialty hospitals and practice will continue as direct payment becomes more available and as the economic impact of adding nurse practitioners to the provider mix is acknowledged.

Research on the effectiveness, cost, and quality of advanced practice nursing services will continue and broaden to focus on new models of care and the nature of advanced practice in relation to specific patient outcomes (Brown & Grimes, 1995; Naylor et al., 1999). As advanced practice nurses are reimbursed and become visible parts of large databases, their interventions will be available to examine in relation to patient care outcomes.

Collaboration and Interdisciplinary Practice

The rhetoric regarding the need for greater interdisciplinarity continues despite the lack of resources to support collaborative and interprofessional education and practice. In the past, the drive to collaboration often came from groups regarded as secondary to medicine who used it as a way to gain recognition. The subject of collaboration has been a staple in nursing but is neither well taught nor well practiced. As advanced practice nursing becomes more central and less dependent on medicine for authority and status, it is not clear what the impetus will be to promote interdisciplinary practice unless the imperative of better patient outcomes can leverage collaboration.

Corser (2000) examined two decades of literature from sociologists, anthropologists, and others for insight into the influential elements of the physician–nurse relationship and the implications for practice. He identified five elements: the different patient care orientations of each profession; the institutionalized traditions that reinforce the paradigm of the scientific, male physician and the caring, emotional female nurse; reinforcement by stereotypical media presentations; the real and perceived power differential between medicine and nursing; and a pattern of communication that sidesteps the basic "contradictions that exist between the overall nursing and medicine paradigms." Corser suggested that effective collaboration will be possible only as a result of additional study of the interactions of the two professions and documentation of the related patient and provider outcomes.

Beyond rhetoric, it will be interesting to see what nursing does to continue its stated commitment to interdisciplinary practice and whether the corporate values associated with team work will prevail.

Globalization and the International Extension of Advanced Practice Nursing

Faculties of schools of nursing in countries around the world are increasingly examining the comparability of their basic and advanced programs to American nursing education programs (Modly, 1995) and, in particular, the possibility of adapting advanced practice nursing preparation to their countries' health and education systems. The international extension of advanced practice nursing raises as many issues for American educators and clinicians as it does for nurses in other countries. For American advanced practice nurses, the questions include how aggressively should our models be proposed, how to candidly present a balanced picture of the strengths and weaknesses of our system, how to present our education and health care system so that elements can be adapted by others as opposed to an "all or nothing" approach. For nurses in other countries, a few of the issues are recognition of the wide variations in educational preparation, support of ministers of health and education, and adequate preparation of nurse faculty to teach advanced practice skills. What is the appropriate role for technology-based instruction and practice across national borders?

E-Health

E-health is the electronic exchange of health-related data collected, generated, or analyzed. It encompasses three aspects: business, clinical, and consumer applications. The success of these applications varies. According to DeLuca and Enmark (2000), business e-health, including financial and reporting applications, is the most well developed of the components. This is evident in the success of electronic claims submissions. Clinical e-health is less well developed secondary to the issues of security, privacy, and data standards.

Advanced practice nurses and other providers could gain significant efficiencies and efficacy through e-mail patient communication and education, chronic illness management, and provider Web sites linked with health information Web sites judged accurate and informative. It is estimated that in 2000 approximately 30 to 40 million Americans accessed the 16,000 to 20,000 health-related Web sites—highlighting the need for analyzing, understanding, and reconciling information that may be inaccurate or conflicting (Stefl, 2000). For consumers, access to health information and products is frequently more easily achieved through technology than through face-to-face encounters with providers. In a more fully developed e-health system, consumers would communicate with providers regarding their disease management, gain access to personal health records, order prescription refills, and schedule appointments. Patient satisfaction with telehealth incorporating video has been shown to be good, but patients and families do not want technology-based care to replace human contact (Thurmond & Boyle, 2002).

E-health poses many and policy questions, including the extent to which advanced practice nurses should be prepared for the technologic, ethical, and communication elements of these new systems by their clinical preparatory programs; cross-jurisdictional practice and reimbursement; and e-consultation versus e-practice or telehealth. What role should advanced practice nurses play in developing standards for clinical information and educating Internet users to evaluate provider credentials and product effectiveness (Greene, 2000)?

Response to Disaster

Recent events have prompted efforts by organized nursing to prepare generalist and advanced practice nurses to respond effectively to terrorist attacks and large-scale disasters. Professional organizations and state boards of nursing recognize the following needs: to facilitate nurses' response to disasters by immediately identifying them as license holders, to promote educational programs for nurses about potential threats and agents (P. Anderson, 2001), and to participate in the public's education (Trossman, 2002). The American Nurses Association, in conjunction with the United States Department of Health and Human Services, established a National Nurses Response Team that would call nurses to events to vaccinate and administer medication to the public (http://www.nursing-world.org/news/disaster/response.htm).

To be responsive and effective, advanced practice and generalist nurses need to know how different classes of chemical, biologic, and radiologic agents work; the likely presenting symptoms; and how to diagnose and treat victims of exposure. This content is being incorporated into nurse practitioner and community health programs as well as continuing education offerings and Web-based resources ("Bioterrorism," 2002). Although such knowledge and treatment skills are important (Coleman, 2002; Coleman & Yergler, 2002; Sibley, 2002; "Training of Clinicians," 2000) the system in which advanced practice nurses will function during these events is poorly defined and organized. This is exacerbated by the fact that there is no "surge capacity" in our current public health system to respond to such disasters ("Warning," 2002).

CONCLUSIONS

Advanced practice nursing continues to develop in a highly open and fluctuating health care environment. Optimistically, flux will provide more opportunities for professional recognition, innovative practice models, greater compensation, organizational support, and autonomy. At the same time, the explosive changes in science and technology, demands on individual and institutional providers, and budget constraints on academic and service institutions create a need to anticipate and position the profession while simultaneously affirming the values and standards that have defined nursing.

REFERENCES

Abelson, R. (2002, June 14). Limits on residents' hours worry teaching hospitals. *New York Times,* p. A14.

Agency for Healthcare Research and Quality. (2002a). *Systems to rate the strength of scientific evidence.* Evidence Report/Technology Assessment No. 47 (AHRQ Publication No. 02-E016). Available at http://www.ahrq.gov/clinic/evrpt-files.htm#strength

Agency for Healthcare Research and Quality. (2002b). *Training of clinicians for public health events relevant to bioterrorism preparedness.* Report 51. Johns Hopkins University EPC (contract 290-97-0006). (AHRQ Publication No. 02-E011).

Aiken, L., Clarke, S., Sloane, D., Sochalski, J., & Silber, J. (2002). Hospital nurse staffing and patient mortality, nurse burnout, and job dissatisfaction. *Journal of the American Medical Association, 288,* 1987–1993. Available at http://jama.ama-assn.org/issues/v288n16/rfull/joc20547.html

Aiken, L., & Salmon, M. (1994). Healthcare workforce priorities: What nursing should do now. *Inquiry, 31,* 318–329.

Altman, L., & Grady, D. (2002, June 13). Hospital accreditor will strictly limit hours of residents. *New York Times,* pp. A1, A30.

American Association of Colleges of Nursing. (2002). Communication from Office of Government Affairs, November 20, 2002. Washington, DC: AACN National Office.

American Nurses Association. (2002a). Nursing-sensitive indicators for community-based non-acute care settings and ANA's safety & quality initiative. *Nursing Facts from the American Nurses Association.*

American Nurses Association. (2002b). Nursing-sensitive quality indicators for acute care settings and ANA's safety & quality initiative. *Nursing Facts from the American Nurses Association.* Washington, DC: Author.

Anderson, E. (2002). *The new professoriate: Characteristics, contributions, and compensation.* American Council on Education Center for Policy Analysis. Available at www.acenet.edu/bookstore

Anderson, G., Monsen, R., Prows, C., Tinley, S., & Jenkins, J. (2000). Preparing the nursing profession for participation in a genetic paradigm in health care. *Nursing Outlook, 48,* 23–27.

Anderson, P. (2001). Are you prepared for terrorist action? *The Online Journal of Knowledge Synthesis for Nursing from Nursing Spectrum.* Available at http://www/stti.iupui.edu/library/ojksn/diaster/diaster_bib_article_6-anderson.htm

Berlin, L., Stennett, J., & Bednash, G. (2002). *Enrollment and graduations in baccalaureate and graduate programs in nursing.* Washington, DC: American Association of Colleges of Nursing.

Betancourt, J., Green, A., & Carillo, J. (2002). *Cultural competence in health care: Emerging frameworks and practical approaches.* The Commonwealth Foundation. Available at www/cmwf.org

Bioterrorism resources on the web. (2002). *American Journal of Nursing, 102,* 86–88.

Blankfield, R., Goodwin, M., Jaen, C., & Strange, K. (2002). Addressing the unique challenges of inner-city practice: A direct observation study of inner-city, rural, and suburban family practices. *Journal of Urban Health, 79,* 173–184.

Brody, J. (2002, October 22). Separating gold from junk in medical studies. *New York Times,* p. F7.

Brown, S., & Grimes, D. (1993). *A meta-analysis of process of care, clinical outcomes, and cost-effectiveness of nurses in primary care roles: Nurse practitioners and certified nurse-midwives.* Washington, DC: American Nurses Association, Division of Health Policy.

Brown, S., & Grimes, D. (1995). A meta-analysis of nurse practitioners and nurse midwives in primary care. *Nursing Research, 44,* 332–339.

Buerhaus, P., & Norman, L. (2001). It's time to require theory and methods of quality improvement in basic and graduate nursing education. *Nursing Outlook, 49,* 67–69.

Bullough, B. (1992) Alternative models for specialty practice. *Nursing and Health Care, 13,* 254–259.

Burd, S. (2002). Accountability or meddling. *Chronicle of Higher Education, 44,* A23–25.

Burnes-Bolton, L. (2001). Nursing research priorities of the National Black Nurses Association. *Nursing Outlook, 49,* 258–262.

Camiah, S. (1997).Utilization of nursing research in practice and application strategies to raise research awareness amongst nurse practitioners: A model for success. *Journal of Advanced Nursing, 26,* 1193–2002.

Centers for Disease Control and Prevention. (2002). Data from the National Health Interview Survey. Available at http://www.cdc.gov/nchc/data/nhis/measure01.pdf

Christman, L., & Grace, H. (1981, September). *Unification, reunification: Reconciliation or collaboration. Modes for collaboration.* Paper presented at the meeting of the Midwest Alliance in Nursing.

Coleman, E. (2002). Anthrax update. *American Journal of Nursing, 102,* 96.

Coleman, E., & Yergler, M. (2002). Emergency: Mass casualty. *American Journal of Nursing, 102,* 44–45.

Corser, W. (2000). The contemporary nurse-physician relationship: Insights from scholars outside the two professions. *Nursing Outlook, 48,* 165–171.

Cukr, P., Jones, S., Wilberger, M., Smith, R., & Stopper, C. (1998). The psychiatric clinical nurse specialist/nurse practitioner: An example of a combined role. *Archives of Psychiatric Nursing, 11,* 2–12.

Cunningham, P., & Kemper, P. (1998). Ability to obtain medical care for the uninsured. *Journal of the American Medical Association, 280,* 921–927.

Debourgh, G. (2001). Champions for evidence-based practice: A critical role for advanced practice nurses. *AACN Clinical Issues, 12,* 491–508.

delaCruz, F., McBride, M., Compas, L., Calixto, P., & VanDerveer, C. (2001). White paper on health status of Filipino Americans and recommendations for research. *Nursing Outlook, 50,* 7–15.

DeLuca, J., & Enmark, R. (2000). E-Health: The changing model of healthcare. *Frontiers of Health Services Management, 17,* 3–16.

DeMarco, R., Horowitz, J., McLeod, D. (2000). A call to intra professional alliances. *Nursing Outlook, 48,* 172–178.

Deshefy-Longi, T., Swartz, M., & Grey, M. (2002). Establishing a practice-based research network of advanced practice registered nurses in southern New England. *Nursing Outlook, 50,* 127–132.

Donaldson, S. (2002). Genetic evolutionary view of health supports nursing research. *Journal of Professional Nursing, 18,* 187.

Downs, F. (1986). Clinical relevance revisited. *Nursing Research, 46,* 3.

Elder, R., & Bullough, B. (1990). Nurse practitioners and clinical nurse specialists: Are the roles merging? *Clinical Nurse Specialist, 4,* 78–84.

Flaskerud, J., Lessere, J., Dixon, E., Anderson, N., Conde, F., Kim, S., Koniak-Griffin, D., Strehlow, A., Tullmann, D., & Verzemnieks, I. (2002). Health disparities among vulnerable populations. *Nursing Research, 51,* 74–83.

Forbes, K., Rafson, J., Spross, J., & Kozlowski, D. (1990). The clinical nurse specialist and nurse practitioner: Core curriculum survey results. *Clinical Nurse Specialist, 4,* 63–66.

Ford, L. (1981). Creating a center of excellence in nursing. In L. Aiken (Ed.) *Health policy and nursing practice* (pp. 430–451). New York: McGraw-Hill.

Ford, L. (1982). Nurse practitioner: History of a new idea and predictions for the future. In L. Aiken & S. Gortner (Eds.), *Nursing in the 1980s: Crises, opportunities, challenges* (pp. 231–247). Philadelphia: Lippincott.

Ford, L. (1986). Nurse, nurse practitioners: The evolution of primary care. Review. Image: *Journal of Nursing Scholarship, 18,* 177–178.

Ford, L. (1997). A deviant comes of age. *Heart and Lung, 26,* 87–91.

Garrard, J., Kane, R., Ratner, E., & Buchanon, J. (1991). The impact of nurse practitioners on the care of nursing home residents. In P. Katz, R. Kane, & M. Mezey (Eds.), *Advances in long-term care (Vol. 1).* New York: Springer Publishing.

Ginsburg, P. (2002). Rough seas ahead for purchasers and consumers. *2001 Annual report, Center for Studying Health System Change.*

Greene, A. (2000). E-Health: Realizing the vision. *Frontiers of Health Services Management, 17,* 33–38.

Hardin, S., & Langford, D. (2001). Telehealth's impact on nursing and the development of the interstate compact. *Journal of Professional Nursing, 17,* 243–247.

Hargraves, J. (2002, June). The insurance gap and minority health care, 1997–2001. *Tracking Report, Center for Studying Health System Change.*

Harrison, J. (1999). Influence of managed care on professional nursing practice. Image: *Journal of Nursing Scholarship, 31,* 161–166.

Hayes, E. (1998). Mentoring and nurse practitioner self-efficacy. *Western Journal of Nursing Research, 20,* 521–535.

Hendrix, T. (2002). The uninsured, tax credits, and crowd-out. *Policy, Politics and Nursing Practice, 3,* 160–166.

Horrocks, S., Anderson, E., & Salisbury, C. (2002). Systematic review of whether nurse practitioners working in primary care can provide equivalent care to doctors. *British Medical Journal, 324,* 819–823.

Institute of Medicine. (2002). *Care without coverage: Too little, too late.* Washington, DC: Author.

Janofsky, M. (2002, May 28). Shortage of nurses spurs bidding war in hospital industry. *New York Times,* pp. A1, A14.

Jenkins, R., & White, P. (2001). Telehealth advancing nursing practice. *Nursing Outlook, 49,* 100–105.

Keckly, P. (2002). *Update 7-28-02*. Available at keckley@ebmsolutions.com

Kippenbrock, T., Stacy, A., Tester, K., & Richy, R. (2002). Nurse practitioners providing health care to rural and underserved areas in four Mississippi delta states. *Journal of Professional Nursing, 18*, 230–237.

Kovner, C., & Rosenfeld, P. (1997). Practice and employment trends among nurse practitioners in New York state. *Journal of the New York State Nurses Association, 28*(4), 4–8.

Lang, N. (2002). Health care: A casualty of competing concerns or priority for 2002. *Journal of Professional Nursing, 18*, 186.

Lewis, M., & Lewis, C. (2002). Nurse practitioners: The revolution produced by a "gender-related destructive innovation" in health care. *Nursing and Health Policy Review, 1*, 63–71.

Lieberman, T. (2002). *The unraveling of health insurance*. Available at www.ConsumerReports.org

Linn, L., & Lewis, M. (1976). Rap sessions for nurse practitioner students. *American Journal of Nursing, 76*, 782–784.

Louie, K. (2001). White paper on the health status of Asian Americans and Pacific Islanders and recommendations for research. *Nursing Outlook, 49*, 255–257.

MacPhail, J. (1972). *An experiment in nursing: Planning, implementing and assessing in planned change*. Cleveland, OH: Case Western Reserve University Press.

Mangan, K. (2002, October 31). Applications to medical schools drop for 6th year in a row. *The Chronicle of Higher Education*. Available at http://chronicle.com/daily/2002 dsaru

McCabe, S., & Grover, S. (1999). Psychiatric nurse practitioner versus clinical nurse specialist: Moving from debate to action on the future of advanced psychiatric nursing. *Archives of Psychiatric Nursing, 13*, 111–116.

McGee, P. (1996). The research role of the advanced nurse practitioner. *British Journal of Nursing, 5*, 290–292.

McGivern, D. (1986). The evolution of primary care nursing. In M. Mezey & D. McGivern (Eds.), *Nurses, nurse practitioners: The evolution of primary care* (pp. 3–14). Boston: Little, Brown.

McGivern, D., Mezey, M., & Baer, E. (1976). Teaching primary care in a baccalaureate program. *Nursing Outlook, 24*, 7–11.

Merzel, C., & Moon-Howard, J. (2002). Access to health services in an urban community: Does source of care make a difference? *Journal of Urban Health, 79*, 186–199.

Mezey, M., & Lynaugh, J. (1989). The teaching nursing home program: Outcomes of care. *Nursing Clinics of North America, 24*, 130–141.

Mitty, E., Bottrell, M., & Mezey, M. (1997). The teaching nursing home program: Enduring educational outcomes. *Nursing Outlook, 45*, 133–140.

Modly, D. (1995). Designing curriculum to advance nursing science and professional practice. In D. Modly, P. Poletti, R. Zanotti, & J. Fitzpatrick (Eds.), *Advancing nursing education worldwide* (pp. 37–44). New York: Springer Publishing.

National Council of State Boards of Nursing. (1992). *Position paper on the licensure of advance practice nursing.* Unpublished manuscript, pp. 1–8. Nurse Licensure Compacts. Available at www.ncsbn.org

The National Organization of Nurse Practitioner Faculties (NONPF), & The American Association of Colleges of Nursing. (2002, April). *Nurse practitioner primary care competencies in specialty areas: Adult, family, gerontological, pediatric, and women's health.* Prepared for the Department of Health and Human Services, Washington, DC: USPHS, DHSS.

Nativio, D. (2000). Robots and nurses. *Nursing Outlook, 48,* 154–155.

Naylor, M., Brooten, D., Campbell, R., Jacobsen, B., Mezey, M., Pauly, M., et al. (1999). A comprehensive discharge planning and home follow-up of hospitalized elders: A randomized controlled trial. *Journal of the American Medical Association, 281*(7), 613–620.

Needleman, J., Buerhaus, P., Mattke, S., Stewart, M., & Zelevinsky, K. (2001). *Nurse staffing and patient outcomes in hospitals.* Available at http://bhpr.hrsa.gov/nursing/staffstudy.htm

Nerenz, D. (2002). *Developing a health plan report card on quality of care for minority populations.* The Commonwealth Fund. Available at http://www/cmwf.org/publist2.asp?CategoryID=11

O'Grady, E. (2002). The nursing shortage: Why nurse practitioners should embrace the problem. *The American Journal for Nurse Practitioners, 6,* 31–36.

O'Neill, E., & Dluhy, N. (2000). Utility of structured care approaches in education and clinical practice. *Nursing Outlook, 48,*132–137.

Paralysis in health care (editorial). (2002, May 28). *New York Times,* p. A18.

Parker, J., Haldane, S., Keltner, B., Strickland, C., & Tom-Orme, L. (2002). National Alaska Native Indian Nurses Association: Reducing health disparities within American Indian and Alaska native populations. *Nursing Outlook, 50,* 16–23.

Portilla, C., Villarruel, A., Siantz, M., Peragallo, N., Calvillo, E., & Eribes, C. (2001). Research agenda for Hispanics in the United States: A nursing perspective. *Nursing Outlook, 49,* 263–269.

Pulchini, J., & Marion, L. (2000). Nurse practitioner education in the new millennium: Challenges and opportunities. *Nursing Outlook, 48,* 107–108.

Rudy, E., Davidson, L., Daly, B., Clochesy, J., Sereika, S., Baldisseri, M., Hravnak, M., Ross, T., & Ryan, C. (1998). Care activities and outcomes of patients cared for by acute care nurse practitioners, physician assistants, and resident physicians: A comparison. *American Journal of Critical Care, 7,* 267–281.

Safran, D. (2002). Seniors and prescription drugs: Findings from a 2001 survey of seniors in eight states. Health Affairs. Available at http://www.healthaffairs.org/WebExclusive/Safran_Web_Excl_073102.htm

Schemo, D. (2002, October 22). Public college tuitions rise 10% amid financing cuts. *NewYork Times,* p. A20.

Shaunghnessy, P., Kramer, A., Hittle, D., & Steiner, J. (1995). Quality of care in teaching nursing homes: Findings and implications. *Health Care Financing Review, 16*(4), 55–83.

Shiels, J. (1999). *Testimony, Subcommittee on Health, Committee on Ways and Means, U.S. House of Representatives, 106th Congress, 1st Session.* Available at http://waysandmeans.house.gov/health/106cong/6-15-99/6-15shei.htm

Sibley, C. (2002). Smallpox vaccination revisited. *American Journal of Nursing, 102,* 26–32.

Sleep-deprived doctors (editorial). (2002, June 14). *New York Times,* p. A18.

Smallwood, S. (2002, September 20). The crumbling intellectual foundation. *Chronicle of Higher Education,* pp. A10–A12.

Smith, D. (1965). Education and service under one administration. *Nursing Outlook, 13,* 54–58.

Starr, D. (2002, September). A team effort that prevents lawsuits. *The Clinical Advisor,* p. 121.

Steele, L. (2001). Incorporating research application into nurse practitioner education. *Online Journal of Knowledge Synthesis in Nursing, Document 3E.* Available at http://www.stti.iupui,edu/library/ojksn/articles/ec_doc3e.htm

Stefl, M. (2000). Editorial. *Frontiers of Health Services Management, 17,* 1.

Thompson, J., Kershbaumer, R., & Krisman-Scott, M. (Eds.) (2001). *Educating advanced practice nurses and midwives: From practice to teaching.* New York: Springer Publishing.

Thurmond, V., & Boyle, D. (2002, April 16). An integrative review of patients' perceptions regarding telehealth used in their health care. *Online Journal of Knowledge Syntheses for Nursing, 9,* Document 2.

Training of clinicians for public health events relevant to bioterrorism preparedness, report 51. Johns Hopkins University EPC (contract 290-97-0006). Report (AHRQ Publication NO. 02-E011).

Trossman, S. (2002). ANA, CMAs help nurses become better prepared to respond to disasters. *The American Nurse, 34,* 1, 10–11.

University of the State of New York, The State Education Department. (2000). Policy discussions on horizon issues impacting the practice and regulation of the 38 professions in the 21st Century. New York.

U.S. Congress, Office of Technology Assessment. (1986). Nurse practitioners, physician assistants, and certified nurse-midwives: A policy analysis. (Health Technology Case Study 37, OTA-HCS-37). Washington, DC: U.S. Government Printing Office.

U.S. Department of Health and Human Services. (2000, November).With understanding and improving health and objective for improving health. (Vols. 1–2). In *Healthy people 2010* (2nd ed.). Washington, DC: U.S. Government Printing Office.

U.S. Department of Health and Human Services. (2000): *The registered nurse population: findings from the national sample survey of registered nurses 2000.* Washington, DC: Health Resources and Services Administration, Bureau of Health Professions, Division of Nursing. Available at www.bhpr.hrsa.gov/dn

U.S. Department of Health and Human Services. (2002). *The health care workforce in eight states: Education, practice and policy, interstate comparisons.* Washington,

DC: Health Resources and Services Administration, Bureau of Health Professions, National Center for Health Workforce Analysis.

Walsh, S. (2002, October 29) Study finds significant increase in number of part-time and non-tenure-track professors. *Chronicle of Higher Education.* Available at http://chronicle.com/daily

Warning: The state of public health in America not healthy. (2002). *Advances, 1,* 1–2.

Wilson, R. (2002, November 1). Faculty members care more about students, less about prestige, study finds. *Chronicle of Higher Education.* Available at http://chronicle.com/news

Winslow, R. (1997, February 7). Nurses to take doctors duties, Oxford says. *Wall Street Journal,* p. A3.

Chapter 2

PHILOSOPHICAL AND HISTORICAL BASES OF ADVANCED PRACTICE NURSING ROLES

Ellen D. Baer

Since almost the inception of modern nursing in America toward the end of the 19th century, certain nurses practiced in ways considered more independent and advanced than the usual nursing activities. Drawn to such practice by their own inclinations, inspired by progressive ideals, and paid by society to acculturate its newest and neediest members, public health and visiting nurses tended to the sick, the poor, the young, the old, in their homes. In addition to providing physical ministrations, these nurses introduced immigrant mothers to illness prevention techniques, taught them sanitary ideals, and encouraged their use of nutritious foods. For the most part, such independent nursing practices developed in fields not yet noticed by physicians, such as midwifery and anesthesia, or outside of mainstream settings, such as among the rural populations served by the Frontier Nursing Service.

By the middle of the 20th century, America's success in World War II had changed the way Americans viewed the world. All things seemed possible, even the eradication of disease. Advances in technology, chemistry, atomic energy, transportation, manufacturing, and a host of other fields developed to assist the war effort, were turned to civilian uses. Health care was a major beneficiary of these new discoveries. Nurses shared in the

37

expansive view of health care possibilities both as providers of many new, expanded services and as beneficiaries of its largesse. Nurses left World War II with officer rank, some federal funding for nursing educational programs, and access to free university education through the G. I. Bill. Many went to college, obtained basic and advanced degrees, and began to think of themselves and their practices in new, expanding ways.

In hospitals, nurses began grouping patients recovering from anesthesia, or suffering from specific maladies such as heart disease, in clusters that ensured them the most concentrated or intensive nursing care.[1] These nurses became expert in managing the care of special populations of hospitalized patients, many of whom were critically ill. Titles like clinical nurse specialist developed to differentiate these expert specialists from their nursing colleagues who functioned in more traditional, general practice roles. Almost simultaneously, visiting and public health nurses increased their expertise in managing the care in clinics, schools, and homes. As the major agents of the nation's widespread public health efforts, these nurses promoted health and prevented disease through patient teaching, immunization services, and widespread public education programs. In the late 1950s and early 1960s, several noteworthy nurse/physician collaborative teams developed in places like Colorado and Rochester, New York, in which physicians mentored experienced nurses to deliver primary care services in clinics. Medical centers like The New York Hospital offered Primex programs to teach nurses the basics of physical assessment and clinical decision making central to delivering primary care services.

The passage of Medicare/Medicaid legislation in 1965 created an expanded demand for health services. The supply and distribution of primary care physicians was unable to meet this demand. In addition, the services demanded were broader in scope than those contained within the domain of medicine prior to the 1960s. Newly empowered consumers organized into advocacy coalitions, such as Grey Panthers, civil rights, and women's movements, sought expanded supportive functions once considered the province of multigenerational families, clergy, and the like. The nursing profession stepped into the breach. Asserting that it possessed the necessary history, organization, and educational facilities, nursing acted to supply knowledgeable and licensed individuals to meet the growing and broader demands in primary care practice.

In subsequent years, it became equally evident that clinical nurse specialists contributed, quantitatively and qualitatively, to meeting a large portion of patients' needs in hospitals and acute care. With the explosion of managed care post-1995, inpatient and acute-care facilities have begun substituting physician care with clinical nurse specialists, now unified with nurse practitioners under the generic term "advanced practice nurses." The major objection raised about the utilization of nurses in independent and autonomous roles came from those in medicine, hospital administration, and government who believed that nurses did not have the expert authority and its derivative, autonomy, on which independent practice rests.

Application of the principles of authority and autonomy to any human activity is problematic. In the context of the dynamic interactions of human experience, authority and autonomy fluctuate as do all processes that involve people. No one is always and absolutely autonomous, just as no one is completely devoid of autonomy. What is at issue is a continuum of authority and autonomy and the contextual boundaries of that continuum. In a subsequent chapter, Sullivan-Marx and Keepnews argue that the debate about authority and autonomy is really a debate about money; that the subtext regarding "authority" is that "how much do you know" really means "how much are you worth," that is, who will be paid, and how much.

Nursing[2] as an occupational category is also problematic. In the generic sense, it encompasses multiple levels of philosophy, educational preparation, and practice that have developed over time as society's complexity increased. Because newer nursing education and practice models did not totally replace earlier ones, and because nursing has resisted mandatory university-based preparation that society recognizes as legitimating all other professions, multiple nursing levels exist. These levels, by definition and quasi-design, occupy different positions on the continuum of authority and autonomy, and their differences are not clear to the public. Organized nursing's inability to enforce stated desired educational entry levels for basic nursing practice understandably raises questions about its ability to ensure the practice quality of yet another kind of nurse. However, although variations in the education of nurses seeking to practice in advanced roles exist, by the 21st century almost all advanced practitioners will be master's prepared and ANA advanced practice certification examinations will require master's preparation.[3]

Therefore, the focus of this chapter is the nurse who may have begun nursing education at the diploma or associate degree level, but ultimately received professional nursing preparation at the baccalaureate or higher degree level, and additional specific graduate education to practice in primary care or other advanced practice roles. Because primary care practice by nurses sparked most of the debate about nurses taking independent practice roles, most of the public commentary focuses specifically on primary care. However, over time, the descriptive language that limited primary care practice to outpatient or ambulatory settings has been replaced by general practice and specialty care descriptions of advanced practice, as is evident in various state nurse practice acts.[4] This chapter, therefore, takes the position that all variations of advanced nursing practice rest on the same authoritative base as does primary care practice.

Within the limits so described, this chapter will discuss some philosophical issues raised by nursing's assertion of its claim to occupy independent provider roles in advanced practice and primary care. The discussion will be biased in the direction of endorsing appropriately prepared nurses practicing in independent practice roles.

DEFINITION

In 1994, the Institute of Medicine's Committee on the Future of Primary Care defined primary care as ". . . the provision of integrated, accessible health care services by clinicians who are accountable for addressing a large majority of personal health care needs, developing a sustained partnership with patients, and practicing in the context of family and community" (Institute of Medicine, 1996, p. 1).

Further, the Institute's (1996, p. 3) Committee identified the nature of primary care as including six core attributes:

1. Excellent primary care is grounded in both the biomedical and the social sciences.
2. Clinical decision making in primary care differs from that in specialty care.
3. Primary care has at its core a sustained personal relationship between patient and clinician.
4. Primary care does not consider mental health separately from physical health.
5. Important opportunities to promote health and prevent disease are intrinsic to primary care practice.
6. Primary care is information intensive.

These definitions represent the views of this author and will serve as reference points from which some philosophical issues can be discussed. The definitions suggest three general, fundamental assumptions regarding the primary care role: (1) It is not specific to any one health profession; (2) it is not limited as to population served, health problems encountered, or duration of practitioner-client relationship; and (3) it requires from its practitioners independent and autonomous decision making based on professional knowledge. It is the assumption regarding autonomy[5] that causes the major delays and dilemmas encountered by nursing when it attempts to occupy the primary health care role.

Despite some model legislation,[6] nursing has most commonly been defined legally as a dependent practice that delivers health care services under the supervision of a duly authorized physician or dentist. As the demand for primary care services expanded, many institutions inaugurated solutions in which nurses, under titles such as nurse practitioner, act in primary care roles, but operate under a system of protocols designed in advance in conjunction with physicians. Such compromises cloud the autonomy issue, because protocols are external constraints that suggest the inability of the nurse to choose correctly among "alternative possibilities of action . . . in accordance with [appropriate] inner motives and ideals. . . ." (Runes, 1942, p. 112). Protocols merely extend the distance between the nurse in practice and the physician in supervision. They act essentially as "standing" or "PRN" orders and implicitly reinforce a dependent model of practice for nursing. However true this criticism of protocols might be, expanding managed care programs and the ever-present threat of litigation have spawned protocols in all sorts of clinical arrangements that affect the practice of all clinicians, not only nurses.

The central issues blocking widespread use of appropriately prepared and truly autonomous nurses to meet people's health care needs in a variety of independent, advanced practice roles are political and are hidden behind protests of whether or not nursing is a true profession, capable of safely caring for patients in an independent manner. This chapter will address both the stated and the hidden issues.

AUTONOMY, AUTHORITY, AND NURSING KNOWLEDGE

Independent, autonomous practice rests on the assumption that the agent of such a practice has the expertise from which that agent derives the authority to act.[7] In the case of autonomous practice, this reliance on authority is essential to the protection of citizens in situations where knowledge is utilized about which the lay consumer has little understanding.

There is a substantial body of literature that discusses the notion of authority.[8] Issues of power, morality, the consent of the subject, the limits to authority and the interactions among the concepts of authority, reason, and freedom form the core of centuries of philosophical debate that cannot be addressed adequately in this chapter. The piece of the debate that seems most applicable here is that which addresses the legitimacy of authority, that is, how an individual or group justifies its claim to an authoritative position on certain bodies of knowledge and the behaviors or actions that derive from that legitimating base. Sociologist Max Weber's conceptual base will be utilized in this chapter to clarify nursing's authority.

Weber described three basic legitimating models for the construct of authority. Legal authority: "the legitimacy of the powerholder to give commands rests upon rules that are rationally established by enactment, by agreement, or by imposition." (Gerth & Mills, 1946). Charismatic authority: the legitimacy of the powerholder rests on "an *extraordinary* quality of a person, regardless of whether this quality is actual, alleged, or presumed" (Gerth & Mills, 1946, p. 295). This personal model has been exemplified by "the prophet with the mark of grace" and has its basis in theological experience (Benn, 1967, p. 216). Traditional authority: the legitimacy of the powerholder rests on "the psychic attitude-set for the habitual workday and . . . the belief in the everyday routine as an inviolable norm of conduct (Gerth & Mills, 1946, p. 296). This basis of authority rests on the principle that certain authority has always existed or is alleged or presumed to have always existed. The most important example of this model is patriarchy.

Medicine possesses an authority aura that encompasses all three types described, whereas nursing's authority base is less broad. Nursing is recognized as having legal and traditional authority to a point. It has charismatic figures such as Nightingale, Dock, Wald, and Sanger, but its overall aura is not charismatic in the same life-saving dramatic sense that characterizes the aura of medical practice.[9]

When nursing asserts its claim to practice independently, it invites comparisons to medicine in the extent of its authority to act in that manner. In that comparison, in the context of the previously described types, nursing is seen as having less authority. But that is a false issue. In comparison to medicine, every profession is seen as having less authority. The important question is does nursing have appropriate, or enough, authority to act independently? Returning to the definition of primary care as the exemplar, the foci of the primary care role are (1) providing integrated, accessible health care services by clinicians who are accountable for addressing a large majority of health care needs; (2) developing a sustained partnership with patients; and (3) practicing in the context of family and community. Further, the core attributes emphasize the social as well as the biomedical sciences; the personal relationship between clinician and patient; the opportunity for health promotion and disease prevention activities; and the integration of mental and physical health care concerns.

These health care goals have been part of modern nursing since its Nightingalean origins. At the 1893 World's Fair, Nightingale's (1894) paper described "Sick Nursing and Health Nursing . . . nursing proper is . . . to help the patient suffering from disease to live—just as health nursing is to keep or put the constitution of the healthy child or human being in such a state as to have no disease (p. 446). At the same meeting, Isabel Hampton (1893/1949, later Robb) spoke of the nurse's ". . . three-fold interest in her work—an intellectual interest in the case, a (much higher) hearty interest in the patient, a technical (practical) interest in the patient's care and cure" (p. 3). Nightingale's focus on environmental conditions, and their manipulation to ensure health, was responsible for her legendary work as a reformer of England's sanitation laws. Nurses were defined as the "ministers of health" who were ". . . not only caring for the sick, but teaching the principles of cleanliness, ventilation and economy" to their patients and the families of patients (Sutcliffe, 1894, p. 511). The district nurse of 19th-century England and the visiting nurse of early 20th-century America clearly provided primary care services to underserved populations.

The same objectives characterize certain current standards of university nursing education and state Nurse Practice Acts.[10] Therefore, the stated foci of the primary care role have historical, educational, and legal bases in nursing practice, and are substantiated as within the context of nursing's legal and traditional authority. The question therefore must lie not with the existence of nursing authority, but with people's recognition of that authority.

A distinction is drawn between de facto and de jure authority: ". . . de jure presumes a set of rules, according to which certain persons are competent (authorized) to do certain things, but not to do other things. . . ." De facto exists when one person "*recognizes* [sic] another as *entitled* [sic] to command him" (Benn, 1967, p. 215).

Medicine and nursing each possess elements of both de jure and de facto authority. What matters to the practice of each is the extent to which each is accepted by the public, and the point at which the practice of each profession is seen as reaching the limits of its authority. Yet within each profession there are recognized differences in preparation and responsibility. In medicine, a general practice physician is not expected to perform neurosurgery, but would be considered competent to suture a small wound. Similarly, nurses prepared in advanced practice must perform within the limits of their specific preparation. However, as nurses have expanded their expertise into independent practice roles such as primary care, they are seen as pushing the perimeter between the professions of medicine and nursing. Sociologist William Goode (1960) described this process as "encroachment," whereby "a new occupation claims the right to solve a problem which formerly was solved by another." The claim of the new group is interpreted by the old as an "accusation of incompetence, and the outraged counteraccusation is, of course, 'encroachment'" (p. 902).

Nursing's reasons for its advanced practice role should be effective in defusing the "accusative" nature of its claim to the role. Historically certain nurses always practiced in this way. Currently, nursing is identifying independent practice more clearly because:

1. Nurses now know better how to assert their rights and claims, and that they must make overt those practices that have been covert for generations of the "doctor–nurse game";

2. Nurses have the expertise to meet the expanding health care needs of society in the face of the declining numbers, not incompetence, of primary care physicians;

3. Advanced practice presents nursing's qualified members with practice roles more consistent with their rigorous preparation; and,

4. By providing a competitive delivery system, nurses can help contain health care costs (Choi, 1981; Fagin, 1982, 1990).

The restrictions on nursing's de facto authority derive largely from the public's lack of knowledge about what nursing is, what nurses know, do, and are capable of doing. Nurses' expanded educational preparation, research-based knowledge, and highly sophisticated practice roles are not generally recognized by the public, which still thinks of nurses at the bedside, in the maternal, handmaiden role of a much simpler era. Development of expert authority occurs interactionally between the group needing a service and the group providing that service. Medicine has been the group recognized as interacting with society's need for primary care. Nursing's role has been seen as necessary, but secondary and dependent, not primary and independent. When educated nurses present themselves as a group prepared to fill the gap in many health care services, cognitive dissonance may occur for those who have older views of nursing. A new group without nursing's historical image might have less difficulty occupying the role, but would lack the trust that nurses have earned from the public. The term "Nurse Practitioner" has been successful because it manages to keep the nurse-trust component, yet simultaneously presents a new image for nurses in new roles.

Accountability Operationalizes Authority

One way to demonstrate authority is through accountability.[11] One cannot, in justice, be held answerable for behaviors, actions, and events over which one has no authority or control or for which one is not responsible (Adkins, 1979). Therefore, nursing is documenting its perceived areas of accountability through conceptual model development, nursing diagnosis taxonomies, quality assurance programs, nursing audits, outcome criteria measurement, and legal and legislative action.

These measures demonstrate some areas for which nurses accept accountability. They do not answer other questions regarding account-ability, such as to whom is one accountable? When reference groups or issues conflict, to which is one accountable under which circumstances? Must one act counter to one's own beliefs in order to be accountable to the goals of a particular group for whom one is the service provider? Nurses often find themselves in conflicts of accountability. Philosopher Newton described a model[12] that helps to clarify conflictive accountability, based on one's definition of health care:

1. If health care is a commodity for sale in a hospital, the patient is a customer, the physician is an outside contractor, and the nurse is a straight employee with responsibility only to the institution and the immediate supervisor.

2. If health care is a series of medical cases, then.the physician is the scientist in charge of the project, the hospital is a laboratory, and the nurse is a subproject participant or assistant who is accountable only to the physician.

3. If health care is seen as the patient's right to relief from pain or ill-ness, and the hospital is the locus of that relief, then the nurse is account-able to the patient.

4. If health care is defined as promoting the general well-being of per-sons, ". . . the patient, nurse and physician form a triad around the single enterprise of furthering that patient's well-being. The patient is the focus, but is expected to . . . aid in his own recovery; the physician is primarily a scientist, oriented towards the body's disease; and the nurse is a com-pletely different professional, holistically oriented toward the patient's entire growth as a person. . . . In this conception, the nurse cannot be accountable for her performance as a nurse to any but her own professional standards" (Newton, 1979, p. 9).

Professional standards begin with the personal ethical system of the nurse as an individual. These standards develop in individuals in the context of their membership in many groups within the larger society. People are socialized culturally in various ways and carry those customs with them into other parts of their lives. Most nurses are women. Their gender carries cultural demands for behavior that affects later, professional behavior. Many nurses are members of groups that have varying experiences of child rearing, socioeconomics, national origin, education, and other factors that influence nurses before they begin the professional socialization process. In addition, each nurse is a member of a social system that legally defines accepted behavior of the nurse as a citizen, resident, and nurse.

The nature of accountability, therefore, is multileveled and complex, and nursing's heterogeneity increases that complexity. The professional level on which nurses hold themselves accountable is most often the last area of accountability to develop. It may carry a weaker personal commitment when in competition with earlier developed senses of accountability, for example, women's accountability as mothers versus women's accountability as nurses. In addition, the nature of accountability changes over time in relationship to changes in the person, the society, and the profession. Conflicts among and between various aspects of accountability have been part of nursing since its earliest years, as this 1893 statement demonstrates: "The superintendent of a training school is under a threefold obligation: first to the hospital in which she works; secondly, to the patients who are entrusted to her care; and thirdly, to the women for whose education as nurses she is responsible (Hampton, 1893, p. 17).

Although Hampton (1893) encouraged all persons connected with the hospital to "resolve that they will work harmoniously together . . . [that] justice may be done to all" (p. 17), the historical evidence is abundant that accountability to the hospital dominated the others. As times and gender customs changed, nurses became more aware of these conflicts, and more skillful in asserting their professional rights, but the conflicts still exist. A major source of such conflict is the difficulty in quantifying what nursing is, what nurses do, in a system that relies heavily on quantifiable data. The essence of nursing, caring, defies measurement, and quality of life does not take precedence when survival is at stake, which is often the case in acute-care settings. In primary care delivery circumstances, immediate survival threats are not as likely, which allows "care" and "quality of life" foci to take precedence. Additionally, as the population ages, and increased numbers of people need supportive care for chronic illnesses and acquired immune deficiency syndrome (AIDS), nurses' broader range of practice is in greater demand.

Nursing as a Discipline

The major argument put forth by those who oppose independent nursing practice is that because nursing uses knowledge from the physical, behavioral, social, and biomedical sciences, it cannot be regarded as having its own unique, independent, and professional knowledge base. There is no question that nursing integrates knowledge from other disciplines. But nursing adds its own special knowledge to the gestalt and applies it in practice in a manner uniquely its own. Nurses do for people what people would do for themselves if they had the will, the strength, and the knowledge that the nurse has.[13] Therefore, as a discipline, nursing's recurrent themes and concerns focus on the wholeness of people, the interaction between people and their environments, and nursing's management of people and environment to enhance comfort, quality of life, and general well-being during, and beyond, illness.[14] In fact, and with irony, it must be noted that this very breadth of background is what makes nursing so clearly suited to the primary health care provider role. It is breadth not possessed by any other health care delivery group because, though medicine also integrates knowledge from other fields, the fields are more limited to the biochemical and physical sciences. While the advances created in medicine by the merger of these sciences cannot be denied, concurrent losses of the supportive, caring functions of healing have been significant.[15] Though increased technology has also affected nursing, the supportive, caring functions of healing have continued to be central to nursing. Since doctoral preparation has become more common for nurses, and a corps of nurses have been prepared as researchers, rigorous scientific inquiry into the knowledge that validates nursing action has reduced the relevance and legitimacy of arguments raised against independent nursing practice. Such arguments must rest then, not on concerns for science or authoritative knowledge, but on power considerations.

POWER, PROFESSIONALISM, AND PROTEST

A social process, professionalization, evolved at the end of the 19th century to organize knowledge growing out of the scientific and industrial revolutions. Developed as a means to protect uninformed citizens required to place their trust in expert authorities, professions also controlled valued information and access to that information, which gave them power. Able to choose and socialize new members, the professions became regulating bodies for their practices and reference groups to which society addressed questions regarding certain areas of knowledge. New professions continue to emerge as technological advances create expert knowledge for those activities formerly conducted according to intuition or trial and error experience. Sociologists describe a continuum of professionalism on which occupations fall by virtue of the extent of their unique knowledge base and orientation to service, the two primary characteristics of professions (Goode, 1957, 1960; Hughes, 1963).

As the "new" professions emerge, the balance of power is disrupted, particularly between groups that share clients, content, and workplaces. The territorial protectiveness stimulated in the older group against the "encroachment" of the newer has already been discussed. A new profession that provides a service to a client once "belonging to" another will derive income from and gain influence over that service and client. This economic and political threat is, not surprisingly, fought by the older group. The incongruity of this reaction by medicine to nursing as nurses enter advanced practice roles is that firstly, most of what is changing is the overtness of nurses' activities, and secondly, the physician practitioners being "threatened" are not those actually delivering the disputed service. Physicians are not providing primary care services in needy areas or in adequate numbers, but they do not want nurses to provide them either—probably because nursing is an increasingly independent profession, with a growing militancy in its refusal to be dominated by medicine. As a consequence, medicine created, and is supporting with its vast resources, physician-extender or assistant groups through which it seeks to maintain control over services and clients without having to use its legitimate professional resources to do so. This creates another irony. Groups clearly labeled "assistant" are given legitimacy to act independently, even to write orders that nurses are pressured to follow.

Such obvious maneuvering led this author toward class and gender interpretations of these power plays. The majority of medical practitioners are more affluent than their nursing counterparts, and constitute an elite, dominant group in American society. Medicine uses its greater economic and influential resources to lobby among legislators and consumers to protect its position. Because medicine is also predominantly male, while nursing is 94% female, sexism, as a societal and historical feature, contributes its piece to what is, in essence, a political struggle. Related to sexism, but derivative of a technologically worshipful society as well, are the different values attached to the two major functions of health care—care and cure. The nurturant, supportive behaviors fundamental to caring and nursing do not engage the American interest or value to the degree that the more instrumental technology of curing and medicine do. Nursing has only begun to address these concerns in the last two decades, as patient outcomes research documents nursing's significant positive impact on patient care. The complex social history of nursing suggests why nurses avoided political issues and activities in prior eras.

Modern nursing emerged as an acceptable occupational alternative for women during the Victorian era. As single women, living away from their homes, earning salaries, and ministering to the bodily needs and functions of both sexes, usually strangers, 19th-century nurses were social revolutionaries who dared not breach too many more conventions for fear of losing their basic footholds. The notions of self-effacement, deference, long hours of toil for small wages, and political reticence, which began as sociopolitical necessities to establish the work in one generation, became habits and customs associated with, ascribed to, and even required of nursing in subsequent generations. With the rise of science and the professionalization of knowledge at the turn of the 20th century, certain individuals and groups of nurses became more politically aware and active. But the majority of nurses avoided issues like sexism, power, and politics.

Nursing, as a group, did not support the 19th Amendment (for women's suffrage) in the early 1900s, equivocated on civil rights in the 1960s, and only belatedly and halfheartedly backed the Equal Rights Amendment of the 1980s. With large numbers that could have exerted noticeable pressure, nurses' reticent behavior cost them the reciprocal support of other disadvantaged groups—women, African Americans, even health care consumers—who might have added strength to nursing's political muscle. Isolated in a "Little world of our own" (Tomes, 1978) and often divided among themselves as to the best action for nursing to take, nurses have not been effective advocates for their own positions.

Some women's groups, attempting to confront sexism in the professions, recommend increasing the number of the underrepresented sex, such as increasing the number of men in nursing and women in medicine. But that is a false solution and has not worked in nursing. The underlying societal attitudes must change, such as increasing the acceptance of assertiveness in nurses and nurturance in physicians. Otherwise, the stereotypes of relative dominance, achievement, independence, and power remain intact, and the traditionally male, White, elite choices continue to be the more desirable ones.

The negative effect of stereotype-driven choices is confounding in multiple ways. Some women who enter the more prestigious field of medicine experience conflict and disillusionment when they discover that physicians do not spend as much time with patients as they had expected. These young physicians' desire to be supportive and nuturant with their clients may be discouraged and even denigrated. Simultaneously, nursing suffers the loss to its ranks of well-qualified and highly motivated women. Similarly, men who enter the more nurturing field of nursing may experience social and economic discrimination. Society is the ultimate loser in this chain of events.

CONCLUSIONS AND SUGGESTED ACTIONS

The question central to this chapter has been: Do nurses have the appropriate authority to act as independent health care providers in advanced practice roles? The evidence presented supports the conclusion that they do—within the context of specific educational preparation for identified nurses, legal sanction by legislative bodies, and public recognition by consumers of health services. Through these three mechanisms, advanced practice roles for nurses will be accepted and legitimated.

Organized nursing must establish specific educational programs and certification criteria on a national basis. A baccalaureate degree to enter general professional nursing practice and master's-degree preparation for advanced practice are essential. Nursing must discriminate among its own levels of preparation and practice in ways that are standard in all other disciplines.

The extension of legislative activity that would permit such practice by properly prepared nurses is necessary in all states. This may require legal encounters that challenge existing restrictions, and it will require some nurses to allow other nurses to earn a different status. Having asserted that some of its members possess specific, independent expertise, nurses cannot then insist that all nurses gain the benefit of that expertise or hide behind physicians when the outcomes of their actions are challenged. In fact, if nurses seek the status of professionals, they must insist on being held accountable for the appropriateness of their actions on all levels.

Public education that alerts consumers to health issues is a well-used and demonstrably successful strategy in the United States. Similar strategies can be employed to familiarize the public with the importance of nursing in health care, and the specific nursing services available from advanced practice nurses. Probably the most important of all actions, nurses must demonstrate the positive health care outcomes and economic value of their practice, and then publicize those results for legislators and consumers through sophisticated use of the media.

Nurses' contributions must be acknowledged, even promoted. How many people know that Margaret Sanger was a nurse; that two previous presidents of Planned Parenthood were nurses (Fay Wattleton and Pam Maraldo); that the Henry Street Settlement was started by a nurse (Lillian Wald); that the first president of the National Organization for Women was a nurse (Wilma S. Heide); that nurses run major government agencies and control $100 million budgets in medical centers? We have allowed the nurse who moves out of the dependent model to cease being identified as a nurse, thereby tacitly reinforcing the public image we now deplore.

A major concern expressed by some nurses who oppose advanced practice by nurses is fear of loss of the nursing role and identity. This is a worthy consideration. Some nurses who enter advanced practice roles become seduced by the power of the stethoscope to provide instant status. This misuse of the model must not be permitted. A stethoscope is only a tool, as is a pencil or a thermometer, with which competent data can be collected and the nursing process activated. The best reason for nurses to provide primary care is because they are nurses. Nursing's focus on people; its blend of medical, behavioral, and social science expertise; and its commitment to caring, teaching, counseling, and supporting patients are the characteristics of nursing that make nurses so uniquely qualified to provide advanced practice and primary health care services to the public.

NOTES

1. Julie Fairman and Joan Lynaugh, *Controlling Crises: A History of the American Critical Care Movement, 1940–1990.* (Philadelphia: University of Pennsylvania Press, 1998). See also, Julie Fairman, "Watchful Vigilance: Nursing Care Technology and the Development of ICUs, 1950–1965," *Nursing Research,* (1992) 1:52–60. See also Joan Lynaugh and Julie Fairman, "New Nurses, New Spaces: A Preview of the AACN History Study," *American Journal of Critical Care* (1 July 1992), 19–24.
2. Florence Nightingale defined nursing as putting the patient in the best position for nature to act upon him. Virginia Henderson defined nursing as doing for patients' those things they would do for themselves if they had the knowledge, the will, and the strength to do them. Dorothea Orem defined nursing as substituting the nurses' actions for the patients own actions to different degrees, partially, wholly, or supportive/educative. The ANA defines nursing as the diagnosis and treatment of human responses to actual or potential health problems.
3. American Nurses Credentialing Center, *Advanced Practice Certification Catalog* (Washington, DC: Author, 1997). See also, Data Sheets prepared for the American Nurses Association by Winifred Carson, Practice Counsel, entitled: States which recognize clinical nurse specialists in advanced practice; Joint regulation of advanced nursing practice; States recognizing advanced practice under independent acts, separate titles of advanced practice acts, or regulations; and Continuing education requirements for prescriptive authority.

   As of this writing (May 1997), various state nurse practice acts reflect public confusion about nursing's roles. Some states (Alaska and Oregon) give full plenary and prescriptive powers to advanced practice nurses. Other states (New York) limit advanced practice nurses' autonomy, by requiring "nurse practitioner(s)" to practice "in collaboration with a licensed physician . . ." (NYS, Article 139, Section 6902 (3a), 1995). Other states do not differentiate between basic and advanced practice nurses. Regarding American Nurses' Association (ANA) certification for advanced practice, as of the end of 1997, applicants for advanced practice certification examinations will be required to have a minimum of master's level preparation. However, because some nurse practitioners were "grandfathered" into the designation prior to that requirement, all advanced practice nurses may not necessarily be master's prepared until well into the 21st century.

4. As an example, in New York State, nurse practitioners are authorized with the following language: "The practice of registered professional nursing by a nurse practitioner, certified under section six thousand nine hundred ten of this article, may include the diagnosis of illness and physical conditions and the performance of therapeutic and corrective measures within a specialty area of practice, in collaboration with a licensed physician qualified to collaborate in the specialty involved, provided such services are performed in accordance with a written practice agreement and written practice protocols" (NYS Education Act, Article 139, Section 6902, Paragraph 3a, 1995). Paragraph 3b authorizes nurse practitioners' prescriptive powers with similar restraints.

5. Dagobert D. Runes, *The Dictionary of Philosophy*. (New York: Philosophical Library, 1942) p. 29, defines autonomy as "Freedom consisting in self-determination and independence of all external constraint."

6. cf., 3.

7. Stanley I. Benn, "Authority." In *The Encyclopedia of Philosophy*, Paul Edwards (ed.), vol. 1 (New York: Macmillan and the Free Press, 1967), p. 215 defines authority as meaning: "to possess expert knowledge and therefore the right to be listened to." Further, "The authority of the expert . . . involves the notion of someone qualified to speak." It presumes standards by which expertise is expressed and recognized, for example, degrees or professional reputation."

8. Ibid., pp. 215–217 briefly reports on this literature.

9. Magali Sarfatti Larson, *The Rise of Professionalism: A Sociological Analysis* (Berkeley: University of California Press, 1977). On p. 31, the author asserts that occupational tasks that are more familiar in ordinary life have less magical allure, and therefore seem to require less expertise.

10. For an example of educational standards, see the University of Pennsylvania School of Nursing Statement of Philosophy and Conceptual Framework: "The faculty believes that nursing is an autonomous profession whose focus is caring for persons throughout the life cycle during periods of wellness and illness" and specifies nursing actions in health maintenance, promotion, and teaching as well as therapeutic interventions. For an example of Nurse Practice Acts, see New York's Education Law, Article 139, Section 6902, 1995: "The practice of the profession of nursing as a registered professional nurse is defined as diagnosing and treating human responses to actual or potential health problems through such services as case finding, health teaching, health counseling, and provision of care supportive to or restorative of life and well-being, and executing medical regimens prescribed by a licensed physician, dentist or other licensed health care provider legally authorized under this title and in accordance with the commissioner's regulations. A nursing regimen shall be consistent with and shall not vary any existing medical regimen."

11. Leon M. Lessinger in *Accountability in Education*. Leon M. Lessinger and Ralph W. Tyler (eds.). Worthington, Ohio: Chas. A. Jones, 1971, p. 29 defined accountability as meaning: "that an agent [agrees] to perform a service [and] will be held answerable for performing according to agreed-upon terms, within an established time period, and with a stipulated use of resources and performance standards."

12. Lisa H. Newton, "To Whom is the Nurse Accountable? A Philosophical Perspective," *Connecticut Medicine Supplement*, 43 (October 1979), pp. 7–9. Presented with permission of the author and the journal.

13. Virginia Henderson's definition of nursing appears in many sources. In this case, I have paraphrased from her quote in: Ellen D. Baer, *Editor's Notes, Nursing in America: A History of Social Reform* (New York: The National League for Nursing, 1990), p. 1.

14. Sue K. Donaldson and Dorothy M. Crowley, "The Discipline of Nursing," *Nursing Outlook, 26,* (February 1978), p. 113: "A discipline . . . is characterized by a unique perspective, a distinct way of viewing all phenomena, which ultimately defines the limits and nature of its inquiry."
15. Edmund D. Pellegrino, "The Sociocultural Impact of Twentieth Century Therapeutics." In *The Therapeutic Revolution: Essays in the Social History of American Medicine,* Morris J. Vogel and Charles E. Rosenberg (eds.) (Philadelphia: University of Pennsylvania Press, 1979), p. 262 identifies the "discontent with medicine today" as related to conflict between ideals of technology and "the Aesculapian physician."

REFERENCES

Adkins, R. D. (1979). Responsibility and authority must match in nursing management. *Hospitals, 53*(3), 69–71.

Benn, S. I. (1967). Authority. In P. Edwards (Ed.), *The encyclopedia of philosophy.* New York: Macmillan and The Free Press.

Choi, M. W. (1981). Nurses as co-providers of primary health care. *Nursing Outlook, 29,* 521.

Fagin, C. M. (1982). Nursing as an alternative to high-cost health care. *American Journal of Nursing, 82,* 56–60.

Fagin, C. M. (1990). Nursing's value prove itself. *American Journal of Nursing, 90,* 17–30.

Gerth, H. H., & Mills, C. W. (Eds. and trans.). (1958). *From Max Weber: Essays in sociology.* New York: Oxford University Press. (Original work published 1946)

Goode, W. J. (1957). Community within a community: The profession. *American Sociological Review, 22,* 194–200.

Goode, W. J. (1960). Encroachment, charlatanism, and the emerging professions: Psychology, sociology, and medicine. *American Sociological Review, 25,* 902.

Hampton, I. A. (1949). Educational standards for nurses. In I. A. Hampton and others (Eds.), *Nursing of the sick 1893.* New York: McGraw-Hill. (Original work published 1894)

Hughes, E. C. (1963). Professions. *Daedalus, 92.*

Institute of Medicine. (1996). *Primary care: America's health in a new era* (M. S. Donaldson, K. D. Yordy, K. N. Lohr, & N. A. Vanselow, Eds.). Washington, DC; National Academy Press.

Lessinger, L. M., & Tyler, R. W. (Eds.). (1971). *Accountability in education.* Worthington, OH: Charles A. Jones.

Newton, L. H. (1979). To whom is the nurse accountable? A Philosophical perspective. *Connecticut Medicine Supplement, 43,* 7–9.

Nightingale, F. (1894). Sick nursing and health nursing. In *Hospitals, dispensaries, and nursing.* Papers and discussions in the International Congress of Charities, Correction and Philanthropy, Section III, June 12th–17th, 1893, under the auspices of the World's Congress Auxiliary of the World's Columbian Exposition, J. S. Billings, MD, & H. M. Hurd, MD (Eds.). Baltimore: Johns Hopkins Press.

Runes, D. G. (1942). *The dictionary of philosophy.* New York: Philosophical Library.

Sutcliffe, I. (1894). The history of American training in schools. In J. S. Billings, MD, & H. M. Hurd, MD (Eds.), *Hospitals, dispensaries, and nursing.* Baltimore: Johns Hopkins Press.

Tomes, N. (1978). Little world of our own: The Pennsylvania Hospital Training School for Nurses, 1895–1907. *Journal of the History of Medicine and Allied Sciences, 33,* 507–530.

Philosophical and Historical Bases of Advanced Practice Nursing Roles

Julie Fairman

llen Baer elegantly and masterfully documents the philosophical and the historical bases of advanced practice nursing roles[1] in her preceding chapter. In the chapter, she sets forth a brief description of the changes occurring in nursing in the first half of the century that created a foundation for the emergence of advanced practice nursing. She then places advanced nursing within a framework shaped by sociology and philosophy, and focuses on the legitimacy of nurse practitioners as primary care providers. Baer chose two constructs—authority and autonomy—to illustrate both the promise and the obstacles advanced practice nurses confronted (and continue to confront) in the health care arena. An examination of these constructs raises a central question: "Do nurses have the appropriate authority to act as independent health care providers in advanced practice roles? (p. 50)"

Baer's central question is not a new one, but has been posed since the 19th century by nurses who worked in expanded roles, from Visiting Nurses serving the poor in urban tenements to the public health nurse visiting an isolated rural family. The question has multiple answers, depending upon the economic, political, and social stake of the inquisitor and the social context of the time. Baer concludes that nurses indeed have the authority to act independently but adds an important caveat: "within the context of specific educational preparation for identified nurses, legal sanction by legislative bodies, and public recognition by the consumers of health care services" (p. 50). It is "through these three mechanisms," she adds, that "advanced practice roles for nurses will be accepted and legitimized" (p. 50).

In this commentary, I reexamine Baer's central question through an analysis of the historical perspective of specific education and legal sanction and offer another compelling and contemporary way of thinking about the power and authority of nurse practitioners (NPs). I argue that NPs already have a strong and legitimate claim to autonomy and authority in their practice, manifested through their relationships with patients. Nurse practitioners' power can be made visible and commanding by crossing medicine's socially constructed boundaries of skill and knowledge.

Legal Sanction

Most scholars will rightly argue, as does Baer, that legal sanction of practice is important, especially when fair payment for services is part of the legislation. Alice Kessler-Harris uses the concept of "economic citizenship" to explicate the relationship between respect for workers, worker's wages, and autonomy. Economic citizenship, Kessler-Harris argues, "suggests the achievement of an independent and relatively *anonymous* status that marks self-respect" (Kessler-Harris, 2001, p. 12)." This is achieved, she continues, with the access to "self-support through the ability to work at the occupation of one's choice, . . . and requires customary and legal acknowledgement of personhood, with all that implies for expectations, training, access to and distribution of resources and opportunity in the marketplace" (Kessler-Harris, 2001, pp. 12–13).

While nurses' claims to moral authority embedded in the provider-patient relationship contribute unquantifiable value to NPs' worth and social power, both tradition and legislation interfere with their autonomy and access to the health care market. Nurse practitioners access the market in various ways: via employment by institutions, other practitioners, or independent practice in some states. However, the key to NPs' unequivocal market access rests in the ability to bill third-party insurers independently and receive equitable pay for their services. Access to the market via this mechanism resides in the political and legislative arena controlled by state and federal bodies and is strongly influenced by organized medicine's ability to control the dialogue and language of reimbursement. For example, the Current Procedure Terminology (CPT), the coding system to process patient claims developed by the American Medical Association after passage of Medicare and Medicaid in 1966 and used by Medicare, Medicaid, private insurers, and the Centers for Medicare and Medicaid

(CMS, formerly the Health Care Finance Administration [HCFA]), still uses physician-focused language (e.g., "The physician provides . . ."). However, in 1997 CMS mandated that nonphysicians (e.g., NPs, nurse-midwives, nurse anesthetists, or physician assistants) who provide services traditionally performed by physicians within the state scope of practice be considered "physicians" and receive equitable reimbursement.

Political power,[2] payment, and autonomy are closely related. Nurses' services in general, with the exception of the services of 19th- and early 20th-century public health and private duty nurses, were traditionally bundled as part of physician or hospital services rather than being individual services (Buhler-Wilkerson, 2001). Patients, insurers, hospital administration, and nursing itself perceived nursing services as inseparable from hospital charges or as an adjunct to physician care, rather than as independent professionals providing a service distinguishable from medicine. This tradition has been extremely hard to overcome for many reasons, including physician dominance in the hospital and in policy-making venues and because of physicians' socially ascribed power. In a very real sense, payment for services is an indication of the power and independence of the provider, and those not paid (e.g., those whose wages are earned indirectly, through payment by either physician or hospital employer) remain invisible and economically dependent upon other groups (Kessler-Harris, 2001).

Education

In health care, the ability to collect payment for services is also closely tied to physicians' claims of authority. Physicians traditionally claimed higher authority in the health care hierarchy and based their claims on their superior education in the sciences (Stevens, 1998). As Eugene Stead, an early proponent of the physician's assistant argued, "the doctor has the largest educational commitment, and society gives him the broadest licensure. The nurse has made a more limited commitment and society has given her a more limited licensure" (Stead, 1967, p. 801). These claims, which supported an empirical, reductionist system of medicine, provided the cultural authority for physicians to claim the role of "captain of the ship" and to create a structure of expectations that they were, indeed, the experts in health care and thus should be paid and ranked accordingly (Birenbaum, 1990). Since the mid-19th century, medicine created its normative status, with all other providers described in language that established hierarchical relationships that constructed and contained reality (Gluck & Patai, 1991; Olson, 2001). The media, medicine, and sometimes nurses themselves used terms such as "secondary provider," "nonphysician," "paramedical," or "mid-level provider" to describe practitioners who were not physicians. Language served to devalue the services provided by practitioners "other" than physicians and created systems of payment tied to medical control.

From their lofty position, physicians claimed not only economic power but also the power to control the knowledge and skills associated with medicine. On closer examination, physicians' claims were not naturally constructed; they were socially constructed by social forces and by physicians themselves. Because of their cultural authority and their gender,[3] physicians had the power to create and recreate the boundaries of medical knowledge and skills. Both medicine and nursing are highly gendered professions, not merely because of the populations that constitute them (most physicians are male and most nurses are female), but because of the assignment of gender—and, therefore, power and authority—to them through the media. Other factors include the use of fetishized objects and specific language, rituals, and images. Both professions reinforce a separation, through protective and self-legitimizing actions, of the technical and scientific as "male" and the emotional and caring as "female," thus creating language and larger cultural infrastructures that are strongly gendered (Longino, 1991). Tools such as otoscopes and even simple devices such as prescription pads have become measuring sticks of medicine's identity, superiority, and difference from other professions and support a gendered division of labor (Oldenziel, 1999; Schiebinger, 1999; Scott, 1988).

Physicians, from their historically privileged position as the "norm" against which to measure all other types of practitioners, develop collective interpretations of their experiences that allow them to constantly recreate their gendered universe of knowledge, skills, and areas of priority—privileging some and discarding others (Oldenziel, 1999; Schiebinger, 1999). In other words, medicine (with strong legislative affinity) defines what is, who is, and who should be (or not be) practicing medicine. Nurses create their own realities and interpretations, but their historical lack of privileged position and control over dominant approaches to health care makes it difficult for them to articulate their own standpoint, their differences from medicine, and their perception of the permeability of professional boundaries (Laslett, Kohlstedt, Longino, & Hammonds, 1996).

Even so, skills and knowledge informally have passed back and forth between nursing and medicine. Most of these skills, such as the use of the thermometer or stethoscope, passed quietly from doctors to nurses when they were no longer considered of high status or were a nuisance (Sandelowski, 2000). On the other hand, sharing of knowledge became a common occurrence in the early critical care units of the 1950s and the dialysis units of the 1960s as nurses and physicians in close quarters taught each other how to care for acutely and chronically ill patients (Fairman, 1998; Fairman & Lynaugh, 1998). Nurse practitioners, however, provided a new model—they chose to take on knowledge and skills that were *not* discarded by physicians. In fact, the skills and knowledge physicians chose to share and nurses chose to take on, for example, the process of clinical thinking, were of high complexity and status.

Clinical thinking includes the skills and knowledge that physicians traditionally used to organize and collect data, including taking a patient history, performing a physical examination, ordering diagnostic tests, creating a diagnosis, formulating treatment options, prescribing treatment, and making decisions about prognosis (Bates, 1995; Englehardt, Spicker, & Towers, 1977; Feinstein, 1967). Physicians used the process of clinical thinking to define themselves and give coherence and validity to the medical role. Physicians' position—their authority and power—was traditionally predicated on their clinical thinking skills, and in fact, contemporary health services, including diagnostic tests and procedures, admitting privileges, and are organized around the clinical thinking process of physicians (Fairman, 1999; Freidson, 1970).

Nurse practitioners took on various pieces of the clinical thinking process at different times, starting with the health history and basic physical examination and moving on, sometimes against great political obstacles, to diagnosis and prescription of treatment. Through piece-by-piece sharing of the whole of clinical thinking, an artificial segmentation and fragmentation of the process occurred that exposed the political character and permeability of the legally and socially constructed practice barriers created by physicians' control of the process. These barriers traditionally defined physicians' practice and authority in society and protected their monopoly over health care (Fairman, 1999).

Power Already Present

There are, to be sure, political forces of education and economics that lend persuasive urgency to nurse practitioners' efforts to gain legal authority and legitimacy. However other frameworks for thinking about the authority and legitimacy of NPs may be equally powerful. Perhaps it is time to refocus on the informal—but no less potent—authority and power NPs already hold. Although, as Baer astutely notes, much effort still needs to be made in the legislative arena to gain legal standing, this is a critical time to acknowledge and celebrate the very visible and compelling authority inherent in individual encounters of NPs and patients (the third mechanism

Baer notes), and to think about a new paradigm of practice—one in which the authority of the NP is conceptualized and contextualized independently from the physician, and as more than an economic clinical substitute for medicine. It may be time to realize, as Scott notes in her analysis of gender and politics, that equality of authority in health care may rest on difference, and that "sameness is not a requirement for equality" (Scott, 1988, p. 177).

Thinking about the authority of NPs in this way avoids the intellectual trap of comparison to the "mean" of the dominant paradigm of medicine, and a new hybrid paradigm of care is created that embraces the power and agency inherent in the knowledge and practice of NPs (J. Fairman & D'Antonio, 1999). NPs are indeed powerful, and their power resonates with the ability to choose and create a new model of health care and to make other groups pay attention (Schwartz Cohen, 1989). Researchers have documented the power of NPs over the last 30 years through numerous studies of their effectiveness and efficiency in comparison to physicians. The seminal study in 1984 by the Office of Technology Assessment (OTA) estimated that NPs safely provided care to over 75% of patients typically seeking the care of primary care physicians (Office of Technology Assessment, 1984). Before and since that report, hundreds of other studies have evaluated the effectiveness of NP care (see chapter 4). Although many of them had limitations—many used the medical model as the "norm" from which to compare the services provided by NPs and physicians—they generally supported the OTA report and documented the safety, quality, and cost-effectiveness of care provided by NPs (Safriet, 1992). The extensive research should be enough to document NPs' legitimate place in the health care arena (and perhaps it is time that analytical efforts be directed elsewhere, for example, to outcome studies between different groups of nurse providers or in different settings).

Indeed, organized medicine has paid attention to the successful studies and the power of NP practice. The American Medical Association's (AMA's) Citizens' Petition on Physician-Nurse Collaboration, launched in June 2000, is just one piece of evidence that organized medicine is paying very close attention to physicians' social and economic prerogatives. The petition, an attempt to rally public support for the AMA's fight against expansion of the scope of practice of "nonphysicians," was couched in the terms of patient safety and the protection of public health, both arguments reflecting medicine's claim to expertise through their scientific education. The AMA contended that the public needed regulations to ensure collaboration between NPs and physicians, including highly restrictive supervisory aspects of collaboration (American Medical Association, 2000).

Instead of stirring public action, the petition illuminated the power of NPs. Although unacknowledged in the petition, NPs and physicians have collaborated in growing numbers over the last four decades, and individual NPs and physicians have created entrepreneurial practice relationships that have not been replicated, even if only in spirit, at the national organizational level (Guthrie, Runyan, Clark, & Oscar, 1964; Lewis & Resnik, 1967; Rogers, Mally, & Marcus, 1968). One-on-one negotiations between nurses and physicians in individual practices can illuminate each profession's source of power—nurses' keen knowledge of their patients or physicians' knowledge of pathology and disease—and integrate them into the everyday realities of providing clinical care. In fact, in such individual negotiations, NPs and physicians push and reframe practice without waiting for legislative definition or approval. National organizations such as the American Medical Association and the American Nurses' Association have focused their concern for patients on the broader-based concerns of economic and organizational dominance.

Although the dichotomy between practice and professional organization is somewhat artificial, it provides a foundation for posing the following questions: How did NPs get to the point where organized physician groups feel the need to appeal to the public to maintain their monopoly on health care? Why have NPs become so threatening to organized medicine? In testimony to NPs power, the AMA petition came too late to assuage organized medicine's fears about physicians' traditional economic, cultural, and social monopoly over health care. Medicine has already felt the effects of political and economic changes occurring in health care, and part of the motivating force was the power and growing number of NPs. By 1998, NPs had claimed larger and larger shares of Medicare reimbursement (see chapter 22).

The petition disappeared quietly by the fall of 2000. Two of the reasons for its lack of success included organized efforts of nursing professional groups and the sheer presence of NPs in the health care arena. Since the mid-1960s, the NP movement grew rapidly and became a source of health care for many of our nation's citizens. In 1970, there were only 250 NPs practicing in the United States. By 1980, however, there were 20,000 NPs; by 1996, 70,993 NPs; and by 2000, 102,829 NPs (Cooper, Laud, & Dietrich, 1998; Spratley, Johnson, Sochalski, Fritz, & Spencer, 2000). In many states, NPs practice independently: they evaluate, diagnose, and prescribe to treat common or uncomplicated chronic illnesses. Nurse practitioners also have become economic competitors with physicians as the supply of both professions continues to increase exponentially and practice opportunities shrink.

The rapid growth in numbers of NPs occurred during a period of physician surplus and will continue in tandem with a projected 24% increase in physician supply between 1995 and 2005 (Cooper et al., 1998; Lang, Sullivan-Marx, & Jenkins, 1996). In addition, although NPs initially were conceptualized to practice in primary care settings serving relatively poor clients without access to physician services, state regulatory codes, such as those requiring physician supervision of collaborating NP practice, require them to work in areas where there are larger numbers of physicians. As a result, more NPs practice in acute care urban health systems than in rural or community-based clinics, thereby creating the possibility and reality of confrontation and competition with physicians.

CONCLUSIONS

Baer concludes that "nursing's focus on people . . . makes nurses uniquely qualified to provide advanced practice and primary care to the public" (p. 51)" At this point in the history of NPs, we must move beyond continued efforts to justify the legitimacy and effectiveness of NP practice; this is a battle already fought and won. We should, instead, harness the power inherent in the patient encounter as the foundation of NPs' authority base. Armed with this perspective, and with the added power of economic autonomy and the appropriate knowledge to provide care, NPs are in an extraordinary position to shift the paradigm of care to one where differences between professions do not necessarily imply inequality or justify exclusion from the marketplace. In many ways, the shift is already underway, as seen in the focus on community-based care, women's health, and health promotion—all areas firmly within the capabilities of both NPs and physicians—and in the shifting language of the reimbursement system.

In the growing intersection of the knowledge and skills shared by both physicians and nurses, the political and social construction of medical authority is writ large. Indeed, the greatest challenge facing both NPs and physicians (in fact, neither profession exists in a vacuum) is negotiation of the "borderlands," in this case, the interface of shared knowledge and skills. First described by Gloria Anzaldua (Anzaldua, 1987) and elaborated on by Liz Stanley (Stanley, 1997), the borderlands serve as the cultural space in which "difference becomes the point at which fundamental epistemological disputes surface around seismic linguistic and ideations shifts. The frontier thereby provides 'the space between' for debate, contention, disagreement" (p. 1), and finally, resolution. Barbara Bates (Bates, 1973) predicted the challenge almost 30 years ago when she noted:

Perhaps the problems of doctor and nurse are not so much professional, as simply human. We [physicians] must learn to share—to share rewards. Both psychological and economic—and to share responsibility in a risk-fraught world where our training has taught us to depend only on ourselves. . . . And we must learn to communicate sufficiently with one another so that each may function effectively, and safely, and reasonably efficiently.

The future of NPs rests on this paradigmatic shift to a greater extent than it does on the journey to legitimacy through legal sanctions and education equivalency. In many ways, these changes will be harder to win, but in the end, they may prove much more enduring.

NOTES

1. Baer addressed "advanced practice roles," which is an inclusive term for nurses in expanded clinical roles and may include nurse practitioners, clinical nurse specialists, and nurse-midwives. I have chosen to restrict my analysis to nurse practitioners.
2. I use the concept of political power in its broadest sense, following the lead of feminist scholar Joan Scott (Scott, 1988). *Politics* in this chapter refers to the unequal distribution of power across all relationships, which could include both local, immediate relationships and governmental relationships.
3. Gender, as used here, does not refer to the biological characteristics associated with males and females but the political power associated with certain socially ascribed characteristics associated with men and women (Scott, 1988).

REFERENCES

American Medical Association. (2000). *AMA citizens' petition.* Washington, DC: Author.

Anzaldua, G. (1987). *Borderlands: The new mestiza—la frontera.* San Francisco: Spinsters Press.

Bates, B. (1973). *Nurses, doctors, and patients.* Sybil Palmer Bellos Lecture, Yale University School of Nursing, New Haven, CT.

Bates, B. (1995). *A guide to physical examination and history taking* (6th Ed.). Philadelphia: Lippincott.

Birenbaum, A. (1990). *In the shadow of medicine: Remaking the division of labor in health care.* Dix Hills, NY: General Hall.

Buhler-Wilkerson, K. (2001). *No place like home: A history of nursing and home care in the United States.* Baltimore: Johns Hopkins University Press.

Cooper, R. A., Laud, P., & Dietrich, C. L. (1998). Current and projected workforce of nonphysician clinicians. *Journal of American Medical Association, 280,* 788–794.

Englehardt, H. T., Jr., Spicker, S. F., & Towers, B. (1977). *Clinical judgment: A critical appraisal.* Boston: D. Reidel.

Fairman, J., & D'Antonio, P. (1999). Virtual power: Gendering the nurse-technology relationship. *Nursing Inquiry, 6,* 178–186.

Fairman, J. A. (1998). Alternate visions: The nurse-technology relationship in the context of the history of technology. *Nursing History Review, 6,* 129–146.

Fairman, J. A. (1999). Delegated by default or negotiated by need: Physicians, nurse practitioners, and the process of clinical thinking. *Medical Humanities Review, 13,* 38–58.

Fairman, J. A., & Lynaugh, J. E. (1998). *Critical care nursing: A history.* Philadelphia: University of Pennsylvania Press.

Feinstein, A. R. (1967). *Clinical judgment.* Baltimore: Williams & Wilkins.

Freidson, E. (1970). *Professional dominance: The social structure of medical care.* New York: Atherton Press.

Gluck, S. B., & Patai, D. (Eds.). (1991). *Women's words: The feminist practice of oral history.* New York: Routledge.

Guthrie, N., Runyan, J., Clark, G., & Oscar, M. (1964). The clinical nursing conference: A preliminary report. *New England Journal of Medicine, 270,* 1411–1413.

Kessler-Harris, A. (2001). In pursuit of equity: Women, men, and the quest for the economic citizenship in 20th century America. New York: Oxford University Press.

Lang, N., Sullivan-Marx, E., & Jenkins, M. (1996). Advanced practice nurses and success of organized delivery systems. *American Journal of Managed Care, 11,* 129–135.

Laslett, B., Kohlstedt, S. G., Longino, H., & Hammonds, E. (1996). (Eds.). Introduction. In *Gender and scientific authority* (pp. 1–18). Chicago: Chicago University Press.

Lewis, C., & Resnik, B. (1967). Nurse clinics and progressive ambulatory patient care. *The New England Journal of Medicine, 277,* 1236–1241.

Longino, H. (1991). *Science as social knowledge.* Princeton, NJ: Princeton University Press.

Office of Technology Assessment. (1984). *Nurse practitioners, physician assistants, and certified nurse-midwives: A policy analysis.* Washington, DC: U.S. Government Printing Office.

Oldenziel, R. (1999). *Making technology masculine: Men, women and modern machines in America, 1945–1970.* Amsterdam: Amsterdam University Press.

Olson, H. A. (2001). The power to name: Prepresentation in library catalogues. *Signs, 26,* 639–668.

Rogers, K., Mally, M., & Marcus, F. (1968). A general medical practice using non-physician personnel. *Journal of the American Medical Association, 206,* 1753–1757.

Safriet, B. (1992). Health care dollars and regulatory sense: The role of advanced practice nursing. *Yale Journal on Regulation, 9*(417), 417–488.

Sandelowski, M. (2000). *Devices and desires: Gender, technology, and American nursing.* Chapel Hill, NC: University of North Carolina Press.

Schiebinger, L. (1999). *Has feminism Changed science?* Cambridge, MA: Harvard University Press.

Schwartz Cohen, R. (1989). The consumption junction: A proposal for research strategies in the sociology of technology. In W. Bijker, P. Hughes, & T. Pinch (Eds.), *The social construction of technological systems. New directions in the sociology and history of technology* (pp. 261–280). Cambridge, MA: MIT Press.

Scott, J. S. (1988). *Gender and the politics of history.* New York: Columbia University Press.

Spratley, E., Johnson, A., Sochalski, J., Fritz, M., & Spencer, W. (2000). *The registered nurse population. Findings from the National Sample Survey of Registered Nurses.* U.S. Department of Health and Human Services, HRSA, BofHP, Division of Nursing. Washington, DC: U.S. Government Printing Office.

Stanley, L. (Ed.). (1997). Introduction: On academic borders, territories, tribes and knowledges. In *Knowing feminisms* (pp. 1–17). London: Sage.

Stead, E. (1967). Training and use of paramedical personnel. *New England Journal of Medicine, 277,* 801–803.

Stevens, R. (1998). *American medicine and the public interest: A history of specialization.* Berkeley, CA: University of California Press.

Chapter **3**

PRIMARY CARE AS AN ACADEMIC DISCIPLINE

Claire M. Fagin

INTRODUCTION TO PRIMARY CARE AS AN ACADEMIC DISCIPLINE*

It is now more than 20 years since the first version of "Primary Care as an Academic Discipline" was presented and then published. At that time, it was seen as a very provocative statement, offering a challenge to both nursing and medicine. To nursing, the challenge was to take ownership of an area that was, historically, distinctly nursing. Although there were bureaucratic obstacles to ownership, like problems with reimbursement of providers, I believed that the greater problems were nursing's own readiness to move into an arena that would inevitably lead to conflict with medicine.

To medicine, the challenge was to reconsider its role in primary care, to give up the fantasy that physicians had to be all things to all people, and to relinquish the control of entry to care. This control was claimed even in areas in which physicians had little interest and in which their dominance produced high cost for little gain.

In rereading this chapter, I believe the basic tenets, definitions, and philosophy remain as relevant today as they were when—with some

_____

* This introduction represents the author's current thoughts on her text from the previous edition.

trepidation—the paper was presented in 1988 at the first annual symposium of the Robert Wood Johnson Program Nurse Faculty Fellows in Primary Care. Nurses have made great strides in primary care. There remain, however, significant obstacles and challenges. Some of these obstacles and challenges have to do with nurses themselves and how they view their roles and their historic connection to nursing itself. Others have to do with the systems of care that constrain all health professionals but affect nurses in particular ways. Still others have to do with public perceptions that confirm and support the notion that physicians can be all things to all people and should control health care.

The accomplishments since this manuscript was first written are enormous. Nurses are now reimbursed directly by the major governmental payers and by private insurers in many states. Prescriptive privileges are the norm. While state law may vary in the specifics, constraints on nurses are negligible and do not interfere with primary care practice. At this time, nurse practitioners (NPs) have statutory or regulatory prescriptive authority in all states. In addition, NPs can prescribe controlled substances in all states except Alabama, Florida, Kentucky, Missouri, Mississippi, and Texas (Pearson, 2002, p. 15). Addressing the remaining restrictions requires state action with strong support from national bodies. As a result of payment changes and prescriptive privileges, nurses are now practicing primary care in individual and group practices throughout the United States, and extraordinary examples of holistic and more traditional practices abounding from New York to Alaska. In this introduction, I use *nurse* to mean nurse practitioners and clinical nurse specialists (advanced practice nurses, [APNs]). This usage assumes that the prevailing sentiment among advanced practice nurses in general, and nurse practitioners in particular, is that they are *nurses* prepared at the graduate level to practice in primary care (and secondary and tertiary care).

I raise this issue because I am increasingly unsure that the assumption that APNs view themselves first as nurses still holds. Recently, journalist Suzanne Gordon, arguably nursing's greatest advocate in print media, told me of the response to speeches and seminars she has given at meetings of nurse practitioners. Having been mentored by nurses like, Joan Lynaugh and others, including me, who view advanced practice nurses as part of the spectrum of nursing, Suzanne always describes nurse practitioners using the term *nurse*. In recent talks she has received a barrage of negative reactions when she links nurse practitioners and APNs to other nurses. "We have a nursing background, but we do not function as nurses," one NP commented. When NPs register confusion about what they should call themselves when introducing themselves to patients, Suzanne suggests they call themselves "Nurse Smith." (Gordon & Buresh, 2000). Many NPs respond that they would never use the title "nurse," in front of their name because "I wouldn't want anyone to think I'm just a nurse."

What's in a name? A lot. Now, as in the past, I always introduce myself by saying "I am a nurse." I answer that way because it is true and because announcing that I am a nurse sets the frame of reference for what and who I am. Nursing gave me the knowledge and skill to do what I do and have done, and inferentially, it tells people what I want them to know about nursing and its possibilities and realities. Identifying myself as a nurse also places me within a body of professionals who have gained a strong level of public trust.

It is interesting that poll after poll in America tells us that the public trusts nurses more than any other health professional or health institution. Similar findings are reported by Meadows, Levenson, and Baeza (2000) in the United Kingdom in their King's Fund publication, *The Last Straw.* Nurses do not gain this trust easily. Our care of and advocacy for patients and families is why we have this public trust. And care and advocacy must be viewed as central in all our work if we are to keep this trust. Our care and concern for people must be translated into finding solutions to the pressing problems in health care today. Nurses understand the complexity of the health care environment and the consequences of unresolved and unaddressed health care issues. Nurses have a bird's-eye view of our society and the influence of a broad array of health factors on the problems people face from birth through senescence to death. Nurses understand how health factors influence children's learning and how nutrition affects the way children face their day in school. Nurses understand the effects of sensory deprivation on youngsters and older people and the needs people have for environments that are not only loving, where this is possible, but enriched by activities that promote health. Nurses see what everyone else is doing in the health care field. Because of our experiences in taking care of the sick and promoting health, nurses are able to distinguish quality care and to understand the conditions that either allow quality to flourish or make its provision a "mission impossible."

Does any other profession or observer have the depth of understanding and ubiquitous presence that nurses have in these health and societal issues? I don't think so. Furthermore, nurses have an unusually holistic approach to the way they view health and illness and the interaction of social problems and health, an approach that is unexcelled by other clinicians. It is part of the way we think. The "public face" of nurse practitioners can give concrete examples of the way nurses think as they put their knowledge to work to enhance patient care. This is evident in their day-to-day primary care of patients and in their public roles of advocacy for people's health and welfare. I want people to know what nurses do, and one way to let them know is to proudly attach the title "nurse" to the clinician who performs health care's vital functions.

A few years ago I was working with Warren Steibel, the producer of the shows "Firing Line" and "Debates-Debates." In anticipation of some pilot programs on nurses and health care issues, the question of how to title the show arose. Familiar with the polls showing trust in nurses, we decided to refer to me as Nurse Fagin. Although the show never moved beyond local cable stations, thus aborting my nascent television career, we liked the distinction of calling me Nurse—which I am first and foremost. My full credentials were shown in the credits and in the introductions, but my "title" was Nurse Claire Fagin, and it gave a certain complementarity to my interviews, highlighting nursing, avoiding the familiarity of first names, and skirting confusion.

Why, I then wonder, are nurse practitioners so resistant to using the title "nurse"? To add status? Why do they not grasp that the path to status and social legitimacy lies in what we do with what we know? Calling oneself "Nurse Smith" seems a lot more professional and generates a lot more confidence than introducing oneself to the patient/client with "Hello, I'm Mary."

Previously, it never would have occurred to me that the identification with nursing would become a serious matter to nurse practitioners. But this issue is a major internal challenge to nursing, perhaps a greater challenge even than those we face from the public, from interprofessional strife, and from any remaining legal barriers. Among the reasons for the nursing shortage and the downturn in student interest in the profession is the attitude of nurses themselves to the climate affecting their work. Surely, the lack of pride in the nursing identification has some place in all of this. Some nursing leaders are even proposing (again) abandoning the title of nurse and finding another that appears to signify greater status. This flight from the word *nurse* is not new. It has occurred before and been found wanting. Thus any such action now must be approached with considerable thought and caution.

Focusing on what we call ourselves saps our energy from addressing critical problems affecting nursing and the public. For example, nurse practitioners continue to face challenging issues related to their relationship with members of other professions. Nurses have made great progress in collaboration with physicians in all realms of health care. The degree of independent work advanced practice nurses perform is discussed throughout this book. As is now the case with the majority of physicians, in many cases, nurse practitioners are employees of practices. This work model raises many practice and ethical issues, not the least of which is that it becomes harder to differentiate the independent portion of a nurse practitioner's work from that of an "extra arm" in the physician's office.

Current practice styles and regulations impede the work of nurses in areas of public health, rightly an independent/interdependent domain of nurses with advanced degrees. Public health and home care practice continue to present major obstacles to full enactment of nurses' professional role. The need for physician's orders for the myriad components of home care and to fully assess and manage patients, among others, are major impediments to practice. Such restrictions and regulations must be addressed and removed.

Although challenges remain to the full practice of primary care by nurses, the view of primary care as an academic discipline in nursing has taken hold and advances the profession. The use of the term *primary care* in academia is ubiquitous. It may not be a title in schools of nursing, but it is an integral part of most curricula, and the concepts have, for the most part, been successfully integrated in every area of study. While experience has informed us that integration of concepts frequently leads to the disappearance of the area of study, in the case of primary care, this has not occurred. Primary care, sometimes under a different rubric, is the "meat" of many graduate programs and is pervasive in undergraduate curricula. Nursing established its place in primary care early and, in my view, holds primacy still. The challenges that remain are significant. Unfortunately, as always for us, the most serious challenges will come from within the profession. However, the extraordinary achievements of the nursing profession in primary care should strengthen all nurses as they face the challenges. These achievements are laudable and give us cause for satisfaction and pride.

REFERENCES

Gordon, S., & Buresh, B. (2000). *From silence to voice.* Ottawa: Canadian Nurses Association.

Meadows, S., Levenson, R., & Baeza, J. (2000). *The last straw explaining the NHS nursing shortage.* London: King's Fund 2000.

Pearson, L. (2002). Fourteenth annual legislative update: How each state stands on legislative issues affecting advanced nursing practice. *Nurse Practitioner, 27*(1), 10–52.

The chapter "Primary Care as an Academic Discipline" was originally written at the invitation of the Robert Wood Johnson Foundation
for presentation at their first annual symposium highlighting the
work of the Nurse Fellows in Primary Care. The title was theirs; the
content was mine. I doubt that I would have articulated the view of early
ownership of the primary care arena by nursing had I not had the opportunity to reflect on the meaning of the term, "academic discipline," offered
me by the Foundation.

It was clear then (Fagin, 1977), and it is even clearer now, that nurses
are educated to be superb primary care practitioners; and that the skills
and knowledge required to practice are imparted in most of our undergraduate programs and continued in many of our graduate programs.
Research over the past two decades has proven that nurses can deliver
cost-effective primary care that can substitute for physician care in many
situations. Further, nurses can provide new and important services in
long-term care and nursing homes.

Other chapters in this book bring the numerical record about nurse
practitioners up to date. This is not my aim in this chapter. Rather, I would
like to put several other issues into a contemporary perspective. First, the
issue of direct reimbursement of nurse practitioners: Over the last eight
years two nursing groups have been extremely successful, on a national
level, in achieving direct reimbursement for their work. They are certified
nurse-midwives (CNMs) and certified registered nurse anesthetists
(CRNAs). More recently, advance practice nurses have gained Medicare
reimbursement subject to state nurse practice acts (Capitol Update, 1998).
Moreover, there are some examples where nurses have successfully developed independent practices targeted at middle- and upper-middle-class
patients (Brenna, 1997). During the 1980s two large-scale reviews of the
literature provided evidence that nurses' styles of delivering care are
extremely suited to people's needs in terms of health teaching and counseling, follow-up care, use of fewer diagnostic tests, and per-episode costs
(Office of Technology Assessment, 1986). Yet, in recent national delibera-
tions, the issue of recommending reimbursement did not benefit much
from these exhaustive data. Now new questions are raised as obstacles to
reimbursement. They have to do with "sameness" of work and "human capital" theory. However, human capital theory as it applies to nurses seems,
at this time, to be referring exclusively to opportunity costs of training.
Opportunity costs are not seen as appropriate for differences in physicians'
backgrounds.

It is interesting to note that studies have found that there are diminishing returns to education as it increases: the return on elementary school

education is highest and the return on graduate studies (excluding professional degrees) lowest (Physician Payment Review Commission, unpublished manuscript). The issues of sameness linked with the human capital theory have not been used in establishing relative costs for different specialties among physicians, clinical psychologists, or limited-license practitioners.

It is hard to believe that these are the true issues that stand in the way of recommending direct reimbursement for nurse practitioners. Nurses are the only group that has produced a large volume of convincing evidence about care and outcomes of care. Yet others have achieved the goal of direct reimbursement without such evidence. Clearly, this issue is still a problem.

Over the past decade we *have* brought primary care into the mainstream of nursing education. Preparation begins at the undergraduate level, and most nurses and others accept the view that graduate education is needed to prepare the nurse practitioner for generalist and specialized roles. A critical mass of faculty *have* been prepared for teaching primary care content. Thanks to the Robert Wood Johnson Foundation, the Kellogg Foundation, the Commonwealth Foundation, and the Joshua Macy Foundation (and others), cadres of nurses have been prepared for both practice and teaching.

While organized medicine's stance in relation to collaboration has not changed significantly (Mangan, 1997), there are thousands of examples of collaborative relationships between nurses and physicians that attest to major change at the patient care level.

There are numerous clinical settings appropriate for learning, and educational resources to provide diverse knowledge and skills in teaching, administration, and research have increased exponentially.

Medical school output has increased markedly, and health systems costs, as predicted, have increased dramatically. Both service-based and provider-based reimbursement are being examined, and new payment structures (such as the Resource Based Relative Value Scale) are in place for implementation.

Much work has been done on the relative merits of community care versus institutionalization. Home care alternatives and hospice are part of many third-party reimbursement programs, and home care has been found to be cost-effective as compared with hospital care. Early discharge programs for low birth-weight infants have led to replications with other populations, and nursing has led the way in these studies.

Nurses are increasingly involved with the "power brokers" of the health care and political systems. They do sit on boards and in various national, state, regional, and local policy-making bodies.

A new issue that emerged in the 1990s with regard to primary care and the nurse practitioner is the extent to which the international community has come to recognize nursing's importance in meeting health care needs. Work on the international scene in primary care is increasing in importance. United States' nursing's maturity is permitting it to help meet needs of nurses and health care systems in other countries through collaborative efforts. The World Health Organization is cognizant of nursing's role in primary care and has named several United States universities and programs in other countries as the WHO Collaborating Center. We can expect, therefore, the international activities of nurse practitioners, and CNMs in particular, to increase.

There is more to be done. Given the extraordinary changes that have occurred in the past decade, by the year 2000 it was projected that nursing should be at the point of achievement in primary care where nurses are making the maximum contribution to our nation's health and the international community. This goal has only been partially achieved.

I said in 1978 that primary care is the generic discipline of nursing. Nothing has happened to alter that view. What has occurred is that nursing has proven that statement, in its practice, education, and research, and no longer needs to claim in rhetoric what is readily seen in reality.

Primary care as an academic discipline is a vital issue for nursing and medicine to address for reasons that have to do with intellectual considerations as well as political, social, and financial factors. More striking, however, is its importance as an issue that permits the conceptualization of a distinction between the medical and nursing models. It should be said at the start that the author does not believe that primary care is a separate academic discipline within nursing nor, based on nursing's history and meaning, should it be. Primary care is an integral part of nursing in all its aspects and is the academic discipline of nursing. How the author arrived at this conclusion will be discussed by defining the term, explaining why the issue is of interest to nursing and medicine, taking a brief look at the major relevant historical events of this century, and examining nursing's past and present focus (Fagin, 1992; Fagin & Goodwin, 1972). It is the author's belief that nursing and medicine have followed, and must follow, separate routes to the goal of primary care.

DISCIPLINES, DEPARTMENTS, AND DISTINCTIONS

To begin from a common understanding of this subject, it is necessary to define what is meant by "academic discipline." There are some cases where semantics *do* make a difference, and this is one of them, since reactions to the concept of primary care as an academic discipline will be based on no small part in the terminology involved. The *Oxford English Dictionary* (1990) defines the word *discipline* as "a branch of instruction or education; a department or learning of knowledge," note that there are two parts for that definition.

Donaldson and Crowley (1978) state:

> Disciplines have evolved as a consequence of a distinct perspective and syntax, which determine what phenomena or abstractions are of interest, in what context such phenomena are to be viewed, what questions are to be raised, what methods of study are to be used, and what canons of evidence and proof are to be required (p. 114)

Looking at primary care within the strict context of such a definition as well as that part of the *Oxford English Dictionary*'s definition that describes "a branch of instruction or education," the idea of primary care as an academic discipline seems reasonable. While its body of knowledge has not been fully developed through theoretical exposition and research, the parameters of this area, which lend themselves to investigation and theory development, have been identified by many writers. Thus, the potential for establishing a theoretical body of knowledge that relates to primary care exists even if all of it is not available to us at the present time.

It is the second part of the definition that is a subject for debate, that is, a discipline as a "department of learning or knowledge." In centers of learning, such as universities, there appears to be a natural transition between the identification of a particular area as a discipline and the belief that this discipline should be administratively or organizationally set up as a department. It is in this area that questions must be raised as to the appropriateness of such an organizational structure for nursing. What are the factors that create, defeat, or blur the formation of a content area as an academic discipline, or, in this case, as an academic department? Are these factors dominated by the intellectual force of argument that pertains to the body of knowledge of the area, or are there other considerations?

An examination of the ways in which the basic sciences are organized in medical schools may clarify the point. In examining the organization in medical education of basic science disciplines—"a branch of instruction or education"—one can note from school to school the blurring discipline lines and the lack of commonality of discipline groupings, that is, the lack of "a department of learning or knowledge." In one school, for instance, the department of anatomy was closed, and two new divisions were created in cell biology and cytology. In other schools, biochemistry may be linked with biophysics, while still other institutions maintain all of the above as separate departments (Kohler, 1982).

Why this lack of consistency? Various factors, such as competition for support, prestige, historical circumstances, perception of problems, and social interactions, contribute to this situation. So does the power of external forces, such as financial support from governmental and private agencies, that influence the growth and specific labeling of academic disciplines. Medical schools across the country have responded to these pressures by increasing their emphasis on education for primary care. It is interesting to note that a 1977 survey by the American Association of Medical Colleges of trends in primary care education that indicated no well-defined locus for coordinating efforts for institution-wide, primary care training through specific departmental structures (Giacoloni & Hudson, 1977) still applies. While no corresponding survey for nursing has been published, the author is confident that a similar conclusion can be made.

Thus, while both medicine and nursing have shown increasing interest in the primary care area, in most cases the educational component has been discretely organized without a corresponding organization within the school's administrative structure.

HISTORICAL PERSPECTIVE

Two distinct lines of development can be identified as we examine the professional health care scene of this century: These are the public health movement and the growth of medical school-hospital establishments, each of these developments with its own priorities. By the late 19th century, the public health movement had achieved major success in controlling the spread of infection and in microbiology; early in the 20th century, it began to focus on the health needs of the poor and on maternal-child health care. During this same period, there were a large number of poor-quality programs that prepared physicians. Flexner's report of 1910 had a profound influence on the nature and the content of medical schools and medial education. It set the stage for the stress on research, which later became the *sine qua non* of the quality medical school. The rising professionalism of the medical group coincided with the growing power of the hospital group and the decline in the power of the physicians involved in the public health movement.

In medicine, the forerunner of today's primary care practitioner was, of course, the general practitioner. Although declining somewhat in numbers in the first 30 years of the post-Flexner period, the almost total extinction of the general practitioner on the American scene occurred after World War II. At that time, a variety of developments pushed the health care system into an emphasis on, and power in, the secondary and tertiary care areas. The extraordinary research and technological process during the decade of the 1940s had stunning implications for the civilian population. There was a growing assumption that the development of technology would be tantamount to the control of illness. With the increase in technology and research, there was a subsequent need for physicians and others to become more specialized as they advanced their knowledge base. It became impossible to know all things about all medical problems.

The financing of hospital growth through the Hill-Burton Act, as well as governmental funding for medical education, grew geometrically during this period. Furthermore, the availability of governmental and private funds for research reinforced the already growing development of an academic role model for the physician-scientist. These faculty members, as the status members of the medical school group, had an enormous influence on medical students who were choosing their future paths. Although attempts were made to revise, or at least maintain, a general practice group within the American Medical Association, these attempts were met with little success for reasons such as "the absence of an academic base, the undefined role of the general practitioner in relation to the specialist, and the difference in working conditions and status between the general practitioner and the specialist" (Lewy, 1977, p. 875).

In addition, the decades from the 1940s through the 1960s were dominated by the health care providers, with few consumer efforts to stop the extraordinary growth of the medical and hospital establishment. In later years, however, some countertrends had begun to develop—among them, the notion of the Great Society, with health care seen as a right rather than a privilege. The funding of health centers connected with the Office of Economic Opportunity exposed gaps in health care; in particular, the gap that we now label the "primary care needs of the people."

These developments reawakened medicine's interest in general practice, and during the 1960s several study commissions set out to explore its future. One such commission indicated that the graduate education of physicians for what had now acquired the label of "family practice" required training equivalent to that of other specialties, as well as the development of a specialty board to give certifying examinations (Millis, 1966). The evolution of a new specialty, it was stated, requires a definition of content, the development of graduate training programs, the development of specialty departments in medical school, the establishment of standards, the development of mechanisms to insure adherence to the standards, the development of continuing education programs to insure maintenance of these standards, and the generation of research programs to further the unique body of knowledge. (Lewy, 1977, p. 875)

It was not easy to establish such programs, especially in universities, since there was no uniform process whereby the content of fields such as community medicine and behavioral science could be taught; besides, there was a severe shortage of qualified teachers in family medicine.

NURSING'S DEVELOPMENT

Nursing's role in the two lines of development in the health scene was in sharp contrast to that of medicine's. Whereas medicine developed its power base in the medical school-hospital establishment, nursing became dominated by the same establishment.

Although the early hospital schools of the late 19th century were based on Nightingale's model and were educational apprenticeships, by the 20th century many became what Joanne Ashley calls "successful instruments for women's oppression" (Ashley, 1977, p. 23). As early as 1915, some leaders in nursing were recommending that nursing education be placed on a professional basis with within colleges and universities. Yet well into the 1930s and 1940s, hospitals simply increased the number of students in their schools to meet the demands for immediate nursing service.

There were great leaders in nursing during the first half of the century, but most of these leaders developed outside of the hospital group and were closely aligned with the public health movement, a movement that in nursing is the historical antecedent of the primary care movement. (Lillian Wald, the founder of the Henry Street Settlement and the Visiting Nurse Service, coined the terms *public health nurse* and *public health nursing*).

The first national nursing organization to have a headquarters and a paid staff was the National Organization for Public Health Nursing (NOPHN), which was established in 1912. For quite some time the public health movement in nursing continued to grow in power, to set standards for practice, and to influence education by requiring certain content, including degrees, as a condition of employment. In the 1940s, the National League of Nursing Education established its own accrediting committee, which was a very significant development in the history of nursing. It ended the proliferation of hospital schools and the student labor method of instruction. The influence of NOPHN was very strong on the League, and many leaders in nursing education prior to 1950 came out of the public health movement.

Now, however, it is sometimes difficult to distinguish public health nurses from other university-educated nurses, since more and more nurses work outside hospital walls and nursing education increasingly focuses on a holistic view of patient, family, and community. This can be said despite the fact that nursing followed the medical path in becoming specialized from the late 1940s through the 1960s. The knowledge explosion identified areas of need, such as psychiatric nursing, and federal dollars accelerated specialization in graduate education. But as their knowledge increased, nurses frequently rejected the kind of technical tasks that the new technology created, resulting in an expressed need for different kinds of manpower; that is, technical aides who were task- and physician-oriented. One unfortunate result of this movement was the increase in fragmentation in hospital care; another was the separation of most nursing leaders from the hospital establishment. The absence of bridges from university to nursing service militated against nursing leaders having an influence on improving hospital nursing care. Fortunately, there are new moves in this direction at the present time.

By the late 1960s in fact, nursing programs have become both generalized and comprehensive, stressing public health and mental health. Had it not been for political factors and nursing's resistance to recognizing its own natural progression, nursing could have conceivably moved very rapidly to prepare for primary health care. The few imaginative nurses who carved out roles in primary care were frequently scorned by their nursing colleagues, and other groups jumped in to fill the primary care gap.

Despite this backing and filling within the profession, or perhaps because of it, pressures from governmental and other groups for a rapid method of preparing nurses to meet primary care needs resulted in the establishment of 100 or more "nurse practitioner" programs of varied duration, content, and type. In this situation, as in others before, nursing's adaptation to meet immediate needs solved some problems but created or perpetuated others. Over the past 40 years, 70,000 nurse practitioners have been prepared. Considerable funding has also gone into the preparation of other health care practitioners and into increasing the number and capability of medical schools. By now, nursing has changed its stance and sees itself as playing a major role in the delivery of primary health care.

AN ACADEMIC DISCIPLINE

We are now at a point where there is interest in primary care on the part of both medicine and nursing. But are the two fields comparable in this area? The author has tried to build a case that indicates they are not comparable, and the analysis will now be completed.

It has become increasingly apparent that for real change to occur, primary care must be seen as a respected part of the academic scene. The mass of data attesting to the influence of high-status medical faculty members on the socialization of medical students supports the importance of establishing the academic centrality of primary care. In both nursing and medical education, in other words, primary care must be part of the mainstream, with its content and faculty constituting an integral part of the academic power structure.

In medical education, however, two problems have been cited as greatly inhibiting the growth and development of comprehensive care. These are the assumptions that comprehensive care (particularly primary care) is solely a function of an attitudinal set and a kind of noblesse oblige that does not require specific training, and "the lack of professionalization of the role required to provide comprehensive care in the role of primary physician" (Magraw, 1971, p. 475).

The Nature of Nursing

Despite the admission by medical educators of the need to educate for primary care, the attitude in most medical centers toward this field, as Alpert pointed out, continues to be condescending (Alpert & Charnay, 1974, Mullan, Rivo, & Politzer, 1993). The subspecialist researchers-clinicians are the tail that wags the dog in every academic clinical department, be it medicine, pediatrics, or obstetrics-gynecology. A conceptual move to equalize the status between the primary care physician and the specialist in internal medicine or pediatrics would have been hard enough. However, since specialists are now considered generalists in their respective fields and subspecialists are the predominant powers, the gaps between the subspecialist group and the primary care group is a wide one indeed. It is therefore understandable that pressures exist resisting the establishment of primary care as an academic discipline within the medical profession. If indeed the establishment of an academic discipline, and subsequently a specific department, to coordinate and develop the primary care component of the curriculum would help to solve some of the political and status issues faced by those devoting themselves to primary care, then this may well be a legitimate goal—for medicine, that is.

For nursing, however—given its natural evolution from a concept of public health and a concern for the individual, family, and community to a concept of primary care—the situation is different, and the solution to the problem is almost the antithesis of the medical solution. In nursing, primary care is *not* low man on the totem pole. Rather, it is increasingly recognized as the integral core of nursing rather than one of its specialties.

The nature of nursing as described by Nightingale and others following her has been too close to the nature of primary care as described by almost everyone else for primary care to be conceptualized as a discrete academic discipline within nursing. Primary care is so multifaceted that it cannot be considered the domain of any one group to cover all its aspects. If we were forced to define it as a separate entity, we would be robbing its strength from all other groups in nursing. What is the body of knowledge for primary care, for instance, that can be differentiated from the body of knowledge needed in nursing in general?

As the author sees it then, primary care as an academic discipline within nursing is *the* generic discipline. The care of people with actual or potential health problems and the manipulation of the environment to contribute to optimal health have long been seen as the generic base of nursing practice. Nursing is defined as including the promotion and maintenance of health, prevention of illness, care of persons during these acute phases of illness, and rehabilitation or restoration of health. Are these not also the functions of primary care described by most writers, and do they not also suggest the knowledge required? As Donaldson and Crowley (1978) stated,

> Nursing has traditionally valued humanitarian service. But in addition, the self-respect and self-determination of clients are to be preserved. The goal of nursing service is to foster self-caring behavior that leads to individual health and well-being. These values and goals, which are intrinsic to professional practice, have shaped the value orientation of the discipline. (p. 114)

Primary care has now moved into the mainstream of nursing education. The stopgap measures to prepare nurses as primary practitioners have accomplished short-term goals. There is a need to continue to incorporate teachers and leaders in educational and service programs who have a strong commitment to primary care. To do this, six ingredients must be present in the educational organization: (1) an understanding of the nature and scope of primary care nursing; (2) faculty prepared for teaching in primary care; (3) philosophical commitment to primary care at the core of nursing; (4) appropriate clinical settings with arrangements for faculty practice; (5) collaborative relationships with physicians that provide for consultation and referral; and (6) educational resources that provide diverse knowledge and skills in teaching, administration, and research. Where nursing faculty in primary care seek and do not find these ingredients, they must help to create them.

Although primary care as the appropriate focus of nursing is a comfortable concept, the issue becomes more complex, more difficult, when one considers the complementary and interdependent roles required to flesh out these concepts. The question of the collaborative or collegial relationships of the two major disciplines involved in primary care—medicine and nursing—is important to study. The lack of coordinated planning in primary care has exacerbated this issue and the situation can be expected to worsen unless it is directly addressed. In the guidelines for federal support of primary care residency programs, the definition of primary care content is virtually identical to every nursing description of this area since 1968. Clearly we must come together in education and practice to utilize the best each discipline has to offer, to build on our individual strengths, and subsequently to collaborate in meeting health needs in a rational manner.

Nurses and physicians involved in primary care have not been sufficiently involved in health-policy-making bodies or in health planning. Health planning is an area studied by many. However, as in 1978 (Falkson, 1978), we have neither a national health policy nor a national health plan or planning process. Proof of this can be found in the way primary, secondary, and tertiary care have developed in the past three decades. If a collaborative and rational plan had been drawn up at the start, it is not inconceivable that a different system of health care could have been organized that would have had a major impact on the nature of primary care services as well as total systems costs.

If the readings from the professional and public marketplaces are correct, there are three periods of change that relate to identifying and meeting primary care needs. The first one occurred in the 1960s with the recognition of the need, and there were a variety of solutions planned and implemented. All were without any connection to one another or any consideration of their long-term effects in areas such as the nurse practitioner movement, the development of the physician's assistant, and the infusion of money into medical schools to expand enrollment with a heavy focus on preparation for primary care. The view commonly held during this period was that a nurse practitioner was to be prepared as a physician-extender, therefore, a physician substitute.

The findings from the next period of change have been very clear in indicating that the nurse practitioner in primary care can indeed fill the vast majority of needs commonly identified. Phase two is replete with studies of the effectiveness of nonphysician providers. Toward the end of this period, we begin to see data that indicate that long-term systems costs can be affected by extended community care versus hospitalization; that is, by assisting people to remain in their own homes through supportive services. On the other hand, the question of how long-term systems costs are affected by the relative expense of educating various practitioners has not been explored.

We are now into phase three, which is the realization that physician-students already in the pipeline have caused an oversupply of specialist physicians in this country. What effect this will have on primary care, on the development of the nursing profession, or on health systems costs is unknown. Several hypotheses can be posed. One is that since physicians control the marketplace, we can expect health systems costs to increase with the abundance of physicians. Economists are examining this issue closely, and various alternatives are being posed, such as service-based (Enthoven, 1993) rather than provider-based reimbursement. Further, the extraordinary expansions of the for-profit sector with a concomitant growth in the percentage of salaried physicians may create other employment possibilities for nurse practitioners. At any rate, in phase three it would be well to examine the issues posed by the already known variables and to pressure for participation in policy development.

It is the author's belief that the expansion of the primary care effort in medicine was in error. This, incidentally, is not because of my lack of good memories about the general practitioners of the late 1930s but, rather, because the author's consumer bias is to get her money's worth for dollars spent. If indeed, at a maximum of six years, a nurse practitioner can deliver at least as good, or in some cases better, primary care than a physician—whose educational costs are much higher, length of education close to double, and income expectations correspondingly greater—then serious questions must be raised about this kind of luxurious approach (Fagin, 1990). Further, many of the reasons for medical specialization were cogent. The explosion of knowledge did indeed make it impossible to know all things about all medical problems. Given the nature of medical education and training, it is entirely appropriate to expect this kind of expertise from the physician. However, this kind of thinking is clearly ex post facto and will have little effect on the present situation. This is all the more reason for a clear identification of where we stand in nursing and medicine in relation to primary care and for a more open and complete discussion of these issues in interdisciplinary and consumer groups.

CONCLUSIONS

Primary care within nursing is the academic discipline of nursing. It cannot be separated from the other components of nursing into a new part but is the dominating force of the discipline itself. An examination of the contents and concepts of primary care clarifies the difference between the professions of nursing and medicine in relation to primary care. Primary care is not a focus of nursing; it is nursing's major focus.

REFERENCES

Alpert, J., & Charney, E. (1974). *The education of physicians for primary care.* Rockville, MD: US Public Health Service.

Ashley, J. (1977). *Hospitals, paternalism, and the role of the nurse.* New York: Teachers College Press.

Brenna A. (1997, October 6). Is there a nurse in the House? *New York Magazine.*

Capitol Update. (1998, January 30). Medicare reimbursement: An update. 16 (01), 2. Washington, DC: ANA.

Donaldson, S. K., & Crowley, D. (1978). The discipline of nursing. *Nursing Outlook, 26,* 113–120.

Enthoven, A. C. (1993). A history and principles of managed competition. *Health Affairs, 12,* 24–48.

Fagin, C. M. (1977). Nature and scope of nursing practice in meeting primary health care needs. In American Nurses Association (Ed.), *Primary care by nursing: Sphere of responsibility and accountability* (pp. 35–51). Kansas City, MO: American Nurses Association.

Fagin, C. M. (1990). Nursing's value proves itself. *American Journal of Nursing, 90*(10), 17–30.

Fagin, C. M. (1992). Collaboration between nurses and physicians: No longer a choice. *Nursing and Health Care, 6,* 25–31.

Fagin, C. M., & Goodwin, B. (1972). Baccalaureate preparation for primary care. *Nursing Outlook, 20,* 240–244.

Falkson, J. L. (1978). We need a national health policy. *Journal of Health, Politics, Policy, and Law, 4,* 311.

Giacolioni, J. J., & Hudson, J. I. (1977). Primary care education trends in U.S. medical schools and teaching hospitals. *Journal of Medical Education, 52,* 971–981.

Kohler, R. (1982). *From medical chemistry to biochemistry: The makings of biomedical discipline.* Cambridge, NY: Cambridge University Press.

Lewy, R. M. (1977). The emergence of the family practitioner: An historical analysis of a new specialty. *Journal of Medical Education, 52,* 875–881.

Magraw, R. M. (1971). Implications for medical education. *American Journal of Diseases of Children, 122,* 475–486.

Mangan K. S. (1997). Some medical and nursing schools declare a truce and start to work together. *Chronicle of Higher Education 44*(17), A10–12.

Millis, J. S. (1966). *The graduate education of physicians.* Report of the Citizens Commission on Graduate Medical Education. Chicago: American Medical Association.

Mullan, F., Rivo, M. C., & Politzer, R. M. (1993). Doctors' dollars and determination: Making physician work-force policy. *Health Affairs, 12,* 138–151.

Office of Technology Assessment. (1986). *Physicians' assistants and certified nurse midwives: A policy analysis.* Washington, DC: U.S. Government Printing Office.

Oxford English Dictionary (8th ed.). (1990). R. E. Allen (Ed.), New York: Oxford University Press.

Physician Payment Review Commission (PPRC). Report on non-physician practitioners. Washington, DC (unpublished).

RESEARCH IN SUPPORT OF NURSE PRACTITIONERS

Frances Hughes, Sean Clarke, Deborah A. Sampson, Julie Fairman, and Eileen M. Sullivan-Marx

S ince the 1960s, researchers have published numerous studies to describe, explain, and justify the nurse practitioner role to society. In this chapter, we present a focused review of research examining nurse practitioners and propose new directions that go beyond the traditional approaches of effectiveness, utilization, and comparison. While not an exhaustive review, our approach takes a broad perspective of nurse practitioner research and the prevailing themes of the last three decades, categorized in three eras. We then categorize the eras and themes: Era I (1960–1979) focuses on the theme of proving the worth of nurse practitioners, Era II (1975–1995) describes research on innovations, quality, and cost of nurse practitioners, and Era III (1990–present) examines current themes and the status of research. Researchers have successfully chronicled the value and justification for advanced practice nurses in health care. Following the review of advanced practice nursing research to date, we will discuss strategies to move the research agenda forward and away from traditional themes of justification, efficiency, and comparison and toward evidence-based practice (also chapter 5).

ERA I: PROVING WORTH, 1960–1979

Nurses worked in expanded roles well before the 1960s. The public health nurses of the early 20th century, nurse-midwives in the Frontier Nursing

Service of the 1920s and 1930s, military nurses during World War II, and the early intensive care nurses of the 1950s all practiced in expanded roles. The nurse practitioners (NPs) of the 1960s were not an exception. The foundational differences, however, between the earlier practitioners and NPs of the 1960s were rooted in more formalized education programs and the rapidity with which the idea of expanded practice disseminated, albeit haphazardly.

The Social Context

The research studies of the 1960s and 1970s reflected the social transition and growth occurring in society and influencing nursing practice. Within the context of the women's movement, the civil rights movement, Lyndon Johnson's Great Society programs, and Vietnam War protests, changes in health care and nursing were not surprising. Enactment of Medicare and Medicaid legislation in 1965, and the commensurate increased demand for primary care providers, revealed the inherent deficit of a health system geared for acute care. At the same time, the Division of Nursing of the Department of Health and Human Services and private funding sources such as The Robert Wood Johnson Foundation made incredibly innovative and highly political decisions to provide money both for postgraduate nursing education and for demonstration projects to fill the gaps in care, particularly for women, children, and people in rural settings. From this context, the pediatric nurse practitioner program developed by Loretta Ford and Henry Silver emerged in 1965 at the University of Colorado and focused on caring for rural families and their children. Arising from a foundation of public health nursing, this program was designed to prepare nurse practitioners at the graduate level through a certificate program funded in part with federal dollars (Silver, Ford, & Stearly, 1967).

The Research Context

As the 1960s progressed, more nurses entered academic collegiate settings, and nursing practice focused on patient-centered clinical problems. Nursing research slowly and reluctantly followed the changes in education and practice. Small groups of nursing scholars posed new types of research questions and defined new nursing values that redirected knowledge development from functional studies toward clinical research and scholarly inquiry.

Few nurses had the knowledge and education to conduct or participate in research, and of those very few nurses who completed doctoral work, many earned their degrees in schools of education or departments of anthropology and sociology. Their research focus necessarily was guided by their particular educational framework rather than clinical practice. Until 1976, more than half of *Nursing Research*'s pages were filled primarily with studies about curriculum, methodological issues, or student concerns (Baer, 1997). Similarly, Sigma Theta Tau did not fund a clinically focused study until 1966 (Sigma Theta Tau International, 1996). Even so, nurse researchers, who were primarily clinicians themselves, were eager to focus on the new nurse practitioner role. They asked questions and collected data according to the tools and skills they had at hand, via essays, surveys, or polls, implementing basic descriptive quantitative studies using samples of convenience. Early on they focused their analyses at very basic levels: How many patients did they care for over particular periods of time, what did they actually do, what kinds of skills and knowledge did they add to their nursing repertoire in order to practice in an enlarged role, how did they "get along" with their physician colleagues? Patient-centered studies, other than quantitative analyses of patient satisfaction, came much later. However, when NPs became more commonplace as health care providers and less self-conscious about their place in the health care system, and nurses in general became more nuanced researchers, different types of studies emerged in later decades.

Research Exemplars

The studies conducted during the early 1960s through the mid-1970s were primarily descriptive in nature, reflecting the early state of nursing research. Many studies, when read closely, carried a sometimes not so subtle subtext reflecting nurses' utter excitement and satisfaction with their enlarged roles, as if they finally had escaped the bonds of traditional practice. The studies also implied, again subtly at first, that nurses provided certain kinds of care, such as the well-baby care, and performed certain tasks, such as immunizations or physical examinations, as competently as their physician colleagues (Fairman, 1997; Geolot, 1990).

One of the earliest reported experiments came in 1961, from the Collaborative Study of Prenatal Factors in Cerebral Palsy and Neurological Diseases in Providence, Rhode Island. Specially trained public health nurses conducted screenings of infants to detect physical defects, a task previously performed only by physicians. In this study, public health nurses were found to be as highly effective as pediatricians in screening efforts (Solomons & Hatton, 1961). In 1963, a nursing care clinic was established at the Thomas F. Gailor Out-Patient Clinics, in Memphis, Tennessee, to reduce the excessive workload created by poor, chronically ill patients visiting the hospital outpatient clinics for routine observation and continuation of long-term treatments. Using physician-developed protocols, the nurses independently staffed the clinics, referred patients to specialists, and provided supervision of patients with chronic, stable conditions (Guthrie, Runyan, Clark, & Marvin, 1964). C. E. Lewis and Resnick (1964) reported on the nurse clinic established in 1964 at the University of Kansas Medical Center. Their analysis indicated significant reduction in the frequency of complaints, a marked reduction in patients seeking doctors for minor complaints, and a marked shift in the preference of patients for nurses to perform certain functions. The researchers concluded that the nurses provided competent and effective care comparable to that of physicians to uncomplicated chronically ill patients in outpatient clinics (Fairman, 1999).

Competition and Changing Questions

Many of the reports in the 1970s continued to describe this exciting new nursing role and the various training programs, and touted nurse practitioners as an answer to the problem of lack of primary care providers, particularly in underserved populations (Glover, 1967; N. Martin, 1967; Schiff, Fraser, & Walters, 1969; Walker, Murawski, & Thorn, 1964). And here again, the research questions were socially constructed and designed with an underlying self-consciousness to "prove" to themselves and the rest of the health care world that NPs were safe practitioners in various settings.

A number of reasons accounted for this approach to research questions during this period. First, physician competence was assumed by other practitioners and the public, based upon the strong cultural authority physicians held in the health care system and their professional organizations, such as the American Medical Association. Nurses' competence had to be proven over and over, on a case-by-case basis (Fagin, 1992).

Second, health resource demand continued to grow in the 1970s, particularly among the elderly and families with children, while the number of general practice physicians continued to decline as more and more physicians entered specialty practice (Fairman, 1999). In contrast, the number of NPs continued to grow as generous federal funding for nursing education specifically targeted nurse practitioner education beginning in 1971 (Geolot, 1990). Due in part to restrictive state practice legislation that required direct physician supervision of NPs, and despite the desperation of overworked primary care providers, physicians and NPs found themselves in competition for the ownership of skills and knowledge once firmly in medicine's domain (Safriet, 1992).

The 1970s also saw a rise in the number of physician-generated articles, both in the popular press and in organization journals, questioning the ability of NPs to provide quality care and lending greater support to physician assistants. Articles of this type tended to be polemic, experiential, and opinion pieces. Much of the discussions in the professional journals were, in part, a direct response to the competition physicians began to experience from other types of practitioners such as osteopaths and chiropractors, who achieved reimbursement victories in the late 1960s and early 1970s. Physicians were also undergoing radical and forced changes in their practice philosophies as federal and state health insurance programs began to make the solo practitioner obsolete. The encroachment felt by physicians was perhaps best expressed and forecasted by George E. Ferrar, Jr. (1969), President of the Pennsylvania Medical Society. In an address to Society officers about future challenges, in particular the emerging "doctor assistants," he warned, "this health professional could become the single greatest opposing force that medical doctors have ever faced" (p. 9).

Nurse researchers responded to the growing unease in the medical and nursing press by designing research to show that nurse practitioners could, indeed, practice in a qualified, expert manner (Holt, 1998). In the 1970s, more and more studies and reports emerged that indirectly tried to make sense and legitimize the massive federal investment in NP education, and to enlighten physicians about the roles NPs could play in their practices. Even so, framed by the growing potential for economic and political competition between NPs and physicians, studies comparing physician and nurse practitioner care in certain venues or for specific populations became the most prevalent form of analysis (Bessman, 1974; Heagarty, Boehringer, Lavigne, Brooks, & Evans, 1973; Russo, Gururaj, Bunye, Kim, & Ner, 1975). The reports generally indicated that nurse practitioners could substitute for physicians and that care provided by nurse practitioners was equivalent, if not better, than care provided by physicians. As early as 1974, the research teams of Sackett, Spitzer, Gent, and Roberts (1974), in Ontario, Canada, concluded that NPs were effective and safe and that it was time to refocus attention to the process of care delivery. Although many comparison studies were simply designed and contained considerable bias, policy makers and the public began to take notice and recognize advanced practice nurses as legitimate providers of health care.

Initially in the NP professional movement, NPs were conceived as a means to provide health care to underserved populations. Yet few of the early research studies actually addressed the care NPs provided in the context of the patient in underserved areas, nor were the studies designed with a sound theoretical approach. Nurse practitioner researchers of the 1960s and 1970s self-consciously focused on themselves, a trend that continued into the next few decades. Of course, the early research provided valuable support for the fledgling movement and for individual practitioners hungry for legitimization and tools to support their practices. In the end, the studies proved to the NPs themselves that it was safe for them "to think" rather than just follow orders (Joan Lynaugh, personal communication, 2002).

ERA II: INNOVATIONS, QUALITY, AND COST, 1975–1995

As we have seen, access to care was a key component in the emergence and utilization of nurse practitioners and other advanced practice nurses from the 1930s to the 1970s (also see chapter 13 on nurse anesthetists). William Kissick (1994) notes in his book, *Medicine's Dilemmas: Infinite Needs vs. Finite Resources,* that an Iron Triangle between cost, access, and quality of care permeates the U.S. health care system. In the late 1970s, access to care remained a dominant theme in health care policy, leading to research that focused on this domain, but the cost of access and the quality of care began to emerge as issues in health services research in the 1980s. From the late 1970s to the early 1990s, research examining nurse practitioner services was driven by health care policy changes and clustered around three distinct but not always novel themes: (1) cost and quality, (2) comparison and competition with physicians, and (3) innovative nursing practice models.

In the 1970s, U.S. nurse practitioners emerged as an important focus of service and research (Levine, 1977). Gaining a better understanding about cost containment for services provided by nurse practitioners compared services of physicians began to drive new studies in the 1980s. In a purely substitutive model, health policy experts questioned the continued need for nurse practitioners in primary care when the physician workforce supply was adequate to meet existing demands (Levine, 1977; Spitzer, 1984). However, the recognition that nurse practitioners *as nurses* have a vested interest in preventive care, community care, caring for populations at high risk, and emphasizing family and holistic approaches to care, led to testing innovative and emerging health care delivery models in the late 1980s and 1990s. Studies of innovative models in which nurse practitioners led care teams or participated in interdisciplinary practice demonstrated cost savings and positive patient outcomes (Lang, Sullivan-Marx, & Jenkins,

1996). In this section, we discuss key research studies over a productive 20-year period in categories related to cost and quality, comparison/competition with physicians, and innovative models.

Cost and Quality

Studies of nurse practitioner practice in Era II continued to focus on the structure of NP roles, cost savings or cost-effectiveness of NP practices, productivity or caseloads of NPs compared to physicians, referral patterns, barriers to NP practice, and patient and physician satisfaction with NP care (Levine, 1977; Pender & Pender, 1980; Poirer-Elliot, 1984; J. A. Ramsey, McKenzie, & Fish, 1982). LeRoy's (1982) perspective that to determine "cost-effectiveness of nurse practitioners, it is necessary to know . . . whether these services are substitutive or complementary to those provided by physicians" (p. 298) reflected the assumption that NPs were a cost substitute for physicians. Studies were often criticized for their methodological limitations and inability to demonstrate cost-effectiveness, yet NP practice research was constrained by both the limited structure and scope of practice barriers facing NPs (LeRoy, 1982; Safriet, 1992).

Feldman, Ventura, and Crosby (1987) reviewed the scientific merit of 248 NP practice documents from the 1970s through the mid-1980s for relevance, clarity, and flaws, resulting in a final list of 56 studies that met scientific merit for examining NP effectiveness. Consistently, nurse practitioners demonstrated high-quality and effective care. Such attention to the value of NPs, as well as physician assistants and midwives, also heightened following the Graduate Medical Education, Nursing, and Allied Professions Commission (GMENAC) report (U.S. Department of Health and Human Services [U.S. DHHS], 1980) on access and quality health care needs. The GMENAC report highlighted the economic perspective that NPs functioned as either complements to or substitutes for physicians (Griffith, 1984; Sox, 1979). Moreover, in the GMENAC report, the federal government acknowledged that nursing had an independent sphere of practice (defining NP practice as unique from physician practice), highlighted patient acceptance of NPs, and recommended that NPs and other primary care health professionals should receive direct Medicaid and Medicare reimbursement. This report and other studies focusing on cost and quality appeared in the context of intense discussion in the medical and nursing literature about who should provide primary care and how to define the domain of primary care (Pender & Pender, 1980; Prescott, Jacox, Collar, & Goodwin, 1981; D. E. Rogers, 1981).

Studies of NPs in the early 1980s indirectly examined cost-effectiveness by focusing on NP referral patterns and types of services provided to dispel assumptions that NP practice would be more costly due to increased referrals to physicians and specialists. Brodie and Bancroft (1982), however, found no differences between the number and types of referrals provided by NPs and physicians in a comparative study of 395 patients. Weinberg, Lijestrand, and Moore (1983) also found no difference in referrals/consultation requests. Watkins and Wagner (1982) reported that NPs made fewer referrals than recommended by protocol for hypertensive patients in rural areas, yet blood pressure control outcomes were good.

In 1986, the U.S. Office of Technology Assessment (OTA) issued a landmark report, "Nurse Practitioners, Physician Assistants, and Certified Nurse-Midwives," indicating that NPs could provide 75% of primary care services, 90% of pediatric primary care services, and 65% of anesthesia services (U.S. Congress, 1986). Further, nurse-midwives were noted to be 98% as productive as obstetricians in providing maternity services. The summary concluded that the high quality of care, patient satisfaction, and emphasis on health promotion and prevention made NPs an excellent resource for care in managed care. Impediments preventing use of NPs included the lack of physician acceptance, legal restrictions, inaccessible reimbursement, and limited coverage of unique NP services such as health education and prevention.

Concerns about health costs dominated the health policy arena during Era II. As nurse practitioner numbers increased, from 16,000 in 1979 to approximately 60,000 in 1995, NP and other nursing organizations sought access to mainstream reimbursement and payment methods at state and federal levels. Questions then raised were about the presumed increases in health care costs by the addition of new providers in the payer mix. Despite opposition, NPs, as well as nurse-midwives and nurse anesthetists, made steady, incremental gains in obtaining reimbursement provider status based largely on their ability to meet health care needs for U.S. citizens who were underserved or minimally served. By the end of Era II, NP research demonstrated that innovative practice models led to cost-saving outcomes when NPs were unimpeded in providing their services. However, to move toward rigorous NP outcomes research, NPs had to first examine competition and comparison issues within the dominant structure of health care delivery, physician-defined services.

Competition/Comparison

In the late 1970s and early 1980s descriptive studies focused on the effectiveness of NPs, using physicians as the normal standard, and on the acceptance of NPs by patients and physicians (DeAngelis & McHugh, 1977; Runyan, 1975; Weinberg et al., 1983). One key descriptive study involved a review of NP and physician clinical records in an inner-city teaching hospital clinic. The researchers found that NPs and physicians saw equally complex patients, while residents' patients were somewhat less complex. NPs in this study focused more on comprehensive and comfort approaches to care than did physicians (Diers, Hamman, & Molde, 1986).

In the 1980s, as the physician supply moved from shortage to surplus, NP research shifted from access and substitution to competition issues. A riveting and challenging editorial in the *New England Journal of Medicine* in 1984, entitled "The Nurse Practitioner Revisited: Slow Death of a Good Idea" (Spitzer, 1984), served as a lightening rod for organized nursing to address barriers to NP practice. Spitzer noted that further repeated "rigorous" studies of NP performance did not seem necessary to prove that NPs are safe, effective, and well received by patients. He noted that NPs were an overstudied health profession and had been for years, in part due to assumptions by leaders and practitioners in both nursing and medicine that NP care could only be evaluated using physician care as the standard (J. Lewis, 1975). Interestingly, this issue endures 35 years after the emergence of NP practice (Hooker & McCaig, 2001; Sox, 2000).

Spitzer (1984) raised key questions about the continued growth of NPs: Will parity of payment between physicians and NPs cancel cost advantage arguments? Will frustration with barriers to practice escalate disillusionment among NPs? He concluded that "the prognosis for the long-term viability of the nurse practitioner concept is [was] poor" (p. 1050), and he challenged the nursing profession to settle disputes about the role and education of NPs lest the movement succumb to obsolescence. Despite his provocative questions, research efforts continued to demonstrate NPs' comparability to physicians in patient care—but with a renewed focus on obtaining mainstream payment of health care services (Aiken & Gwyther, 1995; Blendon et al., 1994; Ramsey, Edwards, Lenz, Odom, & Brown, 1993; E. Sullivan, 1992).

Brown and Grimes (1995) conducted a meta-analysis of nurse practitioners, nurse-midwives, and physicians in primary care. They concluded that nurse practitioner and nurse-midwifery care was comparable to, and at times better than, physician care but that controlled trials were needed to make definitive conclusions about the process and outcomes of nurses in primary care. Mundinger et al. (2000) conducted a randomized controlled clinical trial of patients assigned to NP or physician care, demonstrating comparable outcomes of care in the two groups of patients. Criticism of methods used in the study were raised by physician researchers and physician organizations (Sox, 2000) despite the rigor of the study. The two reports (Mundinger et al., 2000; Brown & Grimes, 1995) failed to settle age-old arguments about comparison and competitiveness between NPs and physicians. Instead, these studies may have encouraged nurse researchers to claim yet again that NP care is effective, but with the acknowledgment that more work is needed on the processes and outcomes of NP care.

Innovative Models

As competition with physicians and concerns about the escalating costs of health care grew in the 1980s, NP studies focused on clinical success and cost advantages in ambulatory care. As new patient needs emerged and NP numbers increased, nurse practitioners moved into new roles in solo practice in primary care and in interdisciplinary teams in long-term care, home care and hospitals (Brooten, 1988; Capezuti, 1985; Kepferle, 1983; E. Sullivan, 1992; Wanich, Sullivan-Marx, Gottlieb, & Johnson, 1992).

Research that evaluated the unique contributions of nurse practitioners began with the inception of the NP role (DeAngelis, Berman, Oda, & Meeker, 1983; J. Lewis, 1975; Mendenhall, Repicky, & Neville, 1980; Pender & Pender, 1980). Supported by the GMENAC report of 1980, studies of NP care gradually carved niches for NP practice. Health policy analysts and leaders in nursing, however, raised major concerns about the ability to fully demonstrate effects of NP care in a structured delivery system that paid for and supported only traditional medical care rather than health promotion and comprehensive care approaches (LeRoy, 1982; J. Lewis, 1975, Prescott et al., 1981; U.S. Congress, 1986).

Nursing contributions to care were identified as patient education, coordination of care, holistic and comprehensive approaches to evaluation and management of patient problems, and redefinition of patient problems with emphasis on the meaning of the situation to patients and their families. Examples of these approaches include NP and advanced practice nursing services focusing on teenage pregnancy, quality of life and functional status of older adults, and transitional care. Studies were also conducted to identify the unique contributions that NPs make through examination of established payment databases. Studies demonstrated that NPs and other advanced practice nurses performed many traditional medical services but also provided services that addressed patients' needs comprehensively in social and economic areas, taking advantage of opportunities to educate patients and families (Griffith & Robinson, 1992; Robinson, Layer, Domine, Martone, & Johnstone, 2000; Sullivan-Marx, Happ, Bradley, & Maislin, 2000). K. Martin (1995) found that 15% of 181 nurse practitioners used nursing diagnoses in their practice to address patients' lifestyles and problems in daily living such as social isolation and self-care deficits. In another survey of NPs' use of the Current Procedural Terminology (CPT) billing codes, NPs stated that they performed services not identified in CPT codes, such as comprehensive patient care, attention to social factors, and capturing the teaching moment (Sullivan-Marx et al., 2000).

In addition to examination of the structure and outcomes of NP practice, analysis of innovative models also included the process of NP care. Johnson's qualitative study (1993) examined the discourse between NPs and patients compared to physician discourse. She concluded that NP conversation differed from a strictly medical approach by the perceived concern for the patient by the NP. This concern was evident through use of a shared language with patients, by a stance of NP and patient co-partnership, and through changes in conversation to establish a connection to the patient through questions, transitions, and brief comments.

Advanced practice nurse models emphasizing nursing approaches to patient care problems rather than physician-centered care demonstrated improvements in patient outcomes among high-risk and high-need patient groups (Lang et al., 1996). Reduction in the use of physical restraints in nursing homes, prevention of functional loss for hospitalized elderly, reduced hospitalization stays, reduced use of emergency services, and reduced use of obstetrical anesthesia have been identified in various nursing outcome studies when care is designed, organized, and provided by advanced practice nurse models (Brooten, Roncoli et al., 1994; Evans et al., 1997; Jenkins & Torrisi, 1995; Naylor, Brooten, Jones, et al., 1994; Wanich et al., 1992).

Era II questions remain: Is it necessary to continue to describe and study NP practice from the standard of physician practice when NP care is well established as safe, effective, cost saving, and well received by consumers and other providers? What models work to best enable NP practice and advanced practice nursing to flourish? What process issues lead to good outcomes that can be replicated and mainstreamed in health care delivery?

ERA III: TAKING STOCK AND MOVING FORWARD, LATE 1990s TO PRESENT

As we move into the present, a new constellation of social and economic forces is shaping NP practice and education. Rising health care costs are once again resulting in increased health insurance premiums, and threatening to aggravate the long-standing problems with access to care in this country. Deep public mistrust has led many to question whether managed care strategies are congruent with American social values. Many predict that health care consumers who have purchasing power will increasingly exercise this clout to obtain as much choice and flexibility in their services as possible. Those less fortunate, including millions of Americans for whom employer-provided health insurance may no longer be available, will face a grimmer version of the status quo (J. C. Robinson, 2001).

As of 2002, research indicates that NPs have limited impact on health care finance. Insurance companies are reluctant to empanel advanced practice nurses as independent service providers with billing discretion, except where it has been expedient to do so or has been mandated by state law (Mason & O'Donnell, 2002). The federally subsidized Medicare and Medicaid programs led the way for reimbursement of advanced practice nurses, and indeed regulators have noted increased billings for Medicare services by NPs and other nonphysician providers since the late 1990s (U.S. DHHS & Office of the Inspector General, 2001). For the moment, the volume of ambulatory care services provided by nurse practitioners in the United States remains small (Hooker & McCaig, 2001). However, it is clear that NPs' potential influence in American health care is not fully realized.

New tensions between NPs and the medical profession are building. The American public is becoming increasingly accustomed to NPs. Research findings on acceptability are largely borne out in practice, and across the country physicians and physician practice groups are incorporating NPs into their teams (Horrocks, Anderson, & Salisbury, 2002). Some physicians perceive NPs as a strong threat and voice concerns that an "uninformed" public may choose providers who are liberal with their time and address psychosocial needs. Physicians, on the other hand, cannot be as generous with their time due to expectations of high revenue generation for a practice, the need to focus on medical problems, and extended training that creates a value perception about their time (Gottlieb, 2001). Organized medicine in the United States continues to finance cross-country lobbying efforts to defend physicians against any further perceived encroachment by nonphysicians on the medical profession's self-claimed territory (Mason, 2000). The rhetoric cites loosely characterized "safety" concerns, but it is clear that individual physicians and their professional associations are fighting diminishing financial prospects (Cooper, Laud, & Dietrich, 1998; Gottlieb, 2001).

The nursing profession that spawned the NP movement is also facing new challenges. A combination of demographic shifts and social forces in the United States resulted in yet another shortage of registered nurses (Buerhaus, Staiger, & Auerbach, 2001). The traditional nursing role in hospitals is seen as a high-pressure, undesirable job (Aiken et al., 2001). Graduate education, always the major vehicle for career mobility in nursing, shifted within a decade from the preparation of educators, managers, and clinical nurse specialists (i.e., advanced training to educate, manage, and support the clinical practice of staff nurses in the traditional role) to the education of NPs. Advanced practice nurses increasingly occupy a large place in nursing practice and education. As traditional staff nurse roles become less attractive to new and veteran nurses alike, tensions develop between generalist nurses, advanced practice nurses, nurse leaders, and nurse educators regarding professional growth, contribution to society, and resources.

The research agenda for nurse practitioners and advanced practice nurses needs to move beyond amorphous labels identifying advanced practice nurses as "cheaper but better" providers of care, substitutes for inaccessible medical care, or holistic, family-focused care managers. Research studies that compare NPs with other providers, characteristic of earlier eras, will continue to be done to fully describe the enterprise of advanced nursing practice. However, new types of research are now needed to refine and hone the full potential of advanced practice nursing in health care delivery in the United States and around the world.

Outcomes Research: Asking the Right Questions

If Era II's findings and a vast worldwide pool of anecdotal experience worldwide are to be believed, stretching the boundaries of traditional nursing practice is both feasible and safe. However, Sox's (2000) critique of the study by Mundinger et al. (2000) (that it was a more expensive and tightly-controlled trial of NPs than is ever likely to be conducted again) clearly set an unachievable agenda. Research suggesting equivalence of advanced practice nurses to physicians would never convince those fundamentally opposed to advanced practice nursing. The research achievement represented by the Mundinger et al. study has perhaps taken us to the end of a road.

Benchmarking advanced practice nurses' care against that of physicians on the basis of "hard" outcomes is hindered by a number of factors. First, direct comparisons of advanced practice nursing care with physician care are extremely rare except in research studies. There are often substantial differences in the types of care or the types of patients seen by advance practice nurses and physician providers in clinics and hospital settings due to billing regulations requiring physician oversight. In many settings, and often for very practical reasons, care is organized to assign complex or unstable patients to physicians and primary care aspects of practice to non-physicians. From a research point of view, the end result is that the natural order provides little opportunity for comparing physician and non-physician providers' outcomes in providing similar services to similar patient populations. Artificial study conditions are needed to perform the comparisons.

Second, easily tracked hard outcomes such as mortality and life-threatening complications may occur so rarely and be so marginally influenced by process of care that, in practice, they are not particularly useful for evaluating advanced practice nursing. If direct comparisons of care are intended to highlight or rule out safety problems, they will also always fall short. It is clear that any problems with the outcomes of patients treated by advanced practice nurses are subtle enough to have escaped detection by the research designs used to date. However, critics are quick to point out that this may reflect shortcomings of the studies rather than true equivalence of outcomes between physicians and NPs. The lack of routinely collected data in areas that may, in fact, be sensitive to advanced practice nurses' practice patterns (e.g., fine-tuned measures of patient quality of life) is distressing. While patient quality-of-life measures and rehospitalization rates, to choose two examples, have intuitive appeal as outcomes, connecting these variables to measurable doses of advanced practice nurse care is often extremely difficult. Beyond this, there are often practical issues involved in collecting such data from enough patients over a long enough period for researchers to stand a reasonable chance of showing differences across patient groups treated under different models of care.

Clearly, the search for sensitive outcome measures to illuminate NPs' contributions must continue. However, instead of restricting attention to questions of comparability and safety, perhaps a better strategy involves addressing the contexts of care and circumstances under which nurse practitioners are the best choice for meeting client needs. For many employers, NPs are a means of lowering the cost of medical care, rather than a way of providing new or qualitatively different services or addressing the needs of underserved client groups. Outside academic settings and organized nursing groups, scope of practice debates deal with legally permitted tasks and acceptable levels of involvement in the care of different types of patients. A coherent, conceptually defensible role for NPs in meeting the health needs of well-defined populations supported by empirical evidence is lacking.

The role of the nurse practitioner in acute care grew during Era III to become a certified specialty in the nursing profession and particularly relevant in tertiary medical centers (Ostrea & Schuman, 1975; see chapter 6). The research literature evaluating acute-care nurse practitioners is early, small, and characterized by data-driven descriptions of the NP role in tertiary settings. Some single-site studies have described cost-effectiveness of acute-care inpatient medical services provided by nurse practitioners in comparison to physician and physician-in-training staff (Howie & Erickson, 2002). While many of the same methodological issues seen in research on primary care practice also appear in tertiary care studies, the literature to date is clear that implementing the NP role in acute care is quite feasible and may entail cost savings and improvements in patient satisfaction.

If randomized trials are considered the standard of evidence to define a scope of practice, will a new study like that of Mundinger et al. (2000) need to be conducted in each setting where the legitimacy of nurse practitioner care is questioned? The Mundinger et al. study suggests that, for a group of mostly medically indigent women with stable chronic illnesses seen in primary care settings, NP care has outcomes indistinguishable from those of physician care. Are the findings of this and other research being extrapolated beyond reasonable limits by NPs in various settings, as some physicians have claimed? Can the findings of Mundinger and colleagues be used to bolster claims that NP care is safe and effective in tertiary care settings? Can the findings be extrapolated to primary care settings where caseloads typically involve more episodic and urgent care? Again, this is a question of politics and values as much or more as it is about fact or testable hypotheses. However, researchers may assist in answering it by gathering data about the multifaceted context and outcomes of care, thereby opening up advanced practice nursing to the inquiries typical of nursing outcomes research (Mitchell, Ferketich, & Jennings, 1998). Specifically, what are the best models of care and the best mix of providers in different settings? Do different models of care produce varying outcomes across clienteles and settings? Defining a niche that NPs can sell to the public and the health care system as their own (as distinct from those of physicians, physician assistants, and generalist nurses) can only be a positive development.

Even if there are clear areas where NPs can claim superior outcomes, simple comparisons of cost-effectiveness between physicians and other providers cannot factor in complexities of reimbursement and the social and organizational realities of health care. In order to achieve their goals of consolidating and expanding their place in the health care system, NPs must assemble evidence that addresses the factors foremost in the minds of decision makers. Findings from methodologically pristine randomized trials may well fall flat in introducing health care system change without a fully developed evaluation model that accounts for the nature of advanced practice nursing and physician practice and the multiple consequences of differences between them.

Another research option beyond direct comparisons is to go back to some of the approaches characteristic of Eras I and II but with research tools and perspectives that were previously not applicable or applied. In some respects, recent studies of advanced practice nurses that examine outcomes using carefully chosen instruments and driven by reflections on the nature of advanced practice (Baradell & Bordeaux, 2001; Hamric, Worley, Lindebak, & Jaubert, 1998) may represent a real advance, even though (or perhaps, especially because) they involve no physician comparison groups and are not randomized trials. A focus on the process of care and patient outcomes rather than on the caregivers themselves is sorely needed and will eventually lead to frameworks that will shape settings of care and the education of NPs. In Era III, researchers will direct their efforts squarely at measuring the outcomes of NP care, but with a clear understanding of the limitations of the much-vaunted "gold standard" of the clinical trial in developing the science of advanced practice nursing and in moving advanced practice nursing's political agenda forward.

Looking Back and Moving Forward: Historical Context

The second major type of research taking shape in Era III deals with broader questions of context. With nearly 40 years of evolution now behind us, it is time to revisit roles of historical, societal, and health system forces in the evolution of the NP movement in the United States and elsewhere. With the growing place of NP education in schools of nursing and with gathering evidence of yet another shortage of generalist nurses, it is time to examine the ties of the NP movement to the parent nursing profession so that both groups can better chart their futures.

Historical research on the NP movement is providing important insights about the future (Fairman, 1999. See also commentary to chapter 2). Viewed through the lens of professional domination and control, the struggles of advanced practice nurses are not new or unique; they are the only the latest in a series of gender- and class-driven fights that nurses have faced over the past century (Group & Roberts, 2001). Understanding NP practice as an outgrowth of the clinical autonomy that nurses claimed for the good of patients in settings such as critical care and public health connects NPs to the profession and its past, and points NPs and NP leaders to effective solutions for dilemmas they currently face.

In many senses, the NP movement is approaching the end of its stormy adolescence. Many forces will influence whether and how it moves into a more secure "adult" identity. Outcomes research and historical and contextual research that pose "big picture" questions hold great promise for helping NPs to take full measure of the accomplishments of the movement and to chart its future.

ERA IV: EMBARKING ON QUESTIONS FOR THE FUTURE

Nurse practitioners and other advanced practice nurses rose from a need to address access to care, and ensuing practice and research continuously responded to external societal pressures to prove advanced practice nurses' worth, safety, and cost savings. Yet nurse practitioners and others are sometimes puzzled about why the plethora of research on the safety and value of nurse practitioners has so little impact on their entry into mainstream U.S. health care. Internationally, nurses are employing the U.S. nurse practitioner model to meet needs in many countries. As the NP literature is used for various purposes, nurse practitioners and health policy makers need to be aware that current NPs are educated, motivated, and shaped by a different set of forces within and outside nursing than their historical contemporaries of 20 and even 10 years ago. Research regarding nurse practitioners in the past was driven more by the need to defend positions in health care and less by a need to know what constituted optimal patient care. However, the movement continues to encounter barriers that cannot be overcome with findings from well-conducted research studies alone. These barriers involve core societal and health care system values. Questions for the future encompass several key areas: (1) optimal patient care through evidence-based practice, (2) organizational models of advanced practice nursing, (3) barriers to advanced practice nursing practice in primary and specialty care, (4) representation of advanced practice nursing practice in public and private databases, (5) translation of U.S. nurse practitioner models internationally, and (6) historical themes and social context of advanced practice nursing.

The questions guiding research in Era IV will be formulated in the context of economic and political arenas in both the United States and the world in ensuing years. That there will be a strong and steady market for health care is a certainty; however, the architecture of the system in which patients will receive care in 20 years is not known. Therefore, it is only by articulating a clearer identity and a better understanding of the larger context in which they operate that NPs can lay claim to a part of this future. We believe that research using a variety of methods and perspectives can help NPs do this, but that research alone will not determine the movement's future. Nurses have been taught for a half century to view research as the key to professional emancipation and self-governance and to see differences in opinion as being best resolved with empirical data. Perhaps in Era IV we will start to see a more realistic assessment of what research actually has to offer in an interprofessional struggle. This struggle is as much about economic realities as it is about empirical fact, and as much (or more) about politics as about public safety.

CONCLUSIONS: AN INTERNATIONAL AGENDA

Nurse practitioners and other advanced practice nurses turn to historical roots and research to legitimize their practice and may be puzzled about why the research has had so little impact. Further, when they search for an understanding of the present by reading about the origins of the NP movement, they are not always aware that they are educated and motivated differently than are physicians or other nurses. Nurse practitioners today are shaped by a different set of forces than their historical contemporaries of 20 and even 10 years ago. Opportunities and barriers in the national and international arena involve core societal and health care system values that may not be overcome with research studies alone.

Well-thought-out arguments that are based on outcomes research evidence and that address political, policy, and financial circumstances are critical to move advanced practice nursing forward. Determining under what models of care patient and systems outcomes will be better with care provided by advanced practice nurses will require considerable cooperation between clinicians and researchers. Advanced nursing practice in other countries, where advanced practice nurses and NPs often have training and scopes of practice radically different than in the United States, can provide some fresh opportunities for gaining insights in this area. In the countries that have attempted to expand the scope of practice for nurses, where is it working well and where is it not? In which countries is there a good fit between the implementation of advanced practice nurse roles and societal values and health care politics? Where is the U.S.-inspired model encountering serious resistance? Where are other models working better? What are the "outer limits" of roles that can be effectively assumed by advanced practice nurses under the right circumstances? An ambitious international consortium of researchers, clinicians, and policy makers may one day be able to look across borders and continents to answer research questions involving models of care that, for fundamental structural and operational reasons, cannot be addressed in the United States. International studies of NPs have an added urgency for other obvious reasons as well. Government officials and leaders in clinical agencies worldwide are attempting to adapt the NP role to address problems in their health care systems. They read literature on U.S. nurse practitioners and are frustrated by the absence of roadmaps for implementing the expanded roles and have no insight at all into whether the U.S. model may work elsewhere.

Only articulating a clear identity and by better understanding the larger context in which they practice can nurse practitioners lay claim to a part of a global future. We believe that research using a variety of methods and perspectives can help NPs do this, but that research alone will not determine the movement's future. Research will contribute to an understanding of the role of NPs nationally and internationally within a wider context of the players and agenda.

REFERENCES AND BIBLIOGRAPHY

Aiken, L., & Gwyther, M. (1995). Medicare funding of nurse education. *Journal of the American Medical Association, 273,* 1528.

Aiken, L. H., Clarke, S. P., Sloane, D. M., Sochalski, J. A., Busse, R., Clarke, H., Giovannetti, P., Hunt, J., Rafferty, A. M., & Shamian, J. (2001). Nurses' reports of hospital care in five countries. *Health Affairs, 20*(3), 43–53.

Baer, E. D. (1997). Values that drove nursing science in the 1960s. *Reflections, 23*(3), 42–43.

Baradell, J. G, & Bordeaux, B. R. (2001). Outcomes and satisfaction of patients of psychiatric clinical nurse specialists. *Journal of the American Psychiatric Nurses Association, 7*(3), 77–85.

Bessman, A. N. (1974). Comparison of medical care in nurse clinician and physician clinics in medical school affiliated hospitals. *Journal of Chronic Disease, 27,* 115–125.

Blendon, R., Mattila, J., Benson, J. M., Shelter, M. C., Connolly, F. J., & Kiley, T. (1994). The beliefs and values shaping today's health reform debate. *Health Affairs, (Spring),* 275–284.

Brodie, B., & Bancroft, B. (1982). A comparison of nurse practitioner and physician costs in a military out-patient facility. *Military Medicine, 147,* 1051–1053.

Brooten, D., Brown, L. P., Munro, B. H., York, R., Cohen, S. M., Roncoli, M., & Hollingsworth, A. (1988). Early discharge and specialist transitional care. *Image: Journal of Nursing Scholarship, 20*(2), 64–68.

Brooten, D., Roncoli, M., Finkler, S., Arnold, L., Cohen, A., & Mennuti, M. (1994). A randomized trial of early discharge and home follow-up of women having Caesarean birth. *Obstetrics & Gynecology, 84,* 832–838.

Brown, S. A., & Grimes, D. E. (1995). A meta-analysis of nurse practitioners and nurse midwives in primary care. *Nursing Research, 44,* 332–339.

Buerhaus, P. I., Staiger, D. O., & Auerbach, D. I. (2001). Implications of an aging registered nurse workforce. *Journal of the American Medical Association, 283,* 2948–2954.

Capezuti, E. (1985). Geriatric nurse practitioners: Their education, experience, and future in home health care. *Pride Institute Journal of Long Term Health Care, 4*(3), 9–14.

Cooper, R. A., Laud, P., & Dietrich, C. L. (1998). Current and projected workforce of nonphysician clinicians. *Journal of the American Medical Association, 280,* 788–794.

DeAngelis, C., & McHugh, M. (1977). The effectiveness of various health personnel as triage agents. *Journal of Community Health, 2,* 268.

DeAngelis, C., Berman, B., Oda, D. & Meeker, R. (1983). Comparative values of school physical examinations and mass screening tests. *Journal of Pediatrics, 102,* 477.

Diers, D., Hamman, A., & Molde, S. (1986). Complexity of ambulatory care: Nurse practitioner and physician caseloads. *Nursing Research, 35,* 310–314.

Etheridge, P. (1991). A nursing HMO: Carondolet St. Mary's experience. *Nursing Management, 22,* 22–29.

Evans, L. K., Strumpf, N. E., Allen-Taylor, S. L., Capezuti, E., Maislin, G., & Jacobsen, B. (1997). A clinical trial to reduce restraints in nursing homes. *Journal of the American Geriatrics Society, 45,* 675–681.

Fagin, C. M. (1992): Collaboration between nurses and physicians: No longer a choice. *Academic Medicine, 67,* 295–303

Fairman, J. (1997). Thinking about patients: Nursing science in the 1950's. *Reflections, 23*(3), 30–32.

Fairman, J. (1999). Delegated by default or negotiated by need? Physicians, nurse practitioners, and the process of critical thinking. *Medical Humanities Review, 13*(1), 38–58.

Feldman, M. J., Ventura, M. R., & Crosby, F. (1987). Studies of nurse practitioner effectiveness. *Nursing Research, 36,* 303–308.

Ferrar, G. E., Jr. (1969). Keynote address, 1969 Officers Conference, Pennsylvania Medical Society. *Pennsylvania Medicine, 6,* 9–10.

Geolot, D. H. (1990). Federal funding of nurse practitioner education: Past, present, and future. *Nurse Practitioner Forum, 1,* 159–162.

Glover, B. H. (1967). A psychiatrist calls for a new nurse therapist. *American Journal of Nursing, 67,* 1003–1005.

Gottlieb, S. (2001, May 14). Low-cost extenders come at a high price. *American Medical News.* Available at http://www.ama-assn.org/sci-pubs/amnews/pick_01/bica0514.htm

Griffith, H. (1984). Nursing practice: Substitute or complement according to economic theory. *Nursing Economics, 2,* 105–112.

Griffith, H., & Robinson, K. R. (1992). Current procedural terminology (CPT) coded services provided by nurse specialists. *Image: Journal of Nursing Scholarship, 25,* 178–186.

Group, T. M., & Roberts, J. I. (2001). *Nursing, physician control, and the medical monopoly.* Bloomington, IN: Indiana University Press.

Guthrie, N., Runyan, J., Clark, G., & Marvin, O. (1964). The clinical nursing conference: A preliminary report. *New England Journal of Medicine, 270,* 1411–1413.

Hamric, A. B., Worley, D., Lindebak, S., & Jaubert, S. (1998). Outcomes associated with advanced nursing practice prescriptive authority. *Journal of the Academy of Nurse Practitioners, 10,* 113–118.

Heagarty, M. C., Boehringer, J. R., Lavigne, P. A. Brooks, E. G. & Evans, M. E. (1973). An evaluation of the activities of nurses and pediatricians in a university outpatient department. *Journal of Pediatrics, 83,* 875–879.

Holt, E. (1998). Confusion's masterpiece: The development of the physician assistant profession. *Bulletin of the History of Medicine, 72,* 246–278.

Hooker, R. S., & McCaig, L. F. (2001). Use of physician assistants and nurse practitioners in primary care, 1995–1999. *Health Affairs, 20,* 231–238.

Horrocks, S., Anderson, E., & Salisbury, C. (2002). Systematic review of whether nurse practitioners working in primary care can provide equivalent care to doctors. *British Medical Journal, 324,* 819–823.

Howie, J. N., & Erickson, M. (2002). Acute care nurse practitioners: Creating and implementing a model of care for an inpatient general medical service. *American Journal of Critical Care, 11,* 448–458.

Jenkins, M., & Torrisi, D. (1995). Nurse practitioners, community health centers, and contracting for managed care. *Journal of the American Academy of Nurse Practitioners, 7,* 1–6.

Johnson, R. (1993). Nurse practitioner-patient discourse: Uncovering the voice of nursing in primary care practice. *Scholarly Inquiry for Nursing Practice, 7,* 143–157.

Kepferle, L. (1983). Projects and demonstrations relating to long-term care. *Journal of Long Term Care Administration,* 54–57.

Kissick, W. L. (1994). *Medicine's dilemma: Infinite needs versus finite resources.* New Haven, CT: Yale University Press.

Lang, N. M., Sullivan-Marx, E. M., & Jenkins, M. (1996). Advanced practice nurses and success of organized delivery systems. *American Journal of Managed Care, 2,* 129–135.

LeRoy, L. (1982). The cost-effectiveness of nurse practitioners. In L. H. Aiken & S. R. Gortner (Eds.), *Nursing in the 1980s: Crisis, opportunities, & challenges* (pp. 295–313). Philadelphia: Lippincott.

Levine, E. (1977). What do we know about nurse practitioners? *American Journal of Nursing, 77,* 1799–1803.

Lewis, C. E., & Resnick, B. A. (1964). Nurse clinics and progressive ambulatory care. *New England Journal of Medicine, 277*(23), 1236–1241.

Lewis, J. (1975). Structural aspects of the delivery setting and nurse practitioner performance. *Nurse Practitioner, 1,* 16.

Martin, K. (1995). Nurse practitioners' use of nursing diagnosis. *Nursing Diagnosis, 6,* 9–15.

Martin, N. (1967). Freeing the doctor from well-baby care. *Medical Economics, 44,* 118–119, 123, 127.

Mason, D. J. (2000). Here we go again. Organized medicine launches an attack on nursing. *American Journal of Nursing, 100*(5), 7.

Mason, D. J., & O'Donnell, J. P. (2002). Nurse practitioners and managed care. In T. G. Cesta (Ed.), *Survival strategies for nurses in managed care.* St. Louis: Mosby.

Mendenhall, R., Repicky, P., & Neville, R. (1980). Assessing the utilization and productivity of nurse practitioners and physician assistants: Methodology and findings on productivity. *Medical Care, 18,* 609–623.

Mitchell, P. H., Ferketich, S., & Jennings, B. M. (1998). Quality health outcomes model. American Academy of Nursing Expert Panel on Quality Health Care. *Image: Journal of Nursing Scholarship, 30*(1), 43–46.

Mundinger, M. O. (2002). Through a different looking glass. *Health Affairs, 21*(1), 163–164.

Mundinger, M. O., Kane, R. L., Lenz, E. R., Totten, A. M., Tsai, W. Y., Cleary, P. D., Friedewald, W. T., Siu, A. L., & Shelanski, M. L. (2000). Primary care outcomes in patients treated by nurse practitioners or physicians: A randomized trial. *Journal of the American Medical Association, 283,* 59–68.

Naylor, M., Brooten, D., Campbell, R., Jacobsen, B., Mezey, M., Pauly, M., & Schwartz, J. (1999). Comprehensive discharge planning and home follow-up of hospitalized elders: A randomized controlled trial. *Journal of the American Medical Association, 281,* 613–620.

Naylor, M., Brooten, D., Jones, R., Lavizzo-Mourey, R., Mezey, M., & Pauly, M. (1994). Comprehensive discharge planning for hospitalized elderly. *Annals of Internal Medicine, 120,* 999–1006.

Ostrea, E. M., Jr., & Schuman, H. (1975). The role of the pediatric nurse practitioner in a neonatal unit. *Journal of Pediatrics, 86,* 628–631.

Pender, N. J., & Pender, A. R. (1980). Illness prevention and health promotion services provided by nurse practitioners: Predicting potential consumers. *American Journal of Public Health, 70,* 798–803.

Poirer-Elliott, E. (1984). Cost-effectiveness of non-physician health care professionals. *Nurse Practitioner, 10,* 54.

Prescott, P. A., Jacox, A., Collar, M., & Goodwin, L. (1981). The Nurse Practitioner Rating Form. Part I: Conceptual development for potential uses. *Nursing Research, 30,* 223–228.

Ramsey, J. A., McKenzie, J. K., & Fish, D. G. (1982). Physicians and nurse practitioners: Do they provide equivalent health care? *American Journal of Public Health, 72,* 55–57.

Ramsey, P., Edwards, J., Lenz, C., Odom, J. E., & Brown, B. (1993). Types of health problems and satisfaction with services in a rural nurse-managed clinic. *Journal of Community Health Nursing, 10,* 161–170.

Robinson, J. C. (2001). The end of managed care. *Journal of the American Medical Association, 285,* 2622–2628.

Robinson, K. R., Layer, T., Domine, L., Martone, L., & Johnston, L. (2000). Capturing the workload of advanced practice nurses. *National Academies of Practice Forum, 2,* 223–230.

Rogers, D. E. (1981). Who should give primary care? *New England Journal of Medicine, 305,* 577–578.

Rogers, K., Mally, M., & Marcus, F. (1968). General medical practice using non-physician personnel. *Journal of the American Medical Association, 206,* 1753–1757.

Rogers, M. (1972). Nursing: To be or not to be? *Nursing Outlook, 20,* 42–46.

Runyan, J. (1975). The Memphis Chronic Disease Program. *Journal of the American Medical Association, 231,* 130–135.

Russo, R. M., Gururaj, V. J., Bunye, A. S., Kim, Y. H., & Ner, S. (1975). Triage abilities of nurse practitioner vs. pediatrician. *American Journal of Diseases of Children, 129,* 673–675.

Sackett, D. L., Spitzer, W. O., Gent, M., & Roberts, S. R. (1974). The Burlington randomized trial of the nurse practitioner: Health outcomes of patients. *Annals of Internal Medicine, 80,* 137–142.

Safriet, B. J. (1992). Health care dollars and regulatory sense: The role of advanced practice nursing. *Yale Journal of Regulation, 9,* 417–488.

Schiff, D. W., Fraser, C. H., & Walters, H. L. (1969). The pediatric nurse practitioner in the office of pediatricians in private practice. *Pediatrics, 44*(1), 62–68.

Sekscenski, E. S., Sansom, S., Bazell, C., Salmon, M. E., & Mullan, F. (1994). State practice environments and the supply of physician assistants, nurse practitioners, and certified nurse-midwives. *New England Journal of Medicine, 331,* 1266-1271.

Sigma Theta Tau International. (1996). Sigma Theta Tau international research fund grant recipients, 1936–1996. Indianapolis, IN: Author.

Silver, H. K., Ford, L. C., & Stearly, S. G. (1967). A program to increase health care for children: The pediatric nurse practitioner program. *Pediatrics, 39,* 756–760.

Solomons, G., & Hatton, M. (1961). The public health nurse as an objective scientific observer. *Nursing Outlook, 9,* 486.

Sox, H. C. (1979). Quality of patient care by nurse practitioners and physician assistants: A ten year perspective. *Annals of Internal Medicine, 91,* 459–468.

Sox, H. C. (2000). Independent primary care practice by nurse practitioners. *Journal of the American Medical Association, 283,* 106–108.

Spitzer, W. O. (1984). The nurse practitioner revisited: Slow death of a good idea. *New England Journal of Medicine, 310,* 1049–1051.

Spitzer, W. O., Sackett, D. L., Sibley, J. C., Gent, M., & Roberts, R. S. (1974). The Burlington trial of the nurse practitioner. *New England Journal of Medicine, 290*(3), 251–256.

Sullivan, E. (1992). Nurse practitioners & reimbursement: Case analyses. *Nursing & Health Care, 13,* 236–241.

Sullivan, J. (1982). Research on nurse practitioners: Process behind the outcomes? *American Journal of Public Health, 72,* 8–9.

Sullivan-Marx, E. M., Happ, M. B., Bradley, K. J., & Maislin, G. (2000). Nurse practitioner services: Content and relative work value. *Nursing Outlook, 48,* 269–275.

U.S. Congress, Office of Technology Assessment. (1986). *Nurse practitioners, physician assistants, and certified nurse-midwives: A policy analysis* (Health Technology Case Study No. 37). Washington, DC: U.S. Government Printing Office.

U.S. Department of Health & Human Services. (1980). *Graduate Medical Education National Advisory Council Report 1980.* Washington, DC: U.S. Government Printing Office. Report 1980.

U.S. Department of Health and Human Services & Office of the Inspector General. (2001). *Medicare coverage of non-physician provider services.* Report OEI-02-00-00290. New York: Author. Available at http://oig.hhs.gov/oei/reports/a525.pdf (Last accessed May 22, 2002.)

Walker, J. E. C., Murawski, B. J., & Thorn, G. W. (1964). An experimental program in ambulatory medical care. *New England Journal of Medicine, 271*(2), 63–68.

Wanich, C. K., Sullivan-Marx, E. M., Gottlieb, G. L., & Johnson, J. C. (1992). Functional status outcomes of a nursing intervention in hospitalized elderly. *Image: Journal of Nursing Scholarship, 24,* 201–207.

Watkins, L. O., & Wagner, E. H. (1982). Nurse practitioner and physician adherence to standing orders criteria for consultation or referral. *American Journal of Public Health, 72,* 22–29.

Weinberg, R. M., Lijestrand, J. S., & Moore, S. (1983). Inpatient management by a nurse practitioner: Effectiveness in a rehabilitation setting. *Archives of Physical Medicine and Rehabilitation, 64,* 588–590.

Chapter 5

LONG-TERM OUTCOMES OF ADVANCED PRACTICE NURSING

Harriet J. Kitzman and Susan Groth

D etermining the impact of health care interventions on patient outcomes has gained new importance in a health care system characterized by increasing technology, costs, demand for quality, and
disparity in access. Concerns by government and industry about rapidly
rising health care costs have led to increased pressure for containment
and, at the same time, for ever more complex, high-quality service. These
concerns and pressures show no sign of abating. Advanced practice nurses, like other health professionals, are confronted with questions regarding the absolute effectiveness and the relative worth of their services to the
health, illness, and well-being of those they serve. Although significant
progress has been made in the last decade, continued evidence demonstrating the effectiveness of advanced practice nursing interventions is
needed as a sound scientific basis for clinical and programmatic decisions,
for accountability to the public, and for public policy debates. Thus, determining the impact of services on patient outcomes of care, both short and
long term, will continue to challenge advanced practice nursing for the
foreseeable future.

In this chapter the focus is on research related to long-term outcomes
of nursing interventions. The length of time that is required for an outcome
to be designated *long term* is not defined. Instead, examples of research on
outcomes that have the potential to extend beyond the duration of the

primary treatment, or short-term outcomes that serve as pathways to other longer term outcomes are identified. First, examples of research are provided that have examined long-term outcomes of advanced practice nursing interventions, many of which have had a significant impact on health services delivery and health care policy. Selected research reports are reviewed individually to demonstrate the range of methodologies used to determine long-term outcomes and the diversity of the interventions studied. Second, some of the conceptual and methodological challenges related to the conduct of this type of research are examined. Third, examples of changes in information technology and methodologies that will increase future opportunities for rigorous research and evaluation are discussed. Finally, the challenges associated with moving the evidence into practice are addressed. If nursing is to participate with other disciplines in meeting the health needs of the nation and share in the discourse that drives health policy, advanced practice nurses will need to participate at all levels in determining the impact of their services on outcomes.

EXAMPLES OF LONG-TERM OUTCOMES RESEARCH

Interventions for Specific Symptoms or Conditions

Studies of interventions directed toward a specific symptom, event, or condition can expand understanding in a particular area and ultimately lead to evidence-based guidelines for nursing practice. For instance, research related to involuntary leakage of urine, or urinary incontinence, in women has led to the recommended treatment of bladder training and pelvic muscle exercise (Sampselle et al., 1997). Because this base of evidence was available, the Association of Women's Health, Obstetric and Neonatal Nurses focused one of its research utilization projects on incontinence in women (Sampselle et al., 2000). The study's objective was to test the effectiveness of an evidence-based protocol for urinary incontinence using a prospective formative evaluation methodology. Twenty-one women's health care sites were included. The intervention included standardized screening and baseline information forms, along with bladder and pelvic floor muscle-training materials that could be distributed to women. For those women available for follow-up, measures showed significant improvement between baseline and 4 months post-intervention. Women reported significantly fewer episodes and fewer days of leaking in the previous week, decreased volume of leakage, lesser extent of leakage, less bother, and decreased avoidance of activities, and thus an improved quality of life (Sampselle, Wyman, et al., 2000).

Yoos, Kitzman, McMullen, Henderson, and Sidora (2002), in a randomized trial of three levels of interventions for children with asthma and their families, found that adding peak flow meter use, when the children were symptomatic, to a symptom recognition and symptom management education intervention resulted in lower asthma symptom severity, fewer symptom days, and less health care utilization. Use of peak flow meters during asthmatic symptoms was associated with fewer symptoms and fewer emergency department visits for those with higher illness severity at baseline and who were Black. The intervention effectively eliminated the disparity in symptom severity between Black and White children. The investigators posited that the objective data on pulmonary function received from the peak flow meter measurements gave families a language with which to talk about the severity of symptoms that was particularly helpful in situations, such as clinics, where different providers managed the child during illness.

Attaining glycemic control in adolescents with diabetes mellitus is a challenge for care providers. Grey, Boland, Davidson, and Li (2000) conducted a randomized trial seeking to sustain metabolic control and quality of life in adolescents. Diabetic adolescents were randomized to either a group that received coping skills training or a control group that did not. Both groups received intensive diabetes management. After 12 months, the treatment group had lower glycosylated hemoglobin, improved diabetes, and improved medical self-efficacy and experienced fewer effects on quality of life than the control group.

S. Moore and Dolansky (2001) conducted a randomized trial of an intervention with coronary artery bypass graft (CABG) surgery patients based on the theory of self-regulation (Johnson, 1999). They hypothesized that a 15-minute audiotape of discharge information for home use, the "Cardiac Home Information Program," would lower levels of psychological distress, raise levels of physical functions, and reduce adverse symptoms in women and men who had undergone CABG surgery. Although the intervention was effective, they found differential effects for men and women one month post discharge. When compared to men in the control group, men in the experimental group had less psychological distress and fatigue. In contrast, the program only produced positive effects on physical functioning in women. The pathways through which the intervention affected men differed from those that affected women, leading the investigators to question whether women and men respond differently, based on sensory terms, to preparatory information.

Depression is a common problem among elderly nursing home residents. A geropsychiatric nurse intervention that included older adult volunteers as resource persons was determined to be effective in reducing the level of depression in nursing home residents (McCurren, Dowe, Rattle, & Looney, 1999). For those randomized to the treatment, the geropsychiatric nurse performed comprehensive evaluations, formulated plans, and provided interventions in conjunction with volunteers who received training, supervision, and consultation from the geropsychiatric nurse.

Home Support to Replace Hospitalization

Several randomized trials conducted on diverse populations have demonstrated that positive quality of care and cost outcomes can be achieved when patients are treated with frequent nurse visits in the home, rather than with hospital admission. In England, Skwarska et al. (2000) randomized patients who had an exacerbation of chronic obstructive pulmonary disease (COPD) to either hospitalization or home support with nurse visits every 1 to 3 days. They found no significant group differences in likelihood of being readmitted within 8 weeks (25% of the home support group vs. 34% of the admitted group were readmitted). The cost of service for the admitted group, however, was double that of the home support group. Home support patients were satisfied with the care, and there were no additional visits to primary care providers.

McConnochie et al. (2001) randomized acutely ill children presenting in the emergency department and eligible for admission to the hospital, to going home with a nurse or hospitalization. They found that in comparison to parents of those admitted to the hospital, parents of children who received care in the "In-Home Hospitalization Program" had lower stated anxiety scores and perceived the quality of care to be higher. There was no difference in length of recuperation for children.

Investigators, also in England, randomly assigned patients with dystonia (spasmodic torticollis, blepharospasm, or hemifacial spasm) to receive botulinum injections by a nurse practitioner in the home or to obtain injections, administered by medical staff, in the hospital outpatient clinic (Whitaker, Butler, Semlyen, & Barner, 2001). Side effects were similar, except the patients in the home group had significantly less dysphagia. The cost of the service was less than half for the patients treated by the nurse in the home, and most patients (82%) preferred the home treatment modality. One of the advantages of a nurse home intervention is that treatment can be multidimensional. In this study, the nurse practitioner in the home was able to identify a number of additional unmet medical needs and referred externally as needed, thus offering an additional benefit to patients.

Discharge Planning

In the past decade significant attention has been given to creating a continuum of care between hospital and home, thus reducing length of hospital stay and readmission. In a randomized controlled trial, Naylor et al. (1999) studied the impact of a comprehensive discharge planning and 4-week home follow-up intervention by advanced practice nurses (APNs) on readmissions, acute-care visits, costs, functional status, depression, and patient satisfaction. Patients were 65 years of age or older and hospitalized with medical and surgical conditions. In collaboration with the patient's physician, patient management was individualized within the established protocol, which identified the number of APN visits during the index hospitalization and at home as well as APN-initiated telephone contact and availability. The investigators found that those randomized to the intervention group, compared to those randomized to the control group, were less likely to be readmitted, were less likely to have multiple admissions, and were hospitalized for fewer hospital days. In the 24-week posthospital period, total Medicare reimbursements for health services for the control group were nearly double those for the intervention group. There were no significant group differences in postdischarge acute-care visits, functional status, or depression.

Some interventions have specifically targeted reduction in length of hospitalization. Brooten, Kumar, et al. (1986), in a randomized trial, studied the effects of early hospital discharge and home follow-up by clinical nurse specialists on very-low-birth-weight infants. The infants in the intervention group were discharged earlier than usual, and their families received instruction, counseling, home visits, and daily on-call availability of a hospital-based perinatal nurse specialist. There were no significant differences between the early discharge group and the usual care group in the number of rehospitalizations, number of acute-care visits, or growth and development of the infant; however, there was a significant reduction in hospital length of stay. The early discharge group went home 11 days earlier, two weeks younger, and weighing 200 grams less than the control group, with a resultant 27% reduction in hospital charges and 22% reduction in physician charges. This seminal study challenged the usual practice of a requiring a set discharge weight for low-birth-weight infants. Brooten, Brown, et al. (1988), in subsequent work, developed the Quality Cost Model of Clinical Specialist Transitional Care, a model that is applicable to any hospitalized patient population at risk for poor discharge outcomes. Among the populations with which this model has demonstrated positive effects are women posthysterectomy, women with unplanned cesarean births, and pregnant women with diabetes.

In Sweden, von Koch, dePedro-Cuesta, Kostulas, Almazan, and Widen Holmqvist (2001) found that stroke patients, randomized to early supported discharge and continued rehabilitation at home after stroke, had greater independence one year later in activities of daily living than those in the control group, who had routine hospital stays and rehabilitation. There were no differences in mortality and other measured outcomes. However, in addition to a reduction in hospital days by nearly one half, they found significant differences in patterns of utilization postdischarge. Control group patients had more occupational therapist, physical therapist, and day-hospital visits, while the intervention group had more visits to nurses in primary care and home rehabilitation.

Primary Care

A randomized trial (Mundinger et al., 2000) compared outcomes for patients randomly assigned to nurse practitioners in a primary care clinic at an urban academic medical center, and to physicians in community-based primary care clinics. It was hypothesized that patient groups would not differ on the outcomes examined. Nurse practitioners independently provided 24-hour coverage of all ambulatory primary care, including decision making regarding hospitalization and referral to specialists. Physicians and nurse practitioners included were subject to the same expectations in terms of productivity, coverage, and number of patients scheduled.

A total of 1,316 patients, who had no regular source of care and who kept their initial primary care appointment after an emergency department or urgent care visit, were enrolled. Follow-up 6 months and 1 year after enrollment found no difference in utilization, overall satisfaction with care, health status, or physiologic measures for patients with asthma and diabetes. Patients in the physician group were more satisfied than those in the nurse practitioner group for only one of four provider attributes (which may have been related to a practice site move during the study period). Patients with hypertension in the nurse practitioner group had lower diastolic values than their counterparts in the physician group. This large-scale randomized trial strongly supports patient outcomes as being similar for nurse practitioners and physicians providing primary care, using the traditional medical model.

Hill et al. (1999) conducted a randomized trial to increase entry into care and reduce hypertension in young, underserved, hypertensive Black men. An educational intervention was given to all participants. In addition, the intervention group also received individualized counseling, monthly phone calls, and a home visit during the 12-month period. The investigators found the educational intervention group and the intensive intervention group did not differ from one another 1 year later. However, both groups experienced a statistically significant reduction in diastolic blood pressure. In addition, this project demonstrated success in meeting the challenges of recruiting and following this population. Further work is needed to determine the best way to deliver care to high-risk populations.

Another area where there is evidence of long-term outcomes is in counseling high-risk alcohol users. The investigators in a randomized trial tested a brief counseling intervention, used within routine primary care, as a means to reduce alcohol consumption of high-risk drinkers (Ockene, Adams, Hurley, Wheelerm, & Hebert, 1999). Practice sites were randomized to provide a special 5–10-minute counseling session for patients identified as high-risk drinkers. The counseling sessions were administered by care providers. The researchers provided education materials and office support. Compared to the control group, the intervention group, which had higher baseline levels of alcohol use, reported significant reductions in alcohol consumption in the 6-month period.

In an attempt to evaluate the effectiveness of in-home geriatric assessments, Fabacher et al. (1994) enrolled veterans, 70 years of age and older, who were living in the community and not receiving health care at the Veterans Affairs medical center. Veterans randomized to the in-home prevention assessment program received a home visit from a nurse or physician's assistant who screened for medical, functional, and psychosocial problems. Participants were informed of findings and recommendations by letter, and trained volunteers provided follow-up visits at 4-month intervals for 1 year. One year follow-up assessments found that, in comparison to the control group, those who received the intervention had higher independent activities of daily living (IADL) scores, less decline in functional status, and higher rates for receiving recommended pneumonia and/or influenza immunization; they were also more likely to have a primary care provider.

Community-Based Interventions

Based on an understanding that the atherosclerotic process begins in youth, Harrell, Gansky, et al. (1998), in a randomized controlled field study, examined the impact of two types of 8-week, elementary school-based interventions on children with multiple cardiovascular disease risk factors. The interventions consisted of a knowledge and attitude program and an adaptation of physical education. One group received a classroom-based intervention presented by regular teachers to all children in the third- and fourth-grade classrooms. The second group, limited to children with identified risk factors, received the intervention in small groups. The third group received usual teaching and physical education and served as the control group. When compared to the control group, both intervention groups had larger decreases in total serum cholesterol at the end of the 8-week intervention. There also was a decrease in body fat, as measured by skinfolds, in both intervention groups, and an increase in aerobic power in the classroom-based group. Additional findings from this study (Harrell, McMurray, et al., 1996) were that the classroom intervention group had significantly greater heart health knowledge and an increase in self-reported physical activity when compared to the control group.

In a randomized trial, Allen (1996) evaluated the effectiveness of a nurse-directed intervention to help patients who had undergone CABG surgery to decrease dietary intake of fat, quit or decrease smoking, and increase exercise. Based on social cognitive theory, the behavioral intervention program began in the hospital prior to discharge and was followed up in the home 2 weeks after discharge. Subsequent sessions took place in the clinic at the 1-month checkup and then by telephone 1 month later. One year after surgery, the intervention group, when compared with the usual care group, had greater reductions in dietary intake of fat and saturated fat, as well as a greater reduction in smoking. The intervention had a modest impact on women reporting that they engaged in regular exercise.

In a randomized trial, O'Sullivan and Jacobsen (1992) studied the effectiveness of a special health care program for adolescent mothers and their infants. The program provided routine care, rigorous follow-up, extra health teaching, and discussions about family planning and educational plans, while the control group received routine well-baby care. Although the drop-out rate was high for both experimental and routine care groups, 91% of study participants were located for follow-up at 18 months. The repeat pregnancy rate was less than half in the health care program group when compared to the routine care group, and infants in the experimental group were more likely to be fully immunized. There was no group difference in mothers returning to school.

In a large randomized trial of a nurse intervention to reduce preterm and low-birth-weight births, M. L. Moore et al. (1998) studied the birth outcomes of 1,554 women receiving prenatal care in a public clinic. All women received a booklet about preventing preterm labor. The intervention group received additional instruction regarding signs of preterm labor. Between 24 and 38 weeks' gestation, the intervention group received telephone calls one or two times per week from a registered nurse. There were no resultant differences in low-birth-weight or preterm births between the intervention and control groups; however, subgroup analysis showed a significant difference in preterm birth rates in Black women over 19 years of age. Although low-birth-weight and preterm birth are relatively short-term outcomes, there are short-term and long-term morbidity implications associated with low-birth-weight and preterm.

In a multisite field study with a complex design, Kang et al. (1995) tested different combinations of interventions in mothers with high education and low education (12 years or less) and their preterm infants. One intervention, state modulation, was a hospital-based program constructed to improve maternal-infant interaction by instructing mothers regarding newborn states of consciousness, infant cues, and arousal techniques to use during infant feedings. The other treatment, Nursing Systems Toward Effective Parenting-Preterm (NSTEP-P) was a comprehensive home visit program. Routine public health nursing and car seat education were included in the design. The high-education mothers received either car seat or state modulation interventions. Low-education mothers were offered (1) car seat/public health nursing, (2) car seat/NSTEP-P, (3) state modulation/public health nursing, or (4) state modulation/N-STEP-P. Follow-up at 5 months corrected age indicated that within the high-education group, the state modulation treatment group had scores superior to the car seat group on the Nursing Child Assessment Teaching Scale (NCATS). Within the low-education group, although not all contrasts were statistically significant, differences in NCATS scores showed a consistent pattern of results: The car seat/public health nursing group had the lowest scores, the state modulation/public health nurse group next, and the state modulation/NSTEP-P group the highest. In contrast to the high-education group, hospital-based state modulation/public health nursing was found to be insufficient for sustained optimal interaction between preterm infants and their mothers with low education. The investigators concluded that intervention programs can be streamlined specific to the needs of the mother but that, for those with greatest needs, duration and intensity of intervention are key regarding long-term outcomes.

A quasi-experimental design was used to test the effect of a middle school and high school-based human immunodeficiency virus (HIV) and sexuality intervention (Siegel, Aten, & Enaharo, 2001). One group received the usual health curriculum. The second group received a curriculum taught by a trained educator; the third group's curriculum was implemented by a peer educator; and the fourth group was the intervention curriculum taught by regular health teachers (only in middle schools). Findings at 12 months postintervention demonstrated that long-term knowledge and sexual self-efficacy were greater in the intervention groups compared to the control group. Intention to stay safe was greater among middle school intervention groups than in the control group. Among middle school females, the initiation of sexual activity was significantly less in the intervention than in the control group.

The field can now draw on 20 years of findings on the long-term impact of a nurse home visitation program that begins during pregnancy and continues through the first 2 years of the child's life. The Nurse Home Visitor—Program, studied through randomized trials in Elmira, New York; Memphis, Tennessee; and Denver, Colorado—has targeted socially disadvantaged women pregnant with their first child. In these trials, women in the intervention group were provided a program of home visiting during pregnancy and the first 2 years of the child's life. The home visiting program was directed toward improving (1) the outcomes of pregnancy (by helping women improve their health-related behaviors), (2) the health and development of the children (by helping parents provide more responsible and competent care of the infant), (3) and the families' economic self-sufficiency (by helping parents plan future pregnancies, complete their education, and find work). The pattern of findings is being replicated in the three sites. In comparison to women in the control group, women in the home visiting group have been found to have improvements in pregnancy outcomes and fewer unintended, closely spaced subsequent pregnancies, and have spent less time on welfare. Children have been found to experience fewer injuries and ingestions (Kitzman et al., 1997) and to be less likely to be abused and neglected (Olds, Henderson, Cole, et al., 1998). Women's partnered relationships have been found to be more stable (Kitzman et al., 2000; Olds, Eckenrode, et al., 1997). In the 15-year follow-up in the Elmira trial, low-income unmarried mothers were found to have had fewer arrests and fewer behavior problems due to use of substances, and their children were found to have fewer arrests, convictions, violations of parole, as well as fewer sex partners and days of consuming alcohol (Olds, Henderson, Cole, et al., 1998). This series of studies is helping us understand how women and families make changes, as a result of home visiting, that have long term implications.

CONCEPTUAL AND METHODOLOGICAL CHALLENGES IN LONG-TERM OUTCOMES RESEARCH

The creation, dissemination, and use of the best possible scientific evidence in decision making is critical in health care delivery (Ellwood, 1988) and in health care policy. Because long-term outcomes have the potential to be the most cost-effective and to have the greatest impact on health and development over time, the evidence that links characteristics of health service to these long-term outcomes, although difficult to obtain, is particularly important.

Designs—Stages in Development of Science

Science is built in phases or steps, at times systematic and at other times resulting from random serendipitous discoveries (Barber & Fox, 1970). The National Cancer Institute has developed a five-phase standard efficacy-effectiveness research model. Although seldom implemented in its entirety, it is an elegant, scientifically defensible model. In the first two phases of this model, hypotheses are constructed based on established concepts, and methods are established and validated. Phase 3 builds on work done in Phases 1 and 2 and consists of carefully controlled intervention trials, during which hypotheses and methodologies are refined. Efficacy trials during this phase determine how well a treatment works in those who actually receive it, under ideal conditions. In Phase 4, the revised intervention is tested in carefully defined subpopulations of the ultimate population targeted. Finally, in Phase 5, through demonstration and implementation studies, the proven intervention is introduced to the community at large, and the health outcomes are measured. Phases 4 and 5, determining how a treatment works in those to whom it is offered, and how it works in the real world, constitute an effectiveness trial. In this phase model, efficacy trials precede effectiveness studies. It is reasoned that if the intervention cannot be shown to be effective when actually administered to persons under ideal conditions, there is little need to go further. If an intervention is found to be effective in an efficacy trial, effectiveness is still not assured and the effectiveness trial is still needed. Once the intervention is performed under real-world conditions and with the broader target population in effectiveness studies, costs, difficulties with implementation of the interventions, and side effects may be identified that in turn render the intervention unacceptable.

Scientifically, a randomized, controlled trial is a powerful technique for determining the efficacy of interventions. The study design allows the investigator to make the most scientifically credible statement about the impact of the intervention. Randomized trials, however, have some practical and ethical limitations when carried out within the natural setting. Effectiveness studies, because of the frequent constraints of natural settings, are likely to be conducted using quasi-experimental designs with different types of analyses, such as cross-sectional analyses, retrospective reviews, and prospective trials.

Although this standard efficacy to effectiveness research model has been recommended by many, programs of research in nursing and in other disciplines often have found the need to reverse, or interrupt, the order. At times, investigators begin with effectiveness studies where they determine the potential viability of the approach when carried out in the natural setting and end with randomized trials. For example, untested multidimensional treatments that are ethically and theoretically sound can be studied in the natural clinical setting and then refined in a randomized, controlled trial (Hoagwood, Hibbs, Brent, & Jensen, 1995). This is a common sequence in nursing research when the investigator wants to try out interventions to establish their ecological validity before investing in the randomized trial. Some investigators have blended elements of the traditional efficacy and effectiveness trials and have used the randomized trial to study the intervention under conditions as close to the natural setting as possible. The study of the impact of the nurse home visitation program for socially disadvantaged women and their children is an example of this blended approach (Kitzman et al., 1997).

Identification of Long-Term Outcomes

When determining the impact of advanced practice nursing services, it is critical to identify the outcomes of interest. Outcomes that have been identified as pertinent to nurses include patient satisfaction with care, physiological status, functional status, health and illness behaviors, symptom control, quality of life, morbidity, mortality, and caregiver burden (Lang & Marek, 1992). These are likely to be sensitive to nursing interventions, and some may be short-term outcomes while others are more often long-term products.

In general, long-term outcomes are of greater value than short-term outcomes, primarily due to the ongoing impact. Clearly, an intervention that reduces distress or improves functioning for a day or week, although important, is of less value than a similar treatment that improves functioning for a year, or even a lifetime. For example, the Nurse Home Visitor program described above had a short-term impact on new mothers during pregnancy and a longer term impact on infants during the first two years after birth. However, of even greater value was the intervention's effect on the life-course trajectory of the women in terms of further spaced pregnancies, decreased use of welfare, fewer arrests, and less substance abuse impairment during the 15-year period after delivery of their first child.

Of all the health care professions, nursing has a particular interest in long-term outcomes. Much of nursing, by its very nature, is designed to assist persons to manage their own health and illness problems in a manner that promotes and maintains the highest possible wellness over time. Health promotion and disease prevention are hallmarks of nursing practice. The American Nurses Association (ANA) indicates health promotion and disease prevention are central to maintaining or improving the health of individuals and communities, and nurses must design and implement interventions to this end (American Nurses Association, n.d.). Health is multi-dimensional, and consists of social, cultural, and behavioral components.

Nurses work with patients to develop strategies to monitor the status of their health and/or illness and to maintain positive health practices that reduce their risk for, lessen the impact of, or prevent further deterioration from disease, while promoting optimal functioning and quality of life. Studies, many of which examine long-term outcomes, have included advanced practice nursing interventions designed to assist persons to care for themselves through life transitions, during illness episodes, and with chronic illness and/or disability.

For example, in the study of discharge planning described earlier, Naylor et al. (1999), found that, although the intervention extended from hospital admission to 4 weeks postdischarge, the number of readmissions for the 6 months after the intervention in the control group was nearly double that in the intervention group. This indicates that the impact of the intervention lasted well beyond the end of treatment. One explanation is that the intervention supported not only recovery from the hospitalized episode, but also better management of participants' overall health. The authors believe the findings are a result of the intervention's focus on the combined effects of primary health problems and comorbid conditions, as well as other health and social issues, in contrast to single disease management.

Measurement of Long-Term Outcomes

To determine the impact of a nursing intervention, outcomes must be selected that have the potential to be affected by the intervention being studied. For example, although there has been significant attention given to evaluating interventions to relieve caregiver burden, a recent meta-analysis (Acton & Kang, 2001) found no overall effect of those interventions on caregiver burden, despite the range of interventions studied. (The interventions were designed to help caregivers cope with the burden of caregiving and included support group, education, psychoeducation, counseling, respite care, and multicomponent methodologies.) Acton and Kang argued that, for the interventions studied, caregiver burden may be too global an outcome measure and investigators may need more precise measures to conduct the evaluations properly. Outcomes need to be sensitive and also need to be measured at the point when the intervention is anticipated to have an effect.

It is important not only to consider the potential to accomplish the immediate outcomes of interest but to know whether the intervention affects the risk status of the persons receiving it. In some instances, the success of the program in producing the projected outcome, for example, weight reduction, can also be expected to reduce the risk status of the person. In the case of obesity, the short-term outcome of weight reduction is evident, but detection of reduction of disease associated with obesity, a long-term outcome, will not be detected in the short term.

Intervention Effectiveness

No intervention is effective for everyone. Thus, identifying those for whom the program is most likely to be effective is critical. At times clinicians, believing that the hypotheses tested were well grounded, are surprised with research findings that indicate an intervention had few or no statistically significant effects. Outcomes are averages for the group, and some patients receive no effects (or even negative effects), while others are significantly impacted. The intervention tested may not work equally well with all persons treated, or under all conditions. Some persons being offered an intervention may have low risk for negative outcomes and, thus, limited room for improvement.

Olds, Henderson, Cole, et al. (1998) found a reduction in the number of arrests and time spent in jail among low-income, unmarried mothers 13 years after the end of a nurse home visitation intervention (which took place during the first pregnancy through the first 2 years of the child's life). This intervention is unlikely to have produced a statistically significant reduction in arrests and time in jail for those who were not at risk for those negative outcomes. Similarly, persons with particular characteristics, or with needs and an opportunity to improve, may respond better to some types of interventions than to others.

In a net cost analysis of the nurse home visitation program, Olds, Henderson, Phelps, Kitzman, and Hanks (1993) found that program costs were recovered by savings in government spending by the time the children were 4 years of age in those families where mothers were low income and unmarried at the time of pregnancy. Thus, if reduction in government spending is the outcome of interest, the intervention needs to be targeted to those who produce high government spending.

Evaluations of home care have generally failed to find improvements in traditional outcomes. Some have posited that improved outcomes might be found if the investigators were to look at subtle condition-specific improvements, which may be better measures of outcomes than traditional outcomes in such high-risk populations as the elderly and chronically ill receiving home care. It has been proposed that better definition of the population to be targeted will be required if cost-effective outcomes are to be detected. Weissert, Chernew, and Hirth (2001), modeling data from the long-term care portion of Arizona's Medicaid Alternative Capitated Acute and Long-term Care Program, proposed that budgeting services could be productively based on (1) risk of adverse outcomes, (2) likelihood that home care could reduce risk, and (3) value of avoiding the outcome. They hypothesized that a system that focuses on improving specific outcomes while reallocating resources to those at higher risk, and/or those most likely to benefit, is likely to improve outcomes and reduce costs.

Intervention: Quality/Intensity/Fidelity

It is important to determine how much intervention (often referred to as dose) and of what quality is needed to produce the outcome. A critical question is whether it is possible to get the same outcomes with fewer services provided by less-prepared individuals. When an intervention has been found to be effective, clinicians are often challenged to provide the intervention at lower cost. Financial constraints result in continued pressures not only to replace expert nurses with less highly trained personnel but to reduce the intensity or duration of the services, thus allowing more patients to be served.

Evidence is emerging, however, that quality and quantity of services are linearly related to outcomes and that there may be a threshold of service that must be reached for the intervention to produce the effect. For example, DeSocio (2000) found that a threshold needed to be reached in the number of home visits to disadvantaged young mothers before outcomes are achieved. In some instances, costs of providing the service can be reduced. However, when the intensity or quality of the service is not adequate to produce the desired outcomes, the service is not cost-effective, regardless of its cost.

Cost-Effectiveness Analysis

Given the health care challenges related to cost and quality, the case for economic evaluations has never been stronger (Russell, Gold, Siegel, Daniels,

& Weinstein, 1996); a cost analysis of some kind is becoming expected in any evaluation of a new program. Although the cost of providing a service may be important for budget preparation, costs alone tell little about whether insurers and consumers should pay for the service. Only when costs are linked to outcomes can it be determined whether the service is cost-effective or worth the investment. In health care, as in other industries, there are opportunity costs associated with every decision about how time and resources should be allocated; and, for programs to be viable, demonstrations of the worth of the services in terms of outcomes are increasingly needed to justify funding.

Historically, data to support the assumed worth of services often have been unavailable, making it difficult to justify the cost allocation during times of financial shortfalls. For example, although innovative and promising nurse-managed centers were developed over the past 20 years, many have closed because they have not achieved financial self-sufficiency (Vincent, Oakley, Pohl, & Walker, 2000). Often the system was not organized so that services fell into those covered by traditional funding streams and new sources of payment were not developed, in part because the centers could produce only limited data on outcomes of services. Linking costs and services to outcomes is crucial for making operating decisions and for marketing a health care system's performance if it is to be competitive in the health care marketplace.

Several well-developed methodologies, some more complex than others, can be used to evaluate the economic impact of health care interventions. Chang and Henry (1999) used the following principles for cost analyses to evaluate cost studies:

> Principle 1: Make explicit the analytic perspective that addresses who pays specific costs and who benefits from an intervention. . . .
>
> Principle 2: Describe the anticipated benefits of an intervention as the value of the health effects. . . .
>
> Principle 3: Specify the components of costs used or considered. . . .
>
> Principle 4: Discount to adjust for differential timing when the costs and benefits studied accrue during significantly different time periods. . . .
>
> Principle 5: Perform a sensitivity analysis to explore the implications of alternative assumptions, preferences, and data. . . .
>
> Principle 6: Calculate a summary measurement of efficiency (i.e., a cost-benefit or cost-effectiveness ratio (pp. 96–97).

Of the studies Chang and Henry evaluated, few (22%) adhered to all six of the principles, and none of the nursing studies did.

In all cost-effectiveness studies, costs are linked to outcomes. Cost-effectiveness analysis uses monetary costs of providing the service as inputs and net improvement in health (nonmonetary) as outcomes (i.e., outputs), such as days in bed. Cost-benefit analysis uses dollar values for both inputs and outputs; patient outcomes are assigned a dollar value. Cost-utility analysis includes both cost and quality-of-life evaluations. Using a patient preference framework, a quality-adjusted life year is used to determine the change that results from the intervention (Weinstein, Siegel, Gold, Kamlet, & Russell, 1996). Although still under debate, quality-adjusted life years is an approach that can be used to compare impacts across clinical areas and health problems. For quality-adjusted life years to be most informative, however, the full duration of the impact of the intervention needs to be captured. This is particularly true for many of the multidimensional interventions of advanced practice nurses that are designed to develop the resources and/or change the methods the person uses to manage health and illness problems over a lifetime. The longer the impact, the greater the cost utility. For example, preventing a lifetime of incarceration is worth more than preventing a short-term period in jail in quality-adjusted life years. And preventing years of life in long-term care is worth more than shortening a disease episode.

As described in the principles above, methodologies to determine cost-outcomes linkages need to be guided by a well-articulated definition of the costs to be considered and how they are determined, the magnitude of the intervention required to obtain the outcomes, and the outcomes that are to be measured (Brooten, 1997). All of these will depend upon choice of perspective, that is, whose costs will be considered—insurers, providers, patients, families, or others. Similarly, they will depend on whose outcomes are important.

Regardless of the approaches to assessing costs, decisions are always based on the relationship between costs of inputs and value of outputs. When a new program costs less than its traditional counterpart *and* produces better outcomes, few would argue that the new program should be implemented. Similarly, when the new program costs more but delivers less than the traditional program, few would recommend its implementation. However, when the program costs more but delivers more, questions emerge about whether the outcomes are worth the opportunity cost foregone by implementing the intervention. Similarly, when the program costs less and produces fewer outcomes, questions may remain regarding whether the lesser outcomes are good enough.

LONG-TERM OUTCOMES: TRANSLATION INTO HEALTH POLICY AND PROGRAMS

Conducting Long-Term Follow-Up Studies

Immediate responses, or short-term outcomes, are easier to measure and document than long-term outcomes. They are also more consistent with the time frame and scope of many research projects. Despite the need for long-term outcomes, follow-up studies that evaluate the continued impact of an intervention long after that intervention has been completed require sustained effort on the part of investigators and subjects and the commitment of resources from funders. To sustain this effort and the utilization of resources, investigators need a sound theoretical and empirical basis for expecting that the intervention will have a sustained effect, as well as sound, rigorous methods to determine whether or not the effect has been achieved. Although nurses have hypothesized long-term effects and have studied the responses of those in their care from the early development of the profession, rigorous methodologies for the study of nursing outcomes have been advanced only during the past two decades. Some of these methodologies can be mastered successfully by the advanced practice nurse in daily practice; however, others will require collaboration with other intra- and multidisciplinary experts. The knowledge, clinical expertise, and insights of the advanced practice nurse are critical in many phases in the research process, particularly the conceptualization, outcome identification, intervention design and implementation, and interpretation of the findings.

Using Statistical Methods Applicable to Nursing Outcomes Research

In recent decades remarkable advances have been made in statistical procedures that can be used to analyze the kinds of data commonly found in nursing outcomes research. Statistical techniques such as multiple regression analysis and multivariate analysis have allowed nurse researchers to increase the sophistication of research designs, taking an ever-increasing number of extraneous variables into account when estimating the impact of interventions. For example, it is possible to determine that the impact of interventions on outcomes is greater for patients with certain characteristics or for those being cared for in settings with certain characteristics. Understanding the role of patient and setting characteristics allows researchers to identify patients for whom the intervention is appropriate more accurately. Similarly, recent advances in statistics support the researcher in determining the processes through which an intervention effects the outcomes, permitting the refinement of the intervention itself.

Although analysis of change is central to many areas of clinical research, there have been important methodological challenges to capturing that change. Newer methodologies that use multiple repeated measures allow investigators to model change at the individual as well as the group level (Willett, 1988). Repeated measurements of patient status over the course of treatment and maintenance, common to nursing practice, set the stage for thinking about research methodologies designed to examine the patterns of change. Growth curve analysis permits the investigator to determine not only the amount, but also the timing of the impact of the intervention. For example, using growth curve modeling, Cole et al. (2002) compared women who received a nurse home visiting intervention during pregnancy and the first two years of their first child's life, with those who had been randomized to a comparison group and did not receive the intervention. They demonstrated that the differences between the home-visited and the comparison groups on quality of mother's jobs and amount of work did not remain stable. Instead, as the time postintervention increased, the differences between the experimental and comparison groups increased, with the experimental group becoming more likely to be employed and in better jobs. It is interesting to note that although the intervention ended at the time the first child was two years of age, the differences in employment grew larger at about the time that child entered school. In interpreting the findings of this multidimensional intervention trial, the investigators posit that the program allowed women to grow in other ways during the time their children were at home, thus preparing for their entry into the workforce when the children entered school. These findings emphasize the importance of long-term follow-up studies of interventions that have the potential to change life course trajectory.

Technology and Long-Term Outcomes

With the ongoing development of database technologies, outcomes will be more readily monitored and evaluated in large populations, using natural prospective effectiveness studies. Despite the collection of extensive data elements, information is often not organized to provide answers to important questions. For this methodology to be useful in determining long-term impacts of advanced nursing practice, databases will be required that include nurse-sensitive indicators of outcomes among the data elements. To do so, however, advanced practice nurses need to be involved because they are in an ideal position to think prospectively about the data that need to be gathered and to provide input into the construction of data systems.

Although advanced practice nurses have used the telephone as an important tool in the delivery of care, emerging new technologies have the potential to change ambulatory, community, and home care dramatically. Although the Internet, as a source of information and support, has received some attention by nurse investigators, such as Brennan et al. (2001), studies that examine the conditions under which Internet interventions will be successful are limited. Similarly, telehealth equipment now makes it possible to complete fairly extensive home or community site assessments—including physical examinations, laboratory assessments, and natural setting observations—from the convenience of the computer in the provider's office. To date, this technology has been used most extensively in follow-up home health care (Kee & Borchers, 1998). Nevertheless, there has been limited study of the effectiveness of treatments provided under such conditions, and multiple questions need to be answered. For example, does the quality of the nurse-patient relationship change, and is the plan of care developed as mutually as it is in face-to-face interactions?

Translation into Practice

Despite the ultimately irreducible nature of uncertainty that surrounds health care decisions (Mike, 1999), scientific evidence has become the cornerstone for evidence-based care, and increasingly it is considered one of the important building blocks of modern health policy. The creation, dissemination, and use of the best possible scientific evidence in decision making is critical. In 1988, Ellwood argued for outcomes management, "a technology of patient experience designed to help patients, payers, and providers make rational medical-care-related choices based on better insight into the effect of the choices on the patient's life" (p. 1551). For Ellwood this included the establishment and continuous updating of permanent databases and linking interventions with outcomes. This information, after analysis and dissemination, would serve as the basis for standards and guidelines for choice of treatment for individual patients. Although the number of studies that link interventions to outcomes has expanded dramatically in the past decade, we currently have only a small part of the evidence Ellwood's proposal recommends to direct patient care.

Treatment recommendations based on scientific evidence do not equal treatment received. For example, recommendations for effective management of depression include acute, continuation, and maintenance phases.

The recommendations include a 4- to 6-month continuation treatment phase for all patients, followed by a 2-year or longer maintenance phase for patients at risk of recurrence (Frank & Judge, 2001). Large studies in natural settings, however, indicate that only about one third of those treated remain in treatment for 6 months, despite the evidence that those who remain on stable therapy for 6 months have a lower risk of relapse or recurrence. Nursing continues to study factors that affect the patient's decision to follow treatment recommendations. However, understanding how patients and nurses identify patient goals and jointly make decisions and develop plans for treatment will be critical if outcomes acceptable to the patient, as well as the provider, are to be achieved.

Health policy makers and clinicians alike need to be cautious when changing a scientifically proven intervention. They believe, too often, that the modified program can produce the same results—a belief that generally is not well founded, and many times is found to be unsupported by research. Although the impact of the original program may have been evaluated, it is important to know whether the new venue changes its effectiveness. The modified program, provided under the new conditions, may produce very different results. In nursing, evaluation is occurring in some instances when previously established nursing interventions are modified. For example, HeartCare, an information support system for patient home recovery after CABG surgery, is an Internet-based program that is being studied (Brennan et al., 2001). Though the effectiveness of the information has been established, the new method of delivery needs to be evaluated.

Longitudinal studies, particularly those with repeated measurements, clearly show that it is possible for well-conceived nursing interventions to have an impact on important long-term outcomes. These findings are critical to an understanding of clinical practice and to inform discourse that leads to health policy. The idea that the interventions of advanced practice nurses have an impact on long-term outcomes has been recognized. Emerging science has simply demonstrated the validity of this statement. The current challenge is to continue to develop and use this important scientific evidence in planning programs and providing care.

REFERENCES

Acton, G., & Kang, J. (2001). Interventions to reduce the burden of caregiving for an adult with dementia: A meta-analysis. *Research in Nursing & Health, 24,* 349–360.

Allen. J. K. (1996). Coronary risk factors modification in women after coronary artery bypass surgery. *Nursing Research, 45*(5), 260–265.

American Nurses Association. (n.d.). *Position statement: Promotion and disease prevention.* Retrieved April 20, 2002, from http://nursingworld.org/readroom/position/social/scprmo.htm

Barber, B., & Fox, R. (1970). The case of the floppy-eared rabbits: An instance of serendipity gained and serendipity lost. In D. Forcese & S. Richer (Eds.), *Stages of social research: Contemporary perspectives* (pp. 27–38). Englewood Cliffs, NJ: Prentice-Hall.

Brennan, P. F., Moore, S. M., Bjornsdottir, G., Jones, J., Visovsky, C., & Rogers, M. (2001). HeartCare: An Internet-based information and support system for patient home recovery after coronary artery bypass graft (CABG) surgery. *Journal of Advanced Nursing, 35,* 699–708.

Brooten, D. (1997). Methodological issues linking costs and outcomes. *Medical Care, 35*(Suppl.), NS87–NS95.

Brooten, D., Brown, L. P., Monro, B. H., York, R., Cohen, S., Roncoli, M., & Hollingsworth, A. (1988). Early discharge and specialist transitional care. *Image: Journal of Nursing Scholarship, 20,* 64–68.

Brooten, D., Kumar, S., Butts, P., Finkler, S., Bakewell-Sachs, S., Gibbons, A., & Delivoria-Papadopoulos, M. (1986). A randomized clinical trial of early hospital discharge and home follow-up of very low birthweight infants. *New England Journal of Medicine, 315,* 934–939.

Chang, W., & Henry, B. (1999). Methodological principles of cost analyses in the nursing, medical, and health services literature, 1990–1996. *Nursing Research, 48,* 94–104.

Cole, R., Henderson, C., Kitzman, H., Sidora, K., Eckenrode, J., Anson, E., & Olds, D. (2002). *Long-term effects of nurse home visitation on maternal employment.* Unpublished manuscript.

DeSocio, J. (2000). *Testing a model of self-directed change: The Memphis New Mothers' Study.* Unpublished doctoral dissertation, University of Rochester, Rochester, NY.

Ellwood, P. M. (1988). Outcomes management: A technology of personal experience. *New England Journal of Medicine, 318,* 1549–1556.

Fabacher, D., Josephson, K., Pietruszka, F., Linderborn, I. K., Morley, K., Morley, J., & Ruberstein, L. (1994). An in-home preventive assessment program for independent older adults: A randomized controlled trial. *Journal of American Geriatrics Society, 42,* 630–638.

Frank, E., & Judge, R. (2001). Treatment recommendations versus treatment realities: recognizing the rift and understanding the consequences. *Journal of Clinical Psychiatry, 62*(Suppl. 22), 10–15.

Grey, M., Boland, E. A., Davidson M., & Li, J. (2000). Coping skills training for youth with diabetes mellitus has long-lasting effects on metabolic control and quality of life. *Journal of Pediatrics, 137,* 107–113.

Harrell, J. S., Gansky, S. A., McMuray, R. G., Bangdiwala, S. I., Frauman, A. C., & Bradley, C. B. (1998). School-based interventions improve heart health in children with multiple cardiovascular disease risk factors. *Pediatrics, 102,* 371–380.

Harrell, J. S., McMurray, R. G., Bangdiwala, S. I., Frauman, A. C., Gansky, A., & Bradley, C. B. (1996). Effects of a school-based intervention to reduce cardiovascular disease risk factors in elementary-school children: The cardiovascular health in children (CHIC) study. *Journal of Pediatrics, 128,* 797–805.

Hill, M. N., Bone, L. R., Hilton, S. C., Roary, M. C., Kelen, G. D., & Levine, D. M. (1999). A clinical trial to improve high blood pressure care in young urban Black men: recruitment, follow-up and outcomes. *American Journal of Hypertension, 12,* 548–554.

Hoagwood, K., Hibbs, E., Brent, D., & Jensen, P. (1995). Introduction to the special section: Efficacy and effectiveness in studies of child and adolescent psychotherapy. *Journal of Consulting and Clinical Psychology, 63,* 683–687.

Johnson, J. E. (1999). Self-regulation theory and coping with physical illness. *Research in Nursing & Health, 22,* 435–448.

Kang, R., Barnard, K., Hammond, M., Oshio, S., Spencer, C., Thibodeaux, B., & Williams, J. (1995). Preterm infant follow-up project: A multi-site field experiment of hospital and home intervention programs for mothers and preterm infants. *Public Health Nursing, 12,* 171–180.

Kee, C., & Borchers, L. (1998). Reducing readmission rates through discharge interventions. *Clinical Nurse Specialist, 12,* 206–209.

Kitzman, H., Olds, D., Henderson, C., Hanks, C., Cole, R., Tatelbaum, R., McConnochie, K., Sidora, K., Luckey, D., Shaver, D., Engelhardt, K., James, D., & Barnard, K. (1997). Effect of prenatal and infancy home visitation by nurses on pregnancy outcomes, childhood injuries, and repeated childbearing: A randomized controlled trial. *Journal of the American Medical Association, 278,* 644–652.

Kitzman, H., Olds, D., Sidora, K., Henderson, C., Hanks, C., Cole, R., Luckey, D., Bondy, J., Cole, K., & Glazner, J. (2000). Enduring effects of nurse home visitation on maternal life course: A 3-year follow-up of a randomized trial. *Journal of the American Medical Association, 283,* 1983–1989.

Lang, N., & Marek, K. (1992). Outcomes that reflect clinical practice. In *Patient outcomes research: Examining the effectiveness of nursing practice* (NIH Publication No. 93-3411). Bethesda, MD: National Institutes of Health.

McConnochie, K., Kitzman, H., Roghmann, K., Dick, N., Wood, N., McBride, J., Conners, G., Brayer, A., & Liptak, G. (2001). *Randomized trial of home nursing to replace inpatient care for common acute pediatric problems.* Abstract presented at the annual meeting of the Pediatric Academic Society, Baltimore, MD.

McCurren, C., Dowe, D., Rattle, D., & Looney, S. (1999). Depression among nursing home elders: Testing an intervention strategy. *Applied Nursing Research, 12,* 185–195.

Mike, V. (1999). Outcomes research and the quality of health care: The beacon of an ethics of evidence. *Evaluation & the Health Professions, 22,* 3–32.

Moore, M. L., Meis, P. J., Ernest, J. M., Wells, H. B., Zaccaro, D. J., & Terrell, T. (1998). A randomized trial of nurse intervention to reduce preterm and low birth weight births. *Obstetrics & Gynecology, 91,* 656–661.

Moore, S., & Dolansky, M. (2001). Randomized trial of a home recovery intervention following coronary artery bypass surgery. *Research in Nursing & Health, 24,* 93–104.

Mundinger, M. O., Kane, R. L., Lenz, E. R., Totten, A. M., Tsai, W., Cleary, P. D., Friedewald, W. T., Siu, A. L., & Shelanski, M. L. (2000). Primary care outcomes in patients treated by nurse practitioners or physicians: A randomized trial. *Journal of the American Medical Association, 283,* 59–68.

Naylor, M. D., Brooten, D., Campbell, R., Jacobsen, B. S., Mezey, M. D., Pauly, M. J., & Schwartz, J. S. (1999). Comprehensive discharge planning and home follow-up of hospitalized elders: A randomized clinical trial. *Journal of the American Medical Association, 281,* 613–620.

Ockene, J. K., Adams, A., Hurley, T. G., Wheeler, E. V., & Hebert, J. R. (1999). Brief physician- and nurse practitioner-delivered counseling for high-risk drinkers: Does it work? *Archives of Internal Medicine, 159,* 2198–2205.

Olds, D., Eckenrode, J., Henderson, C., Jr., Kitzman, H., Powers, J., Cole, R., Sidora, K., Morris, P., Pettitt, L., & Luckey, D. (1997). Long-term effects of home visitation on maternal life course and child abuse and neglect. Fifteen-year follow-up of a randomized trial. *Journal of the American Medical Association, 278,* 637–643.

Olds, D., Henderson, C., Jr., Cole, R., Eckenrode, J., Kitzman, H., Luckey, D., Pettitt, L., Sidora, K., Morris, P., & Powers, J. (1998). Long term effects of nurse home visitation on children's criminal and antisocial behavior: 15-year follow-up of a randomized trial. *Journal of the American Medical Association, 280,* 1238–1244.

Olds, D., Henderson, Phelps, C., Kitzman, H., & Hanks, C. (1993). Effect of prenatal and infancy nurse home visitation on government spending. *Medical Care, 31,* 155–174.

O'Sullivan, A., & Jacobsen, B. (1992). A randomized trial of a health care program for first-time adolescent mothers and their infants. *Nursing Research, 41,* 210–215.

Russel, L., Gold, M., Siegel, J., Daniels, N., & Weinstein, M. (1996). The role of cost-effectiveness analysis in health and medicine. *Journal of the American Medical Association, 276,* 1172–1177.

Sampselle, C., Burns, P., Dougherty, M., Newman, D., Thomas, K., & Wyman, J. (1997). Continence for women: Evidence-based practice. *Journal of Obstetric, Gynecologic, and Neonatal Nursing, 26,* 375–385.

Sampselle, C. M., Wyman, J. F., Thomas, K. K., Newman, D. K., Gray, M., Dougherty, M., & Burns, P. A. (2000). Continence for women: A test of AWONN's evidence-based protocol in clinical practice. *Journal of Obstetric, Gynecologic, and Neonatal Nursing, 29*(1), 18–26.

Siegel, D. M., Aten, M. J., & Enaharo, M. (2001). Long-term effects of a middle school- and high school-based human immunodeficiency virus sexual risk prevention intervention. *Archives of Pediatrics & Adolescent Medicine, 155,* 1117–1126.

Skwarska, E., Cohen, G., Skwarski, K. M., Lamb, C., Bushell, D., Parker, S. & MacNee, W. (2000). Randomized controlled trial of supported discharge in patients with exacerbations of chronic obstructive pulmonary disease. *Thorax, 55,* 907–912.

Vincent, D., Oakley, D., Pohl, J., & Walker, D. S. (2000). Survival of nurse-managed centers; The importance of cost analysis. *Outcomes Management for Nursing Practice, 4,* 124–128.

von Koch, L., dePedro-Cuesta, J., Kostulas, V., Almazan, J., & Widen Holmqvist, L. (2001). Randomized controlled trial of rehabilitation at home after stroke: One-year follow-up of patient outcomes, resource use and cost. *Cerebrovascular Diseases, 12,* 131–138.

Weinstein, M., Siegel, J., Gold, M., Kamlet, M., & Russell, L. (1996). Recommendations of the Panel on Cost-Effectiveness in Health and Medicine. *Journal of the American Medical Association, 276,* 1253–1341.

Weissert, W., Chernew, M., & Hirth, R. (2001). Beyond managed long-term care: Paying for home care based on risk of adverse outcomes. *Health Affairs, 20,* 172–180.

Whitaker, J., Butler, A., Semlyen, J. K., & Barner, M. P. (2001). Botulinum toxin for people with dystonia treated by an outreach nurse practitioner: A comparative study between a home and clinic treatment service. *Archives of Physical Medicine & Rehabilitation, 82,* 480–448.

Willett, J. B. (1988). Questions and answers in the measurement of change. In E. Z. Rothkopf (Ed.), *Review of Research in Education, 15,* 345–422.

Yoos, H. L., Kitzman, H., McMullen, A., Henderson, C., & Sidora, K. (2002). Symptom monitoring in childhood asthma: A randomized clinical trial comparing peak expiratory flow rate with symptom monitoring. *Annals of Allergy, Asthma, & Immunology, 88,* 283–291.

PART **II**

THE PRACTICE ARENA: MANY ROLES, MANY SETTINGS

Change in health care delivery, health disparities, and the development of a pluralistic health care workforce have provided opportunities for nurse practitioners to demonstrate their skills in care coordination, care management, and advocacy for patients. Their contributions are leading to improved outcomes of care that are highly valued in all settings. In Part II, we present a variety of advanced nursing practice roles that evolved from specialty practice and specific settings. In each chapter, the authors focus on the innovative development of each new field for advanced practice nursing and emphasize the importance of standard educational approaches and practice based on evidence.

Four new chapters have been added to this edition. The meteoric emergence of acute-care nurse practitioners in tertiary medical centers is thoroughly described by Becker and Richmond, who give an account of how nurses in these settings have used a nurse practitioner model to develop skills in technological procedures, clinical decision making, and communication with nurses, physicians, patients, and family to move nursing forward in the care of critical illnesses and specialty nursing practice. Fehder brings us through the 70-year history of certified registered nurse anesthetists, who emerged from hospital nursing and critical care practice to provide over 65% of all anesthesia services in the United States currently. In his chapter, the reader will gain a clearer understanding of how accountability for advanced practice nursing develops in students and is sustained by these advanced nurse practitioners. Robinson and Petzel in their chapter describe the full range and depth of advanced nursing practice in the

Veterans Affairs health care system, a federal model that has facilitated the innovation of nurse practitioner models of practice throughout the broad ranges of its health care system. Mariano's chapter discusses graduate prepared nurses in holistic care and addresses the topic of alternative therapies that are so much on the minds of consumers and only now making their way into mainstream health care. Mariano's chapter reflects her national role in developing a preparatory program in complementary and alternative modalities and describes how standards are guiding the construction of academic programs and certification efforts.

Barber and Burke's chapter on advanced practice in managed care appeared originally in the third edition of this book. The authors have dramatically updated the chapter to reflect the changes of the last few years, the current status of managed care, and how advanced practice nurses function in this environment. Managed care is now well established nationally as a clinical and fiscal modality, but the field continues to be in great flux. Barber and Burke lead with the insiders' voice.

Similarly, Naegle has revised her chapter on primary care in advanced practice psychiatric-mental health nursing to reflect the increasing clarity and acceptance of a primary care focus within the long-established field of psychiatric-mental health nursing. Her example of how these specialty nurses would care for patients with alcohol and drug dependency provides a graphic demonstration of the benefits of this role and her own clinical expertise.

Three chapters have been updated to describe the evolution of advanced practice nursing in geriatric, school-based, and nurse-midwifery practice, elucidating how nurse practitioners focus on the patient from their community and cultural perspectives, emphasize socioeconomic aspects of care, and comprehensively view the meaning of the health problem to the patient. Stillman, Strumpf, and Paier remind us of the exponential growth in the older adult population that will require nurse practitioners to have a clinical foundation in health care of older adults and to develop practices that demonstrate quality outcomes for patients in all community and institutional settings. Igoe presents a compelling argument for use of nurse practitioners in school-based health centers to close gaps in health disparities through primary, preventive, and behavioral health care. Thompson's chapter on nurse midwifery presents a compelling argument for the development of regional, national, and international policy supporting health for all women and children through support of an international model of nurse midwifery practice.

These chapters provide a view of the rich history and promising new developments in advanced practice that augur well for patients and signal the profession as to the continued contributions of advanced practice nursing to patient care.

C h a p t e r **6**

ADVANCED PRACTICE NURSES IN ACUTE-CARE SERVICES

Deborah E. Becker and Therese S. Richmond

O ne of the hallmarks of a profession is its responsiveness to societal needs. The intensifying acuity of patient needs and the reduction in the health care workforce has resulted in a mismatch of needs and resources, thus limiting the ability of the existing system to adequately meet patient needs. Early in the 1990s, leaders in the profession recognized the changing needs for patient care providers in the rapidly evolving health care system. It became evident that advanced practice nurses had a scope of practice that could be maximized to meet both the medical and nursing needs of vulnerable, acutely ill patients (American College of Physicians, 1994; Miller, 1998). Today, acute care nurse practitioners (ACNPs) deliver direct and advanced patient care to patients with acute and critical illnesses and injuries. This chapter describes the emergence of the ACNP as a direct caregiver and the role the ACNP plays as a member of the interdisciplinary team.

ACNP SCOPE OF PRACTICE AND STANDARDS

The response by visionary nurse leaders to prepare advanced practice nurses to meet patient needs in the changing health care system culminated in the introduction of the ACNP, by building on the achievements

135

of nurse practitioners (NPs) in primary care settings coupled with in-depth specialty preparation. The ACNP fills the gap in patient care services that had been acknowledged nationwide (Miller, 1998).

The American Nurses Association (ANA) and the American Association of Critical Care Nurses (AACN) delineated the scope of practice for adult acute care nurse practitioners in 1995. This inaugural scope of practice was particularly important in providing a broad definition of the nature and boundaries of professional practice for the ACNP (American Nurses Association & American Association of Critical Care Nurses, 1995). The scope of practice is dynamic, evolving over time to fulfill the needs of patients and society in a changing health care environment (Richmond, Dubendorf, & Monturo, 1999).

According to the scope of practice for adult ACNPs, "the purpose of the ACNP is to provide advanced nursing care across the continuum of acute care services to patients who are acutely and critically ill" (ANA & AACN, 1995, p. 11). The provision of care by ACNPs is not setting dependent, but rendered in any venue in which patients have acute, specialized health care needs. ACNPs focus is on stabilization of the acute medical problem, prevention and management of complications, comprehensive management of the injury and/or illness, and restoration to maximal levels of health within an interdisciplinary and collaborative health care team (ANA & AACN, 1995).

The standards of practice (ANA & AACN, 1995), together with the scope of practice for adult ACNPs, inform the ACNP certification process and examination. There is a mutuality of interaction among the scope and standards, individual state nurse practice acts regulating ACNP practice, and the evolution of educational programs preparing advanced practice nurses as ACNPs. Each serves to inform the others, indicating the importance of the scope and standards and the dynamic interaction and evolution of the ACNP role over time.

EDUCATIONAL PREPARATION

The ACNP is an advanced practice nurse prepared at the graduate level. The curriculum incorporates a combination of didactic and guided clinical experiences to broadly educate the ACNP to manage patients with acute and critical illness and injury. Because the care of these patients entails the use of technology for assessment, diagnostic workup, and management, the infusion of content concentrating on the development of critical thinking skills related to technology is an important thread throughout the curriculum.

The didactic content encompasses core basic sciences and research and an intense focus on evaluation, diagnosis, and management of the acutely ill patient with diverse illnesses, injuries, and comorbidities. A system-based disease focus stressing a physiologic and psychosocial approach to diagnostic decision making and management forms the core. These didactic courses integrate nursing and medical approaches to patient care. Incorporation of clinical guidelines and evidence-based practice facilitates the students' understanding and application of external scientific evidence to the patient care situation (Glanville, Schirm, & Wineman, 2000).

A major focus is to incorporate advanced technologies in the assessment and management of acutely ill patients. Instruction on the ways in which technologically derived information is infused into diagnostic reasoning and how these technologies are used in patient management complements the acquisition of psychomotor skills in using technology in practice (El-Sherif, 1995).

The clinical portion of the program begins with an advanced clinical decision-making course that builds on the physical assessment proficiency of generalist nurses and prepares them to perform comprehensive histories, employ expanded physical assessment techniques, amplify critical thinking, and identify complicated abnormalities.

The clinical practicum includes guided clinical fieldwork with experienced practitioners in a diversity of settings. ACNP students have a broad theoretical base in disease management, patient assessment, and clinical decision making. Based upon this firm foundation, students' clinical rotations permit them to concentrate on a particular patient population of acutely or critically ill or injured patients. Despite individualization of clinical experiences, core competencies (common to all students) must be met to complete the clinical rotation successfully. The nature of the clinical rotation takes into account the strengths and weaknesses of students, their unique background, and their professional aspirations.

The selection of clinical preceptors has evolved over time. Early in the development of the ACNP, physicians were the primary preceptors. Now that there are experienced ACNPs in richly diverse practice arenas, there are more opportunities for students to partner with nurse practitioners and/or physicians for the clinical practicum. The clinical preceptor is an invaluable asset to the educational program. It is essential to have a group of expert clinicians that are willing to invest their time and effort to the development of assessment, diagnostic, and management skills of the ACNP student. The clinical preceptor must be a content expert and must also be able to assess the student's level of knowledge. The preceptor capable of doing this can facilitate an exceptional clinical experience based on the student's individual needs (Ligas, 1997).

To facilitate students' clinical rotations and to maximize their learning experiences, it is important to have clinical faculty who are intimately familiar with the objectives of the clinical practicum and who can ensure that students are obtaining the relevant experiences to meet those objectives. The clinical faculty act as a liaison between the clinical preceptor and the faculty and between the student and the preceptor. Having clinical faculty available to the clinical preceptor throughout the student's clinical practicum reassures the clinical preceptor that a valued preceptor partnership exists. Both clinical preceptors and clinical faculty provide feedback to the students concerning their clinical performance. For example, the preceptor provides feedback to the student that is structured by the program objectives, but also evaluates the student in terms of the clinical practice's needs as well as their individual expectations of practice. The clinical faculty provides consistent application of the expectations according to developmental level and across diverse clinical placements.

ACNP ROLE CONCEPTUALIZATION AND IMPLEMENTATION

ACNPs fulfill the diverse needs of acutely ill and vulnerable patients across the continuum of services in diverse geographic locations. The term *acute* has usually been associated with the type of facility in which patient care is provided or has been used to describe the patient who is experiencing either a new onset or an exacerbation of an existing illness (Miller, 1998). The diverse care settings include, but are not limited to, emergency departments, critical care units, step-down units, and medical/surgical floors. In addition, acutely ill patients are also managed in outpatient facilities such as surgical centers, facilities for ventilator-dependent patients, and specialty centers such as those designed for congestive heart failure or renal-dialysis patients. Indeed, ACNPs frequently manage patients through the transition from acute and critical care to community reintegration (Reel, 1999). In a survey of ACNPs, one researcher stated that respondents continue formulating roles to fulfill identified needs for an advanced practice nurse to manage aspects of patient care in a variety of settings (Kleinpell, 1998; Kleinpell-Nowell, 2001).

ACNPs assume positions in a variety of organizational placements. The two major placements are unit based or service based. Regardless of the organizational placement, the ACNP may derive salary from the nursing service in a hospital system or through a professional practice plan. If planning to submit to Medicare for direct compensation for care provided, the

ACNP will need to know the source of his or her salary and become fully conversant with the rules regulating reimbursement (Richmond, Thompson, & Sullivan-Marx, 2000).

Unit-Based Acute Care Nurse Practitioner

ACNPs may be employed to manage the care of patients in a circumscribed geographical area, such as an intensive care unit or a medical/surgical floor (Genet et al., 1995). The role of the unit-based ACNP is typically defined by the needs of the patient population and system. The implementation of the unit-based ACNP will be influenced by the type of institution, the presence or absence of residency programs, and the characteristics and complexity of the patient population to be managed.

An example of a unit-based ACNP is the cardiac-surgery intensive care unit NP. ACNPs typically are responsible for the management of all patients who are admitted postoperatively after coronary artery bypass surgery, valve replacement surgery, or transplant. ACNPs are responsible for the initial assessment of patients upon their return from the operating room and for the diagnosis and management of acute problems. Understanding the intraoperative course and the effects of anesthesia is crucial. ACNPs are responsible for establishing and maintaining hemodynamic stability and adequate ventilation. They direct fluid therapy and vasopressor support to sustain this hemodynamic stability during the postanesthesia equilibration and rewarming. Diagnostic decision making is critical to patient outcome and occurs in rapid succession during this vulnerable postoperative period. Management of complications is based on accurate diagnosis and a comprehensive knowledge base of the physiology, presentation, and interventions for problems such as inadequate coronary artery perfusion, postoperative bleeding, or inadequate oxygenation. Typical privileges of the ACNP in this milieu include the right to order additional intravenous fluids, vasopressors, or blood products to be administered based on the evaluation of the hemodynamic values, the laboratory data, and the patient assessment. Invasive techniques such as placement of central lines, pulmonary artery catheters, and arterial lines often are included in the practice scope of the ACNP in this setting. ACNPs oversee patient progression, intervene as required to ensure optimal progression (e.g., such as weaning the patient from mechanical ventilation, removing mediastinal chest tubes), and eventually transfer patients to the medical/surgical floor. All of these activities, and more, are within the scope of practice for a unit-based ACNP.

Service-Based ACNPs

An alternative model is that of the service-based ACNP who manages patients across the continuum of acute-care services. The ACNP may work within a physician practice or be employed by the hospital. In either situation, the ACNP undergoes the credentialing and privileging process at the hospital in which care is provided. If part of a physician practice plan, the ACNP will most often have a collaborative compact or contractual arrangement in which the nature of the role and the patient-centered activities of the ACNP are detailed.

An example of a service-based ACNP is the trauma nurse practitioner. Trauma patients receive care in the prehospital setting, emergency department, resuscitation bay, and intensive care unit, as well as on the medical/surgical floor and in the physician office for follow-up visits. The service-based trauma nurse practitioner typically is responsible for and/or is involved in the care of the patient in all of these areas. When the trauma patient presents to the emergency department via ambulance, the trauma nurse practitioner participates in the resuscitation, performs the comprehensive health history and physical examination, and formulates the admission orders. After the patient is transferred to the intensive care unit, the ACNP manages the multiple facets of the patient's care, including the type of intravenous medications received, diagnostic lab and diagnostic monitoring, and evaluating response to therapy. When medical stability is achieved, the ACNP decides to transfer the patient to the medical/surgical floor and plans for discharge of the patient. The trauma nurse practitioner may also be responsible for the patient's care at the post-discharge office visit.

Practice Privileges

The scope of practice is consistent for all adult ACNPs, but the manner in which the role is implemented and the array of privileges sought and obtained are all shaped by state regulations and the characteristics of the patient population and practice setting. ACNPs are usually credentialed and privileged by the medical staff committee of each hospital in which they practice. Presentation of ACNPs' credentialing application includes, but may not be limited to, two or three references from academic and clinical areas, proof of graduation from an accredited program, copies of the ACNPs' licenses from the state in which they will practice, and national certification (Kamajian, Mitchell, & Fruth, 1999).

The application process for practice privileges varies across institutions. Privileges cannot exceed the scope of practice of the adult ACNP, state-level regulations, or the knowledge and skill preparation of the individual practitioner. As part of the privileging process, a list of privileges that the nurse practitioner requests is generated. This often includes a description of the array of patients that the ACNP will be responsible for managing, the classes of medications that can be prescribed, the diagnostic tests that can be ordered, and the type of procedures, technologies, and interventions that the nurse practitioner can perform. The process that will be adopted to determine the competency of the ACNP in the performance of procedures will also be delineated. Proof that the nurse practitioner is competent in performing procedures and managing technologies must be provided to the credentialing committee before the ACNP can perform them independently.

The ACNP may first receive temporary practice privileges. During this period, the privileges are often limited in scope and require a supervising or collaborating colleague. The need for or level of medical supervision and/or collaboration for the ACNP varies substantially from state to state and is regulated by the states' practice acts and regulations. Ideally, collaborative practice should promote a climate of trust and respect between two professions based on their explicitly defined, mutually complementary roles in patient care. Even if the consulting/supervisory relationship is merely pro forma, the NP's ability to practice relies on an individual physician's willingness to allow it (Lee & Pulcini, 1998). However, for many NPs, the collaborative requirement is a form of legislative restriction on scope of practice and poses a barrier to their efforts to practice independently (Lee & Pulcini, 1998). Optimally, collaboration should be driven by mutual agreement and not driven by mandates.

Collaborative practice between ACNPs and physicians has always been the most essential component in the delivery of quality care to acutely ill and injured patients. A truly collaborative practice eliminates redundancies in patient assessment and management (Genet et al., 1995). Clear communication between disciplines is crucial in order to provide the best quality of care to this particularly vulnerable population (Baggs et al., 1999).

THE ACNP IN THE INTERDISCIPLINARY HEALTH CARE TEAM

The ACNP and Patient Care

The patient is central to the practice of the ACNP, who develops a partnership with the patient and family to mutually develop and fulfill the goals of care. From the nursing paradigm, the ACNP brings to the patient encounter a person-centered focus supported by excellent communication skills (Van Soeren & Micevski, 2001). These skills, coupled with the knowledge of disease management and authority invested in the ACNP, set the stage for developing effective partnerships with patients and families.

The role of the ACNP is relatively new and not one that has always been clearly understood by patients and their families (in addition to other members of the health care team). In the early 1990s when the role was first introduced in tertiary care facilities, many patients thought that the ACNPs who entered their rooms, examined, and treated them were doctors. The early ACNPs spent much of their time educating their patients about who ACNPs were and the collaborative nature of their role with the patient's physician. There are still times when this relationship has to be explained to patients.

Once patients experience care from a team that includes an ACNP, they often express satisfaction, finding the care more comprehensive and holistic (Rudy et al., 1998). Research on the effectiveness of ACNPs includes effects of cost, length of hospitalization, and key quality indicators. Bissinger, Allred, Artford, and Bellig (1997) compared cost and quality outcomes of patients managed by nurse practitioners with those managed by medical house staff in a neonatal intensive care unit. They found that the NPs provided quality patient care equal to that of the house staff, at a lower cost per infant and with greater continuity and consistency. Hammond, Chase and Hogbin (1995) compared the effectiveness of nurse practitioners to that of senior house officers in an oncology practice. Patients who saw NPs expressed higher satisfaction than those who saw a senior house officer, and the NPs were also found to give more information and to ask patients if they had any questions more frequently than did the house officers. Importantly, NPs' decision-making skills were found to be equal to those of senior house officers.

In another study, such dramatic cost savings were found following the implementation of NPs in a surgical practice, due to the improvement in patient outcomes, that NPs were subsequently utilized in other neurosurgery and general surgery practices (Hylka & Beschle, 1995). Similarly Spisso, O'Callaghan, McKennan, and Holcroft (1990) found ACNPs on a trauma service reduced patient length of stay, outpatient clinic waiting time, and patient complaints. Documentation of quality care was also improved.

Rudy et al., (1998) examined differences in provider activities and clinical outcomes obtained between patients who were primarily cared for by ACNPs or physician assistants and those principally cared for by resident physicians. The ACNPs and physician assistants spent significantly more time reviewing chart notes, interacting with patient family members, performing hands-on assessments, and performing research and administrative duties. Patients cared for by resident physicians were older and sicker than those cared for by the ACNPs and physician assistants. There were no differences in outcomes between groups, underscoring the fact that NPs provided comparable care to the medical residents.

Byrne, Richardson, Brunsdon, and Patel (2000) examined the delivery of care in the accident and emergency department and found that the patients were equally as satisfied with the delivery of care by emergency nurse practitioners (ENPs) as they were with care provided by physicians, with ENPs scoring higher on four parameters. Patients rated the ENPs higher than the physicians on the following patient characteristics: Patients were more likely to have received health and first aid advice, were more likely to have been told whom to contact if they needed more help and advice following discharge, were more likely to have received written discharge instructions, and were less worried about their health. Talking to patients and giving information and explanations regarding their health status served to reassure the patients and helped them cope better with their condition.

ACNP practice has always been focused on meeting patient needs. Oermann and Templin (2000) surveyed 239 consumers about 27 attributes of health care and nursing care quality. The most important indicators of quality nursing care to consumers were found to be being cared for by up to date and well informed nurses; being able to communicate with the nurse; spending enough time with the nurse and not feeling rushed during the visit; having a nurse teach about the illness, medications, and treatments, having the nurse help the patients cope with illness and maintain their usual activities; being able to call the nurse with questions; and having a nurse teach strategies to avoid illness and stay healthy.

Many of the studies outlined here have examined ACNP practice relative to the quality nursing indicators identified by Oermann and Templin (2000). It is evident that the patient-responsive care provided by ACNPs is meeting the needs identified by patients. The holistic nature of ACNP practice meets both the physiological and psychosocial needs of patients.

The ACNP and Nursing and Medical Colleagues

As advanced practice nurses, ACNPs prescribe patient treatments that have here to fore been in the exclusive domain of medical colleagues. The shifting boundaries of practice have now resulted in different relationships with generalist nurses who are responsible for providing bedside care to acutely and critically ill and injured patients.

The introduction of the ACNP to the health care team creates challenges and opportunities. Bedside nurses who have been socialized to "take orders" from patients' physicians are now exposed to a new world in which care is prescribed by ACNPs. This challenge, however, is not solely at the individual nurse level; it also includes departments of nursing struggling to establish cultures and policies that incorporate the ACNP's broadened scope of practice. At times resistance arises, and nursing colleagues may not recognize, at first, the contribution that the ACNP can make to patient care.

When the ACNP is first introduced to the nursing staff, the response by many is that the advanced practice nurse is a "doctor-wannabe." However, when ACNPs have the opportunity to demonstrate their clinical judgment and worth to patient care, they become an invaluable partner to the bedside nurse. Often the physician is not readily available to nursing staff when a change in patient condition requires an immediate response. The availability of physicians has traditionally been limited by the competing demands of multiple patients in a variety of settings (often several hospitals) and in surgical practices. The ACNP, as a member of a collaborative team, is available to respond to the patient situation, make medically prudent clinical decisions, evaluate the patient's response, and adjust the plan as needed.

The ACNP and Physician Consultants

ACNPs often need to consult physicians for their expert opinion in specific patient situations. For example, it may be necessary to consult the infectious disease team for recommendations on how best to evaluate and/or treat a patient's infectious process or to consult the renal service for patients with potential or actual renal compromise. Due to the complex nature of acutely ill patients, it is imperative the ACNP obtain a quick response to the request for consultation and maintain clear, direct communication throughout the consultation process. The best way to manage this is to develop collegial relationships with these specialty consultants.

The changing world of health care and the resultant changes in scope of practice of advanced practice nurses have, at times, stretched the mindset of colleagues in other disciplines. Physician colleagues, used to being consulted only by other physicians, may initially be confused by who the ACNP is and how the ACNP fits into this process. This is a substantial departure from years of the traditional medical model of patient care, yet opens a new level of collaborative, patient-centered care in which each discipline can contribute to the quality of patient care.

The ACNP and Allied Health Disciplines

The ACNP frequently collaborates with other disciplines such as respiratory therapy for ventilator management or physical therapy for ways to promote mobility in the bedridden patient. Consulting other disciplines does not reflect poorly on the nurse practitioner's abilities, but rather upholds the belief that other health care team members are experts in their fields. By consulting other specialists, the nurse practitioner can gather expert clinical opinion so that clinical management is optimized.

The ACNP and Other Advanced Practice Nurses

ACNPs often confer with and seek the expertise of other advanced practice nurses who serve in a variety of roles, such as research coordinators, case managers, staff development nurses, and clinical nurse specialists. These advanced practice nurses can provide expert opinions on how to best facilitate patients' care, maximize bedside nursing expertise, and manage specialty patient problems.

ACNPs are likely to collaborate with advanced practice nurses in research-based endeavors. Many acute-care settings have a variety of ongoing research studies that use the services of advance practice nurses as study coordinators. There may be opportunities for the ACNP to participate in the recruitment of participants in a research study and to facilitate data collection. Given the variety and complexity of study protocols, ACNPs need to be aware of protocols for studies in which their patients are participating so that they do not break protocol and so they may be knowledgeable and attuned to potential side effects of the therapies included in the research protocols. Clearly, as a member of research subjects' primary service, ACNPs need to be fully cognizant of all activities that affect the care of their patients so they can optimally provide care and advocate for their patients.

In addition, ACNPs collaborate with case managers. Case managers are advanced practice nurses who focus on ensuring that groups of patients with common diseases or problems are obtaining medically necessary care in a timely manner. Although differing approaches are used, case managers track and facilitate patients' progress on a trajectory that has been jointly developed by the interdisciplinary team. Case managers are likely to consult with ACNPs to ensure that their patients are receiving diagnostic evaluations expeditiously and that the level of care provided is appropriate for hospitalization. When case managers fulfill the role of utilization coordinators, they justify patients' length of stay in the hospital with the payer source. Many times, ACNPs are expected to provide oral or written information that justifies the hospital stay or the intensity of services provided to ensure payment by third-party payers.

Another key role that advanced practice nurses fill is in clinical staff development. In this role, advanced practice nurses systematically conduct needs assessments of the nursing staff to identify and fill learning deficits. They conduct orientations for new staff, renewal programs to maintain knowledge and skills, and provide basic and advanced life-support courses. Further, they ensure nursing staff compliance with completing mandatory in-services required by specialty designation organizations and regulatory agencies such as the Joint Commission on the Accreditation of Healthcare Organizations (JCAHO) and state health departments. Effective working relationships between ACNPs and advanced practice nurses in staff development are mutually beneficial. ACNPs are obliged to maintain basic (and often advanced) life-support certification and can capitalize on existing programs to fulfill these requirements. In addition, ACNPs are knowledgeable experts who can teach staff in educational programs organized by staff development colleagues.

ACNPs and clinical nurse specialists (CNSs) are often involved in the care of acutely and critically ill and injured patients in the same settings. The two advanced practice roles have common responsibilities, but frequently different foci of practice. While ACNPs focus primarily on the direct care of individual patients, CNSs tend to focus primarily on facilitating the care of groups of patients, often working through bedside nurses. CNSs incorporate administrative responsibilities, staff development, quality initiatives, and the continual improvement in care provided by nurses into their array of responsibilities. The CNS, as the clinical expert on the nursing unit or service, identifies nursing needs of patients and families and works with staff to ensure that those needs are being optimally met. Patient and family teaching and support are responsibilities jointly held by the ACNP and CNS.

Patient care and systems of care benefit when ACNPs and CNSs understand their overlapping and unique contributions to the care of acutely and critically ill and injured patients and their families (Richmond, Dubendorf, & Monturo, 1999). Patient care benefits by the presence of ACNPs, who contribute by their ability to meet both the direct medical and nursing needs. Similarly, patient care benefits by the presence of CNSs, who contribute to the development of systems of care that facilitate optimal patient care. Together, ACNPs and CNSs, in cooperation with key members of other disciplines, have the potential to create seamless systems of care.

SUMMARY

Acute-care advanced practice nurses provide services with the main objective of meeting the needs of patients. The method of achieving this goal differs depending on the role. An interdisciplinary approach in which all members recognize their limitations, understand when it is beneficial to consult others, and appreciate the uniqueness of each member's contributions provides the patient with the best opportunity for a quality outcome.

REFERENCES AND BIBLIOGRAPHY

American College of Physicians. (1994). Physician assistants and nurse practitioners. *Annals of Internal Medicine, 121,* 714–716.

American Nurses Association & American Association of Critical Care Nurses. (1995). *Standards of clinical practice & scope of practice for the acute care nurse practitioner.* Washington, DC: American Nurses Publishing.

Baggs, J. G., Schmitt, M. H., Mushlin, A. I., Mitchell, P. H., Eldredge, D. H., Oakes, D., & Hutson, A. D. (1999). Association between nurse-physician collaboration and patient outcomes in three intensive care units. *Critical Care Medicine, 27,* 1991–1998.

Bissinger, R. L., Allred, C. A., Arford, P. H., & Bellig, L. L. (1997). A cost-effectiveness analysis of neonatal nurse practitioners. *Nursing Economics, 15,* 92–99.

Byrne, G., Richardson, M., Brunsdon, J., & Patel, A. (2000). Patient satisfaction with emergency nurse practitioners in A&E. *Journal of Clinical Nursing, 9,* 83–93.

DeMarco, R. F., Horowitz, J. A., & McLeod, D. (2000). A call for intraprofessional alliances. *Nursing Outlook, 48,* 172–178.

El-Sherif, C. (1995). Nurse practitioners—Where do they belong within the organizational structure of acute care setting? *Nurse Practitioner, 20,* 62, 64–65.

Gardner, D. B., & Cary, A. (1999). Collaboration, conflict and power: Lessons for case managers. *Family and Community Health, 22,* 64–77.

Genet, C. A., Brennan, P. F., Ibbotson-Wolff, S., Phelps, C., Rosenthal, G., Landefeld, C. S., & Daly, B. (1995). Nurse practitioners in a teaching hospital. *Nurse Practitioner, 20,* 47–54.

Glanville, I., Schirm, V., & Wineman, N. M. (2000). Using evidence-based practice for managing clinical outcomes in advanced practice nursing. *Journal of Nursing Care Quality, 15,* 1–11.

Hammond, C., Chase, J., & Hogbin, B. (1995). A unique service? *Nursing Times, 91,* 28–29.

Hylka, S. C., & Beschle, J. G. (1995). Nurse practitioners, cost savings and improved patient care in the department of surgery. *Nursing Economics, 13,* 349–354.

Kamajian, M. F., Mitchell, S. A., & Fruth, R. A. (1999). Credentialing and privileging of advanced practice nurses. *AACN Clinical Issues, 10,* 316–336.

Kleinpell, R. (1998). Reports of role descriptions of acute care nurse practitioners. *AACN Clinical Issues, 9,* 290–295.

Kleinpell-Nowell, R. (2001). Longitudinal survey of acute care nurse practitioner practice: Year 2. *AACN Clinical Issues, 12,* 447–452.

Knickman, J. R., Lipkin, M., Finkler, S. A., Thompson, W. G., & Kiel, J. (1992). The potential for using non-physicians to compensate for the reduced availability of residents. *Academic Medicine, 67,* 429–438.

Kontryn, V. (1999). Strategic problem solving in the new millennium. *AORN Journal, 70,* 1035–1037, 1039–1040, 1042–1044.

Lee, M., & Pulcini, J. (1998). Barriers to independent practice: Mandatory collaboration between nurses and physicians. *Clinical Excellence for Nurse Practitioners, 2,* 172–173.

Ligas, J. R. (1997). Experiences as preceptor to acute care nurse practitioner students: One physician's view. *AACN Clinical Issues, 8,* 123–131.

Miller, S. K. (1998). Defining the acute in acute care nurse practitioner. *Clinical Excellence for Nurse Practitioners, 2,* 52–55.

Morse, S. J., & Brown, M. M. (1999). Collaborative practice in the acute care setting. *Critical Care Nursing Quarterly, 21,* 31–36.

Navuluri, R. B. (1999). Integrated quality improvement program in patient care. *Nursing & Health Sciences, 1,* 249–254.

Neale, J. E. (2001). Patient outcomes: A matter of perspective. *Nursing Outlook, 49,* 93-99.

Nemeth, L. (1999). Leadership for coordinate care: Role of a project manager. *Critical Care Quarterly, 21,* 50–58.

Oermann, M. H., & Templin, T. (2000). Important attributes of quality health care: Consumer perspectives. *Journal of Nursing Scholarship, 2,* 167–172.

Reel, V. K. (1999). Utilization of the acute care nurse practitioner in lung transplantation. *Clinical Excellence for Nurse Practitioners, 3*(2), 80–83.

Rhee, K. J., & Dermyer, A. L. (1995). Patient satisfaction with a nurse practitioner in a university emergency service. *Annals of Emergency Medicine, 26,* 130–132.

Richmond, T. S., Dubendorf, P., & Monturo, C. (1999). Scope & standards of clinical practice. In P. Logan (Ed.), *Principles of practice of the acute care nurse practitioner* (pp. 1-23). Stamford: CT: Appleton & Lange.

Richmond, T. S., Thompson H. J., & Sullivan-Marx, E. M. (2000). Reimbursement for acute care nurse practitioner services. *American Journal of Critical Care, 9,* 52–61.

Rudy, E. B., Davidson, L. J., Daly, B., Clochesy, J. M., Sereika, S., Baldisseri, M., Hravnak, M., Ross, T., & Ryan, C. (1998). Care activities and outcomes of patients cared for by acute care nurse practitioners, physician assistants, and resident physicians: A comparison. *American Journal of Critical Care, 7,* 267–281.

Scott, R. A. (1999). A description of the roles, activities and skills of the clinical nurse specialist in the United States. *Clinical Nurse Specialists, 13,* 183–190.

Spisso, J., O'Callaghan, C., McKennan, M., & Holcroft, J. W. (1990). Improved quality of care and reduction of housestaff workload using trauma nurse practitioners. *Journal of Trauma, 30,* 660–665.

Van Soeren, M. H., & Micevski, V. (2001). Success indicators and barriers to acute nurse practitioner role implementation in four Ontario hospitals. *AACN Clinical Issues, 12,* 424–437.

Zapp, L. (2001). Use of multiple teaching strategies in the staff development setting. *Journal for Nurses in Staff Development, 17,* 206–212.

Chapter 7

ADVANCED PRACTICE NURSES IN MANAGED CARE

Patricia M. Barber and Marina Burke

This chapter discusses the role of advanced practice nurses (APNs) in managed care by first reviewing how managed care has evolved in the last few years, what the current trends are, and how advanced practice nursing continues to impact the delivery of health care. The chapter also examines the strides that APNs have made in expanding their clinical practice, since this is important in understanding their role in managed care and health care in general. The chapter also touches on some of the challenges that APNs confront as they continue to make their mark as contributors to the health care industry.

THE DEFINITION OF MANAGED CARE

Understanding the organized delivery system (ODS), the current structure of health care delivery in the United States, is critical in defining managed care. It is a system that includes hospitals, groups of medical providers, and in some cases insurers, organized to meet all of the health care needs of a community (Madden & Reid Ponte, 1994). Organized delivery systems have emerged due to the rising cost of health care, competition in the health care market, and the consolidation of hospitals and providers into networks. Ideally, the ODS can provide for more coordination by providers, less confusion for patients, and the delivery of quality care that contains costs.

According to experts, managed care—or managed competition, as it is sometimes called—embodies an effort by employers, the insurance industry, and some members of the medical profession to establish priorities and decide who gets what from the health care system (Robinson, 2001). At first glance, this definition may appear somewhat limited; however, it does capture the essence of managed care over the last quarter of a century. We should elaborate further and add the intent or theory behind the concept of managed care provided by Uwe Reinhardt, PhD, the James Madison Professor of Political Economy at Princeton University: Managed care is (or should be) a delivery of coordinated care focusing on prevention and treatment of acute episodes to prevent health catastrophes and improve patients' health during their lifetimes, while controlling costs (Mitka, 1998).

BACKGROUND OF MANAGED CARE

The passing of the health maintenance organization (HMO) Act of 1973 initiated a change in thinking about how our health care system should be structured and laid the groundwork for the evolution of the managed care system. Managed care in the 1970s was characterized by very restrictive requirements and was not readily accepted until the 1980s when those restrictions were relaxed. At that time, employers were anxious to accept the concept of prepaid health care as an alternative to fee-for-service care as a way to deal with escalating health care costs that had reached double-digit annual growth rates. Employers, as well as insurers and some physician groups, bought into the concept and helped to further the development of managed care as a way to avoid government regulation of the health care industry. The early structure of managed care was a staff model HMO such as Kaiser-Permanente. As managed care expanded, physicians, insurers, and the "more educated consumer who desired choice" became involved. This resulted in the demand for broader networks of physicians resulting, in PPOs (preferred provider organizations) and IPAs (independent physician associations), the formation of disease management programs and companies, and other forms of managed care.

HEALTH CARE INDUSTRY TRENDS

Health care spending reached $1.3 trillion in 2000, growing at a mean annual rate of 7.3% during the forecast period 2001–2011. During this period, it is expected that health spending will grow 2.5% per year faster than nominal gross domestic product (GDP) so that by 2011 it will constitute approximately 17% of GDP, up from the 2000 level of 13.2%. Projections for the year 2011, or shortly thereafter, bring that total to $2.8 trillion in health care costs (Heffler, Smith, & Won, 2002).

The evolution of both managed care and the ODS continues to have an impact on the business of health care delivery, and the major health insurance plans are reacting to this evolution. Insurers are offering alternative benefits and revising their benefit plans and payment mechanisms in order to ensure the maximum profit and stay competitive. Cigna, for example, is expanding its Healthy Rewards discount program to include cosmetic surgery, laser vision correction surgery, eyewear, and hearing care services (Goldman Sachs, 2001). Employers continue to play an active role in health care, shopping for bargains for their employees and exerting their influence on providers of care. The Central Florida Health Care Coalition, formed by large employers such as Lockheed Martin, Walt Disney World, and Universal Studios, announced that it would devise an incentive program to reward doctors who improve quality of care (Goldman Sachs, 2001). Health plans have relaxed some of the very restrictive utilization review requirements that were typical in prior years, and they are working with the government to find creative solutions to address the increased health care costs for our nation's elderly and poor. For example, United Health has discontinued its requirement for prior authorization for a referral across the board. In addition, after a series of discussions with the Centers for Medicare and Medicaid Services, the health plan has agreed to lower its proposed deductible increase for hospital stays on its PrimeCARE Gold Medicare product in Wisconsin (Goldman Sachs, 2001). Managed care profit margins declined in the 1990s. In 1994 and 1995, over 90% of most for-profit managed care plans were profitable; in the later 1990s, less than 40% were making a profit (Ginzsberg, 1998).

MANAGED CARE TODAY

Managed care now dominates health care in the United States. By 1999, only 8% of persons with employer-sponsored health insurance had traditional indemnity insurance (Dudley & Luft, 2001). In 1996, the percentage of revenue received by all physicians from managed care was 38%. In 1999, that proportion had risen to 49%, and most physicians had managed care contracts and one third had capitation (prepaid on a per capita basis for a specified list of services) contracts (Dudley & Luft, 2001).

Most experts, however, would agree that managed care is in a transition phase. The average U.S. consumer continues to believe strongly in the right to unrestricted access to high-quality health care. The gatekeeping concept, in which a primary care physician coordinates and determines all care, including when to seek the advice of a specialist, is becoming less popular. The current climate of managed care can be characterized by more choice in selecting a physician, less restriction in accessing care, and a return to fee-for-service reimbursement and, in some cases, options for indemnity coverage.

Enrollment in managed care plans reflects this change: More consumers are switching from HMOs to plans where there is more choice, less control by a gatekeeping provider, no prior approval for referrals, and less utilization review. Some managed care practices are proving to be ineffective, and some insurers in the private sector are discontinuing practices. For example, Harvard Pilgrim Health Care, in New England, discontinued its use of gatekeepers in 1997 because of patient complaints and because no evidence was found that gatekeeping had an impact on referral patterns. In addition, as indicated above, United Health no longer requires prior authorization review to obtain a referral because it was determined that requested referrals were denied in less than 1% of cases (Dudley & Luft, 2001).

Some of the factors that have contributed to the current structure of managed care and that will continue to have influence in the future are (1) costly new technology and drug therapy; (2) an expanding definition of health with a focus on prevention and screening; (3) monitoring of managed care plans by state and federal government; (4) expansion of the Internet, providing more information about health care to the general public; and (5) well-informed consumers who are not hesitant to voice their needs.

ADVANCED PRACTICE NURSING IN MANAGED CARE

Traditional roles of the advanced practitioner are research, education, consultation, and practice. Interventions focus on individuals, families, and communities. As managed care and the ODS continue to evolve and change, the opportunities for advanced practice are varied. APNs can contribute to organized delivery systems by building primary care capacity, producing high-quality outcomes, achieving competitive costs, coordinating care across delivery systems, and providing comprehensive care (Lang, Sullivan, & Jenkins, 1996). The interdisciplinary team approach to patient care, which is characteristic of managed care, allows APNs the flexibility and opportunity to be valuable contributors because of their scope of practice, and their contributions can help to strengthen managed care delivery systems.

PHYSICIANS, EMPLOYERS, HOSPITALS, AND HEALTH CARE PROVIDERS

The role of physicians and other health care professionals as providers of care and the role of employers as purchasers of care continue to change as managed care changes. The hospital, once the primary setting for health care delivery, is also undergoing transition as the ODS evolves and more care is delivered in ambulatory settings and in the home.

Physicians

The managed care philosophy of shifting the risk from the insurer to the physician has had a major impact on how physicians deliver care. Managed care encourages physicians to focus on preventive care and early diagnosis rather than costly episodic care, theoretically leading to a better quality of care. Physicians are also being monitored by insurers for utilization patterns and quality of care through the use of peer review. A trend in managed care is the decline of physicians in solo practice and the development of hospital-physician organizations and practice management companies. Developing business affiliations and instituting strict management of practices are activities that physicians view as survival strategies in an environment where there is less revenue and higher administrative costs.

Employers

Employers are developing coalitions to negotiate discounts with managed care companies to curtail rising health care costs, and they are offering incentives to physicians for better utilization. In addition, employers are introducing creative strategies (tax reimbursement mechanisms) for out-of-pocket health care expenses for their employees.

Hospitals and Health Care Providers

The role of the hospital has and will continue to change dramatically in the 21st century. After a peak in 1980, inpatient admissions declined by 20%, despite an increasing and aging population, and average length of stay continues to decline (Ginzberg, 1998). Most patients now require care in clinics, at home, and in specialized ambulatory treatment centers, and care is provided by a variety of health care providers. Looking forward, it is likely that most patient care will be physician directed; however, non-physician health care professionals will increasingly provide more of the services, utilizing an interdisciplinary team approach. This trend offers APNs, who are the largest and fastest growing group of nonphysician clinicians, the opportunity to coordinate and provide more primary care in all settings. Most APNs are trained in various areas of primary care, such as adult health, pediatrics, family health, women's health, or gerontology, although increasing numbers are choosing critical care, emergency department care and other specialty pathways (Cooper, 2001).

THE FUTURE FOR MANAGED CARE

To address rising health care expenditures in the 21st century, the U.S. Congress and the executive branch reached agreement to reduce prospective outlays for Medicare by $115 billion during the years 1998 to 2002. In addition, in recent years both Congress and the state legislatures have been exploring and enacting new legislation that would control the degrees of freedom that managed care has enjoyed during the last years. The American public has also become more involved in the legislative arena to limit the managerial autonomy of the plans (Dudley & Luft, 2001). This trend will continue to exert pressure on health plans to manage costs, ensure quality, and meet the demands of legislatures and consumers.

To survive economically, health plans must remain responsive to consumer and purchaser (employer) preferences, as well as to the ever-changing regulatory environments in which they operate. Consumer demand for less restriction and greater choice in health care has encouraged the dramatic growth in open-ended managed care products such as preferred provider products and point-of-service plans. This demand is also driving growth among plans that give patients direct access to certain types of specialists without referrals or other preapproval requirements (Roper & Mays, 1998). According to Paul Ellwood, who coined the phrase *health maintenance organization,* the HMO Act and other proposals have permanently revolutionized medical care in the United States. It is his opinion that the first phase of managed care has shifted power from physicians and insurers to large-group purchasers of medical services. This shift in power has reduced the growth of health care expenditures by about $500 billion. The purchasers of health care neglected to consider the other component of the original HMO proposal: quality and competition. The next phase of managed care will involve another power shift from insurers and physicians to consumers and patients, who will exercise choices based on objective comparisons of quality (Mitka, 1998).

STATISTICS AND PROJECTIONS FOR ADVANCED PRACTITIONERS

Advanced practitioners deliver care, manage patients and families, teach, consult, research, and do a range of other activities based on the needs of patients and the environment in which they practice. They are expert practitioners. They work in hospitals, communities, and homes, with individuals and with groups (Madden & Reid Ponte, 1994). APNs are growing in number and are increasingly independent, as the following list indicates:

- It is estimated that, as of 2000, there were 139,394 APNs in the United States (Pearson, 2002).
- From 1995 to 2005, the primary care APN workforce is projected to increase from 55,000 to 115,000, while the number of primary care physicians will increase by about 10% (Cooper, 2001).
- A recent APN education enrollment survey indicates that, as of 2000, there were 18,465 full- and part-time Master's-level nurse practitioner and nurse practitioner/clinical nurse specialists enrolled in programs nationally, and 110 completed post-RN certificate programs (Berlin, Bednash, & Stennet, 2001).
- During the last 20 years, 22 states have granted independent practice status to APNs. In all but one state, the supervising physician need not be present during the delivery of care (Sox, 2000); however, collaboration is required.
- The Balanced Budget Act of 1997 expanded Medicare reimbursement to APNs in all sites (Sox, 2000).

SETTINGS OF ADVANCED PRACTICE IN MANAGED CARE

The goals of managed care continue to evolve in the 21st century. Health promotion, disease prevention, and continuity of care are still emphasized, but delivering quality care while containing cost has proven difficult to achieve. The APN role in clinical, research, and managerial areas is developing and will continue to be viewed as one way to help achieve this goal of delivering quality, cost-effective care.

Hospital Setting

Advanced practitioners continue to flourish in the acute-care setting, caring for patients and families in a variety of roles. Most APNs have worked as bedside nurses for many years and often have more than one area of expertise. Their nursing experience and understanding of the hospital system have proven to be very beneficial to the acute-care environment. The hospital setting can be attractive to APNs who like the autonomy and challenge it offers. Drawbacks to some are the lack of patient continuity, minimal opportunity to practice primary care, and increasingly sicker patients.

Hospitals continue to bear the brunt of managed care cost-containment efforts. Since APNs are still less expensive than attending physicians, management views them as attractive providers. For this reason, academic medical centers in particular are becoming much more open to the concept of utilizing APNs in a variety of roles. The 1997 Balanced Budget Act has proven to be an additional incentive. Because acute-care APNs can now directly bill Medicare for their services, hospitals are using them as permanent direct care providers, rather than medical residents or attending physicians, to help reduce expenses that result from extended lengths of stay and multiple readmissions. Their goal is more rapid patient turnover and an increase in revenue. APNs as case managers expedite in-hospital treatment and discharge planning and can have a direct impact on length of stay. In addition, hospitals are having difficulty filling residency programs in medicine and surgery and APNs provide a competent workforce.

As the concept of the organized delivery system expands and hospitals merge, the focus continues to be on financial survival. More patients are being treated in the ambulatory setting, and hospitals must continue to be concerned with length of stay and patient turnover. Patients who are admitted for extended stays are usually quite sick and need an interdisciplinary team approach to care. Academic hospital systems are finding that the APN, as an integral part of the team, is able to act as a liaison between physicians and nursing and coordinate care for these patients, which can ultimately impact length of stay.

In some academic medical centers, APNs directly manage patients as substitutes for medical residents and fellows. From a managed care perspective, with its emphasis on the interdisciplinary team approach, the APN is better equipped to provide comprehensive continuity of quality care that involves the patient, other disciplines and the family. In addition, APNs are increasingly found in specialty areas, like surgery and bone marrow transplant units, working as complementary providers, performing admission physicals, episodic care, and extensive patient education.

Hospitals are making an investment in data analysis in order to take a critical look at the roles of APNs and outcomes. The Heart Failure Program at Vanderbilt Medical Center and School of Nursing hired an acute-care APN to assist in managing their uncomplicated heart failure patients. The one-year study's purpose was to determine whether adding the APN to the complement of staff would decrease overall costs of hospitalization. Patients managed by house staff during the year before the addition of the APN were compared to those managed after the APN was added to the staff. Total hospital costs and lengths of stay were significantly lower after recruitment of the APN; approximately $100,000 was saved after accounting for the APN's salary and benefits. Interestingly, most of the savings were in total ancillary costs—laboratory costs and electrocardiograms. Despite the fact that the study was not randomized, the APN functioned at the full clinical scope of practice by admitting, treating, and discharging patients in a collaborative model (Kleinpell-Nowell & Weiner, 1999).

Ambulatory Setting

The care of older adults in outpatient settings attempts to integrate nursing, medicine, social work services, and other health care disciplines. Advanced practice nurses contribute to this goal by providing a mix of direct patient care, delivering primary and specialized education to patients and families, and bridging gaps between several disciplines. Medicaid managed care programs are growing as states continue to shift that risk to health plans and advanced practitioners continue to care for this population. One study in Texas looked at patient satisfaction and perceived health in an adult and geriatric Medicaid managed care clinic. Patients with a diagnosis of hypertension and/or diabetes were followed by either an APN or a physician. Using two validated instruments, one that assessed perceived health and another that assessed satisfaction with the provider, they found no significant difference in perceived health between the groups cared for by APNs or physicians. This finding supports other studies that have shown equal patient satisfaction whether the care is given by an APN or physician (Pinkerton & Bush, 2000).

Outpatient geriatrics continues to integrate nursing, medicine, social services, and other disciplines to serve this needy population. The Program of All-inclusive Care for the Elderly (PACE) is an example of a long-term, managed care model that has been reproduced in several places nationally. Its enrollees live at home or in skilled nursing facilities. The program is an HMO, receiving capitated payments for high-risk, dually eligible (Medicare and Medicaid) older adults. Using interdisciplinary teams, which include APNs in some cases, it seeks to prevent hospitalizations and coordinates all necessary services, including inpatient care, for its enrollees (Eng, Pedulla, Eleazer, McCann, & Fox, 1997). Such programs need to track outcome data to improve their delivery of care and stay afloat. One PACE study developed a quality assessment tool at eight centers in an effort to standardize quality to patients across settings. Tracers such as dementia, wounds, terminal illness, and depression were evaluated. Records were reviewed by geriatric nurse practitioners and geriatric physicians, who found overall high quality with several areas for improvement. The study is important in that cutting-edge geriatrics is using the expertise of APNs to improve geriatric care (Pacala, Kane, Atherly, & Smith, 2000).

Columbia Advanced Practice Nurse Associates (CAPNA) is an adult primary care practice in New York City associated with Columbia University School of Nursing and New York Presbyterian Hospital. The practice has expanded since its inception in 1997 and now has contracts with several payers, including Oxford, United Health Care, HealthNet, and Aetna. The APNs, all of whom are Columbia School of Nursing faculty, are credentialed by each plan as PCPs (primary care providers) and are listed on the rosters as available to patients for primary care. Currently, APNs see 150–200 patients per month. The payers conduct their own utilization and health plan employer information data set (HEDIS) measures with CAPNA in the same manner as with physician practices. The 2000 randomized trial by Mundinger et al. is one of the only trials that evaluate APNs and physicians who share similar responsibilities and patient panels. The study is limited in that it only lasted six months; however, it can positively impact the role of APNs in primary care and in managed care contexts. The results showed no difference between APNs and physicians in outcome measures of patient satisfaction, health status, physiologic test results, and service utilization.

Kaiser-Permanente has been utilizing a physician-APN model to care for mostly long-term care residents. In southern California, this model has been in existence for 14 years. APNs and physician assistants (PAs) work in collaboration with physicians in the community and in nursing homes and serve approximately 750 long-term care and 140 subacute care residents in 45 skilled nursing facilities. The goal is to keep frail elderly, as healthy as possible and out of the hospital. Although there are several years of experience in the APN-physician model, very little outcome data have been measured.

Another APN model utilized to transition discharges from hospital to home for elderly cardiac patients resulted in a cost savings of $4,212 per patient. Advanced practice nurses coordinated and provided the discharge planning and home follow-up for these patients, and the savings resulted from 61% fewer hospital admissions and 70% fewer inpatient days for readmissions 6 weeks postdischarge (Lang et al., 1996).

Home Care

More APNs are working in home care, often bridging hospital and home to provide seamless discharge and to maximize efficient continuity of care. Again, the 1997 Balanced Budget Act now allows nurse practitioners to be directly reimbursed for home services. VNS CHOICE, a program of the Visiting Nurse Service of New York, is a capitated, managed long-term care Medicaid program. Advanced practitioners follow the frail elderly at home, coordinating services and attempting to prevent unnecessary hospitalizations. They function as primary care providers and as consultants to physicians and registered nurses.

The Visiting Doctors Program at Mount Sinai Hospital in New York City is a collaborative practice, caring for homebound elderly. Approximately half the panel are covered by Medicare, and the other half are dually eligible under Medicare and Medicaid. There is an equal mix of APNs and physicians, and each has independent patient panels. All providers serve as preceptors for APN students and internal medicine residents for home care rotations. Although there are no managed care health plans involved in this program—most patients are covered by Medicare and Medicaid—it is a very good illustration of APNs serving in a particularly autonomous role. The philosophy of the program in many ways is in line with that of managed care: prevention of inappropriate emergency department visits and hospital admissions and providing as much care at home for chronic and acute illness as possible.

THE NEED FOR ADVANCED PRACTICE NURSES IN LONG-TERM CARE

Advanced practice nurses, particularly geriatric nurse practitioners (GNPs), have emerged as ideal health care personnel to assess, monitor, and manage the physical, functional, and psychosocial status of elderly persons through the continuum of long-term care (Ebersole, 1983). In nursing homes, GNPs provide access to and continuity of medical management that may otherwise be unavailable. The ability to deliver primary care as an independent provider is what most APNs desire and what motivated them to pursue continued education, and primary care of the elderly in the skilled nursing facility (SNF) provides an opportunity to be independent and care for individuals who have very complex needs. In some cases, GNPs have been shown to focus more on primary and preventive care of residents and to attend better to geriatric syndromes and health issues in long-term care settings than do primary care physicians (Burl, Bonner, Rao, & Khan, 1998).

Can our current health care delivery system and managed care environment accommodate the health care needs of our aging population? One of the challenges we face as a nation, and one that will certainly put the health care industry to the test, is the growing number of elderly people in our society. By the year 2030, 20% of the American population will be age 65 and over, and between the years of 2000 and 2030, the number of people age 85 or older will increase by 4 million (University of Illinois, 2001). Approximately 4% of people over the age of 65 reside in nursing homes; 40% of nursing home residents are age 85 and older (U.S. General Accounting Office, 2001), and the number of individuals residing in nursing homes is projected to grow from 275,000 to more than 350,000 in 2030 (Strahan, 1997).

These projections, coupled with the workforce shortage in the nursing profession, present a challenge to our current health care infrastructure. Most efforts to address the nursing shortage focus on the hospital setting, but little is being done specifically to address the nursing workforce in the long-term care setting. The role of the APN in long-term care is being explored as a possible stabilizing and strengthening influence in the geriatric workforce.

Since the middle of the 1990s, the number of APNs working in SNFs has increased. In addition, the number of companies that employ APNs to deliver primary care in SNFs has increased in the last 5 years. EverCare, a subsidiary of UnitedHealth Care, is the largest employer of nurse practitioners, with 310 APNs operating in 12 states and caring for 710,000 residents. Advanced practitioners deliver primary, preventive care in collaboration with a primary care physician to the frail elderly in the homes. The EverCare model is a unique approach that provides all medical services to long-stay residents utilizing a capitated package of Medicare-covered services with more intensive primary care provided by the APN. The program's underlying philosophy is that better primary care will result in reduced hospital stay. Although very few outcome data have been formally analyzed (work in progress), it has been shown that the residents have experienced fewer hospital admissions and readmissions and improved management of geriatric syndromes.

Employing APNs to work in SNFs is becoming a very competitive business. In addition to EverCare, approximately a half dozen other companies are competing for market share nationally. Some of their clients are the larger chains of nursing homes that would like to have APNs working in all their homes. A number of smaller physician-owned companies are also hiring APNs to work collaboratively with them in their offices and with their nursing home patients. They are finding daily preventive care and medical control of geriatric syndromes by an APN have prevented hospital admissions and improved the quality of their elderly patients' lives. Nursing homes are also finding this added value and are hiring APN staff to work collaboratively with the medical director and be a resource for the nursing staff. With the increase in the use of subacute care (a short stay in a SNF, typically for rehabilitation posthospital stay), there is also the opportunity to care for sicker, younger individuals who are there for shorter periods. The Fallon Clinic is a for-profit multidisciplinary group practice in Worcester, Massachusetts, and is affiliated with the Fallon Community Health Plan, a nonprofit HMO with a Medicare risk contract that has been in effect since 1980. The clinic began using geriatric nurse practitioner–physician teams in 1989 to provide primary and preventive care to long-term care residents. The effectiveness of the GNP-physician team was examined by reviewing emergency department transfer rates, hospital lengths of stay, and specialty visits for patients covered by GNP-physician teams, compared to patients covered by physician only. Acute-care and emergency department costs were significantly lower for the GNP-physician team patients. In addition, there was a gain of $72 per resident per month with the team care compared to a loss of $197 per resident per month for physician care alone. Nursing home drug costs, skilled nursing days, and primary care visits were higher for those covered by the teams, but the difference was not statistically significant. Overall costs of the GNP-physician team were 42% lower for the aggregate pool (skilled nursing plus intermediate care) and 26% lower for long-term stays (Burl et al., 1998).

CHALLENGES

As managed care and the organized delivery system continue to evolve, advanced practice nurses face a number of challenges because the APN role in the health care industry is evolving as well. Tangible restrictions on prescriptive authority and scope of practice dictated by some states are hurdles that are being overcome as states expand their practice acts. Lack of hospital privileges for experienced and well-known APNs in a hospital setting continues to be a difficult barrier and will prove more difficult in the coming years with the increasing number of APNs who function as primary providers. Inability to break into the commercially insured market is a challenge for APNs who work in managed care settings. These practitioners, who often have a large educator role or see physicians' patients, have described feeling like invisible providers (Neale, 1999).

One of the biggest challenges that APNs face is the lack of outcome data. Outcome analysis is critical to promote APN practice, and APNs should not be hesitant to have their clinical practice evaluated and measured. Managed care organizations routinely evaluate physicians in their network by measuring utilization outcomes such as hospital admission rates, lengths of stay, readmission rates, discharge planning, and continuity of care. Positive outcomes will advance APNs' ability to function more effectively in a system that is changing and in need of efficiencies and quality providers. Indeed, they must spearhead outcome studies in all the settings in which they work. Positive APN outcome studies can be marketed to managed care organizations and the public (Buppert, 2000).

OPPORTUNITIES AND THE FUTURE

Advanced practice nurses have assumed varied roles in managed care. Their numbers are growing, and the concept of the APN is becoming the norm in most environments. Many opportunities exist, and APNs should capitalize on the changes taking place in the health care market. Managed care has brought changes and a new focus on the delivery of quality care. Advanced practitioners are trained to provide comprehensive quality care that includes not only diagnosis and treatment but also a holistic approach to patient care, including patient and family education. They have unique skills to offer an industry that continues to evolve and change. Change brings opportunity, and advanced practitioners have always been amenable to emerging changes and will continue to be.

REFERENCES AND BIBLIOGRAPHY

American Health Care Association News Release. (2001). The nurse staffing crisis in nursing homes—Consensus statement of the Campaign for Quality Care. 3/16/01.

Bakewell-Sachs, S., Carlino, H., Ash, L., Thurber, F., Guyer, K., Deatrick, J. A., & Brooten, D. (2000). Home care considerations for chronic and vulnerable populations. *Nurse Practitioner Forum, 11,* 65–72.

Berlin, L. E., Bednash, G. D., & Stennet, J. (2001). *2000–2001 enrollment and graduations in baccalaureate and graduate programs in nursing* (pp. 49, 55–56). Washington, DC: American Colleges of Nursing.

Buppert, C. (2000). Measuring outcomes in primary care practice. *Nurse Practitioner, 25,* 88–98.

Burl, J., Bonner, A., Rao, M., & Khan, A. (1998). Geriatric nurse practitioners in long-term care: Demonstration of effectiveness in managed care. *Journal of the American Geriatrics Society, 46,* 506–510.

Cooper, R. A. (2001). Health care workforce for the twenty-first century: The impact of nonphysician clinicians. *Annual Reviews of Medicine, 52,* 51–61.

Dudley, R. A., & Luft, H. (2001). Managed care in transition. *New England Journal of Medicine, 344,* 1087–1092.

Ebersole, P. (1983). Long-term care currents. *Ross Timesaver, 6*(3) 11–14.

Eng, C., Pedulla, J., Eleazer, G. P., McCann, R., & Fox, N. (1997). Program of all-inclusive care for the elderly (PACE): An innovative model of integrated geriatric care and financing. *Journal of the American Geriatrics Society, 45,* 223–232.

Farley, D. O., Zellman, G., Ouslander, J. G., & Reuben, D. B. (1999). Use of primary care teams by HMOS for care of long-stay nursing home residents. *Journal of the American Geriatrics Society, 47*(2), 1–12.

Fisher, H. M., & Raphael, T. G. (2000). Building home care into managed long-term care: The VNS CHOICE model. *Caring, 19*(6), 8–11.

Ginzberg, E. (1998). The changing US health care agenda. *Journal of the American Medical Association, 279,* 501–504.

Goldman Sachs. (2001). Public company news. *Managed Care Weekly,* 11–23.

Heffler, S., Smith, S., & Won, G. (2002). Health spending projections for 2001–2011: The latest outlook. *Health Affairs,* 3/4.

Kane, R. L., Flood, S., Keckhafer, B., & Rockwood, T. (2001). How EverCare nurse practitioners spend their time. *Journal of the American Geriatrics Society, 49,* 1530–1534.

Kertesz, L. (1997). The new world of managed care. *Modern Healthcare, 5,* 11–13.

Kleinpell-Nowell, R., & Weiner, T. M. (1999). Measuring advanced practice nursing outcomes. *AACN Clinical Issues, 10,* 356–368.

Lang, N. M, Sullivan, E. M., & Jenkins, M. (1996), Advanced practice nurses and success of organized delivery systems. *American Journal of Managed Care, 2,* 129–135.

Lynn, M. M., Achtmeyer, C., Chavez, C., Zicafoose, B., & Therien, J. (1999). The evolving role of advanced practice nursing within the new veteran's health administration. *Health Care Management Review, 24,* 80–93.

Madden, M. J., & Reid Ponte, P. (1994). Advanced practice roles in the managed care environment. *Journal of Nurse Administrators, 2,* 56–62.

Mitka, M. (1998). A quarter century of health maintenance. *Journal of the American Medical Association, 280,* 1223–1231.

Mundinger, M. O., Kane, R. L., Lenz, E. R., Totten, A. M., Tsai, W., Cleary, P. D., Friedewald, W. T., Siu, A. L., & Shelanski, M. L. (2000). Primary care outcomes in patients treated by nurse practitioners or physicians. *Journal of the American Medical Association, 283,* 59–68.

Neale, J. (1999). Nurse practitioners and physicians: A collaborative practice. *Clinical Nurse Specialist, 13,* 252–258.

Pacala, J. T., Kane, R. L., Atherly, A., & Smith, M. A. (2000). Using structures implicit review to assess quality of care in the Program of All-inclusive Care for the Elderly (PACE). *Journal of the American Geriatrics Society, 48*(8), 1–15.

Pearson, L. (2002). Annual legislative update. How each state stands on legislative issues affecting advanced nursing practice. *Nurse Practitioner, 27*(1), 7–13.

Phillips, D. Erecting an ethical framework for managed care. *Journal of the American Medical Association, 280,* 2062–2064.

Pinkerton, J., & Bush, H. A. (2000). Nurse practitioners and physicians: Patients' perceived health and satisfaction with care. *Journal of the American Academy of Nurse Practitioners, 12*(6), 210–217.

Robinson, J. C. (2001). The end of managed care. *Journal of the American Medical Association, 285,* 2622–2628.

Roper, W., & Mays, G. (1998). The changing managed care-public health interface. *Journal of the American Medical Association, 280,* 1739–1740.

Rueben, D., Schnelle, J. Buchanan, J., Kington, R., Zellman, G., O'Farley, D., Hirsch, S., & Ouslander, J. (1999). Primary care of long-stay nursing home residents: Approaches of three health maintenance organizations. *Journal of the American Geriatrics Society, 47,* 131–138.

Sox, H. (2000). Independent primary care practice by nurse practitioners. *Journal of the American Medical Association, 283,* 106–108.

Stahl, D. A. (2000). Subacute care for seniors: Implications of the Balanced Budget Act of 1997. *Clinics in Geriatric Medicine, 6*(4), 1–16.

Strahan, G. W. (1997). *An overview of nursing homes and their current residents: Data from the 1995 National Nursing Home Survey.* (Advance data from Vital and Health Statistics, no. 280.) Hyattsville, MD: National Center for Health Statistics.

University of Illinois. (2001). *Who will care for each of us? America's coming health care crisis.* A Report from the Panel on the Future of the Health Care Labor Force in a Graying Society, The Honorable Lynn Martin, Chair.

U.S. General Accounting Office. (2001). *Nursing workforce—Recruitment and retention of nurses and nurses aides is a growing concern.* Statement of William J. Scanlon, GAO-01-750T.

Chapter **8**

NURSE PRACTITIONERS IN THE SCHOOL-BASED HEALTH CARE ENVIRONMENT

Judith B. Igoe

School-based health care offers nurse practitioners and nurses an exceptional opportunity to combine and create new forms of primary health care (population-focused programs and services), as well as primary care (personal health services). For example, the Individuals with Disabilities Education Act (IDEA) provides access to a free and appropriate education in school to millions of children and youth with disabilities and other special health care needs. These students come to school with a variety of primary care needs that must be managed throughout the day if they are to remain in school, such as catheterization, gastric feedings, medication administration, and nasogastric suctioning. This care presents a challenge to all nurses because these students must also learn to care for themselves with greater independence. *Healthy People 2010,* the nation's primary health care agenda, calls for nurses in schools to offer population-focused disease prevention and health promotion programs with self-care themes in order to improve the lifestyles of Americans beginning in childhood and adolescence (U.S. Department of Health and Human Services, 2000).

The importance of having health services available at schools cannot be overstated. A significant number of children are at risk of school failure due to social, emotional, or health problems. Seven percent of children ages 5 to 17 are limited in their activities because of chronic health conditions.

Thirteen percent of public school children and youth are enrolled in special education programs. Students identified as learning disabled are 6% of total enrollment (National Center for Education Statistics, 2002).

Poverty, homelessness, substance abuse, violence, and suicide continue to plague young people and interfere with their well-being and school success. Children and youth in low-income families have significantly higher rates of activity limitation due to chronic conditions (Federal Interagency Forum on Child and Family Statistics, 2002). In addition, increasing numbers of children and youth with special needs from multicultural backgrounds are attending schools. The number of school-age children who spoke a language other than English at home and who had difficulty speaking English doubled from 1979 to 1999, representing 5% of all school-age children in the United States. In the western United States, 29% of children had difficulty speaking English (Federal Interagency Forum on Child and Family Statistics, 2002).

At the same time, the number of nurse practitioners and other nurses practicing in schools has increased over the last 5 years (Centers for Disease Control and Prevention, 2000). School-based student health centers have demonstrated impressive results in terms of the quantity and quality of health services available to students who are poor, without access to primary care, and at high risk. Indeed, investigators have reported 8 out of 10 students enrolled in school-based student health centers regularly make use of the services and report high satisfaction (Lear, Eichner, & Koppelman, 1999). While the evaluation of generalized nursing services in schools has been more limited, this public health approach is also the subject of growing attention (Igoe, 2000).

This chapter focuses on the education, role, functions, and accomplishments of nurse practitioners in school-based health facilities and on the operation and effectiveness of school-based health centers. Some of the key literature concerning school-based student health centers will be reviewed. References regarding the practice of the school nurse in the delivery of generalized primary health services and management of the overall school health program are plentiful and can be found elsewhere (Iverson & Harp, 1994; Passarelli, 1993; Schwab & Gelfman, 2001).

EDUCATIONAL PREPARATION OF THE SCHOOL NURSE PRACTITIONER

In 1968, Aria Rosner, nursing supervisor for the Denver Public Schools, came to the schools of nursing and medicine at the University of Colorado

Health Sciences Center with a request for an adaptation of the pediatric nurse practitioner (PNP) role for improvement of school health programs in the school district (Rosner, 1973). At that time, findings from a recently released health survey concerning access to primary care for school-age youth in Denver were discouraging. Although Denver Health and Hospitals opened one of the first community health centers in the country in 1965, 25% of students (approximately 15,000 children and youth) were not using these neighborhood facilities. Many of these students were poor, eligible for this care, and had serious health problems.

Plans to develop a school nurse practitioner (SNP) program were soon underway. Tables 8.1 and 8.2 represent the competencies and educational guidelines for the preparation of school nurse practitioners developed in 1977 by the American Nurses Association, the American School Health Association, and the Department of School Nurses/National Education Association (now the National Association of School Nurses) (1978). The American Academy of Pediatrics added its support several years later. At about the same time these guidelines were published, the American Nurses Association established a school nurse practitioner certification program.

Since then, there have been several joint endorsements of the role and functions of the SNP from a variety of professional associations, including the National Association of School Nurses, the American School Health Association, and the American Nurses Association (Institute of Medicine, 1997). Furthermore, the existence of the National Nursing Coalition for School Health—which includes the National Association of Pediatric Nurse Associates and Practitioners, the National Association of School Nurses, the National Association of State School Nurse Consultants, the American School Health Association, and the Public Health Nursing Section of the American Public Health Association—and the establishment of a National Center for School Nurses within the American Nurses Foundation in Washington, D.C., clearly demonstrate that primary care nurses (nurse practitioners) and primary health care nurses (generalist school nurses) are committed to working together for the improvement of student health.

Between 1969 and 1989, nearly 400 school nurse practitioners were prepared at the University of Colorado. Funding to support the program came from the U.S. Department of Health and Human Services, Health Resources Services Administration, Bureau of Health Professions, Division of Nursing. The first nurses admitted into the program came from Colorado schools, but by the mid-1970s there was a growing demand for this program from school nurses throughout the country.

A summer program was established in Colorado with distance learning arrangements so that nurses came to Colorado for two summers for didactic

TABLE 8.1   Guidelines on Competencies of the School Nurse Practitioner

On completion of a formal course of study, school nurse practitioners should demonstrate their competency by performing the following activities:

1. Serve as a health advocate for the child.
2. Assist parents in assuming greater responsibility for health maintenance of the child, and provide relevant health instruction, counseling, and guidance.
3. Contribute to the health education of individuals and groups, and apply methods designed to increase each person's motivation to assume responsibility for his or her own health care.
4. Assess and arrange appropriate management and referrals for children with health problems who require further evaluation and care by their personal physicians or others, and collaborate with them in decision making involving health care and services.
5. Help families who are devoid of physician services to find a personal physician or other primary care provider who will assume ongoing responsibility for health care.
6. Collaborate with teachers and other school personnel by interpreting pupil health status, and provide guidance regarding adjustments and management of educational and health programs for students with special needs.
7. Identify the health status of the child by securing and evaluating a thorough health and developmental history, and record the findings succinctly and systematically.
8. Assist in obtaining an appropriate physical examination.
9. Initiate, perform, and assess appropriate preventive, developmental, and screening tests, and refer, whenever necessary, through appropriate channels.
10. Participate with other health and educational professionals in the evaluation and management of children with health, learning, and emotional problems.
11. Assist in determining the presence of significant emotional disturbances and psycho-socio-educational problems in childhood and adolescence, and in planning for referral and management of these problems.
12. Provide appropriate emergency health services.
13. Advise and counsel students concerning acute and chronic health problems, and assume responsibility for appropriate intervention, management, or referral.
14. Make home visits when indicated for effective management of health problems.
15. Participate in providing anticipatory guidance and counseling to parents concerning problems of child rearing, including those related to developmental crises, common illnesses, accidents, dental health, and nutrition.

(continued)

TABLE 8.1   Guidelines on Competencies of the
School Nurse Practitioner (continued)

16. Identify community resources.
17. Participate in developing and coordinating health care plans, involving family, school, and community, to enhance the quality of health care to diminish both fragmentation and duplication of services.
18. Assess and evaluate nursing practice in the school setting.

Source: Guidelines on Educational Preparation and Competencies of the School Nurse Practitioners. (1978). A Joint Statement of the American Nurses Association, the American School Health Association, the Department of School Nurses/National Education Association. Journal of School Health, 48(5), 265–266. Reprinted with permission. American School Health Association, Kent, Ohio.

and clinical work. During the other months, the nurses engaged in independent study assignments as well as an intensive year-long practicum with a physician preceptor in their own communities. Physician preceptors were especially important for nurse practitioners in schools because of the isolation of school settings from the medical community. The practicum enhanced the nurses' clinical skills and also provided an opportunity to orient physicians to the SNP role and encourage their support. It was also an ideal time to recruit physicians for more active participation in school health.

Between 1970 and the present, the federal government through the Bureau of Health Professions, Division of Nursing at the Health Resource Services Administration of the U.S. Department of Health and Human Services funded school nurse practitioner programs throughout the United States. Some of these programs, like the Colorado program, moved from certificate to graduate degree programs. Here SNP course work was often incorporated into family, pediatric, and mental health primary care programs. This action resulted in an increasing number of nurse practitioners with a variety of backgrounds entering schools as primary care providers for school-based student health centers. At the same time the number of specialized educational programs for SNPs decreased.

The SNP program led to the development of a certification program for graduates that was offered first through the American Nurses Association and subsequently the Nurse Credentialing Center. From the outset, this certification program generated a great deal of debate about whether or not the SNP credential should be separate from the PNP certificate. No consensus was ever reached, and the SNP certification program was eventually closed to new applicants during the 1990s because of a limited demand for this credential.

TABLE 8.2   Guidelines on Educational Preparation
of the School Nurse Practitioner

The course of study of the school nurse practitioner program should add to the nurse's existing base of nursing knowledge and skills and should provide an opportunity to increase the nurse's ability to make discriminative assessments of the health status of the school child.

The following general areas should be covered in the curriculum:

Growth and Development—A comprehensive review of physical, perceptual, cognitive, and psychological growth and development and their normal variations, including the use of appropriate screening instruments.

Interviewing and Counseling—The principles of the interviewing process and basic approaches to counseling pupils and their parents, including utilization of psychotherapeutic, behavior modification, and anticipatory guidance techniques.

Family Dynamics—A study of the attitudes that affect member interactions and the critical periods in family life, including the effect of family dynamics and sociocultural patterns on health.

Positive Health Maintenance and Health Education—
a) The study of the knowledge and techniques necessary for school nurse practitioners to obtain adequate health appraisal to assess nutritional status and dental health.
b) The common emotional adjustment problems of each age group.
c) Principles of health education, including disease and accident prevention.

Childhood Illness—Review of the common pediatric illnesses, their prevention and management, and the early recognition of complications.

Exceptional Child—Study of physical, emotional, and environmental factors that influence a child's ability to function in the school setting.

Mental Health—Review of the factors that affect the emotional and psychological development of the child and his or her relationship to others.

Community Resources and Delivery of Child Health Care Services—Review of community resources, health delivery systems, and the referral process.

Family/Nurse/Physician/School Relationship—Interpretation of the goals of the team and required role changes. Review of the elements required to effect change.

Clinical Experience—Planned field experiences and practice in schools and other settings under the direction of competent instructors and practitioners that provide a transition from theory to clinical application.

Source: Guidelines on Educational Preparation and Competencies of the School Nurse Practitioners. (1978). A Joint Statement of the American Nurses Association, the American School Health Association, the Department of School Nurses/National Education Association. *Journal of School Health, 48*(5), 265–266. Reprinted with permission. American School Health Association, Kent, Ohio.

ROLE, FUNCTIONS, AND EFFECTIVENESS OF THE SCHOOL NURSE PRACTITIONER

A compelling argument for differentiating the SNP from the PNP role and functions, initially, was the desire to prepare SNPs in depth for this specialized practice within a limited period of time. Several characteristics distinguished the SNP role and educational program from the PNP role and program. Nurse practitioners for schools had to know how school districts operated, in contrast to health delivery systems, including their structure and organizational culture, approach to policy making, financing, capacity and resources for school health, program management models, staffing arrangements, and communication styles. Second, the nurses had to learn how to set up and manage a primary care center in a nontraditional health setting. They also need to know how to obtain access to resources for simple laboratory procedures, how to expand data systems to accommodate more health information about individual students, and how to address more complicated issues of student confidentiality that have recently intensified as primary care providers in schools find themselves struggling to comply with the Health Insurance Portability and Privacy Act (HIPPA) and the Family Educational Rights and Privacy Act (FERPA). Furthermore, school nurse practitioners would need to be able to bridge the gap between health and education systems for referral, follow-up, and case/care management of students receiving primary care in the schools. Finally, issues of role conflict between school nurses, other school and community personnel, and SNPs required additional understanding and skill.

In schools, the chief informant is often a child rather than an adult. Consequently, the child, as well as his/her parents, has to be informed and involved in the delivery of any health service. Acknowledgment of this fact means that SNPs must be extremely skilled in communicating at the child's level of understanding. Some programs have met this challenge over the years by hiring school-age youth as patient models to work side by side with nurses enrolled in the SNP program. Another instructional strategy involves the use of a special group of preceptors. Elementary school teachers have role-modeled and coached nurses during their interactions with young school children with successful results.

School nurse practitioners prepared at Colorado received special neurodevelopment instruction and closely supervised clinical practice so that they had a clear understanding of how students process information and learn. Eventually, all SNPs were prepared to administer and interpret a number of neurodevelopmental, mid-level assessment tools, including those developed by Levine.

By the mid-1970s, the Handicapped Children's Act (now the Individuals with Disabilities Act, reauthorized in 1997 as P.L. 105-117) had passed. Nurses qualified to deliver primary care in schools now also required the skills necessary to provide complex nursing care to students with disabilities and special health care needs. The key objective now was that nurses know and be able to explain the link between the health service to be delivered and the child's ability to learn. The nurse became part of an interdisciplinary team of school psychologists, social workers, counselors, teachers, speech pathologists, and physical and occupational therapists. School nurse practitioners had to familiarize themselves with developmental and educational assessments as well as therapeutic tools and approaches used by a wide range of professionals.

Since emotional and behavioral disorders were as prevalent among students as physical health complaints, SNPs received instruction and closely supervised clinical practice in the assessment and management of children and youth with such disorders. Although the extent of their skill was never intended to match that of the clinical psychiatric nurse specialist, SNPs were prepared to perform mental health status exams and initiate simple interventions and referrals.

The initial anecdotal studies of school nurse practitioners yielded several practice models. In one model, the SNP was responsible for the entire school health program in one or two schools. In another model, the SNP floated between several schools where assigned school nurses did the subsequent follow-up case management. In a third model, the SNP worked from school-based as well as mobile student health centers.

Early studies of the SNPs in the 1980s by Goodwin (1981) and Meeker, DeAngeles, Berman, Freeman, and Oda (1986) indicated the nurses were capable of handling 87% of student complaints. One investigation even reported a 96% problem resolution rate for SNPs. It was also this author's impression that when SNPs functioned as gatekeepers to the rest of the school and community primary care teams (thereby limiting the delivery of unnecessary services), the cost of this care in schools was probably 4 times less than the cost in traditional community health care facilities where students often failed to keep their appointments and to follow through with prescribed therapies. This estimate was based on a comparison of the average national costs of pediatric primary care per child in the community at the time versus the cost of SNP services in a school-based student health center. The assumption here was the nurse practitioner would do the initial workup and, depending upon the findings, decide with the interdisciplinary school team if more diagnostic work was needed and by whom. This approach is in sharp contrast with the arena style of health services delivery that prevails in many school-based student health centers today, where each student sees a number of providers simultaneously (e.g., social worker, psychologist, mental health specialist, etc.).

A CONCEPTUAL FRAMEWORK FOR THE PRACTICE OF SCHOOL NURSE PRACTITIONERS

In 1987, the conceptual framework for SNPs depicted in Figure 8.1 was developed in accordance with the competencies and educational guidelines for SNPs presented in Tables 8.1 and 8.2. The framework borrows heavily from the work of nursing faculty at the University of Minnesota during the 1980s (Wold, 1981), but appears to be still relevant for nurse practitioners in schools today. There were three purposes for developing this framework:

1. to operationalize the role;
2. to foster uniformity of practice;
3. to identify specific areas of practices for which new knowledge and services would need to be discovered, including the development of assessment and intervention tools.

The fact that SNPs work in settings where health and education are closely intertwined and the students, as a whole, are generally physically healthy, has always meant that their practice emerges out of nursing as well as a host of other disciplines in addition to medicine (e.g., psychology, education, speech pathology, counseling). Today that practice is increasingly evidence based.

The perspective presented in Figure 8.1 suggests that the real and potential health problems of school-age youth are heavily influenced by the child/family's (1) self-concept; (2) sense of physical, emotional, academic, and social integrity; (3) problem-solving abilities; and (4) level of energy. Consequently, the subjective and objective segments of the health assessments for these children and youth target these areas. Health histories, for example, are designed to elicit in-depth information about school performance, peer relationships, and family progress with developmental tasks. Children with special health care needs, who are shuttled from one special service to the next and experience a sense of disjointedness rather than solidarity, are carefully evaluated for indications of high stress and poor coping mechanisms that interfere with their ability to learn. SNPs are also especially concerned about students who come frequently to their health

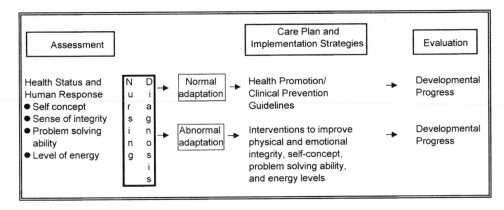

FIGURE 8.1   A conceptual framework for the practice of school nurse practitioners.

office/center with vague nonspecific complaints. These symptoms often are the first signs of school adjustment problems that will eventually place these students at high risk for school failure (Lewis & Lewis, 1989).

Equally important areas of investigation for SNPs are determinations of the child's level of energy as measured subjectively and objectively by a series of questions and tests intended to identify the amount of rest, uninterrupted sleep, and exercise students receive on a regular basis as well as their physical strength and endurance levels.

Physical examinations as well as health history sessions are opportunities for students to actively participate in their evaluation with their parents and the nurse. Overall and specific cerebral functions are key areas of the physical examination to identify processing disorders that may slow down and/or limit the student's academic performance. Mental health status examinations are indicated if the initial assessment indicates problem areas, such as student mastery of age-appropriate problem-solving skills.

Other developmental assessments are often conducted as indicated. The strengths and functional abilities of the child and family, as well as real or potential limitations, are incorporated into the diagnosis.

Interventions are designed to manage acute and chronic physical and mental health complaints as well as difficulties associated with poor self-concept, a diminished sense of integrity, dilemmas with problem solving, and low levels of energy. For students who are uninsured, poor, and struggling with chronic diseases that require medications and special therapeutic services, the case management work is complex and time consuming. Although some of these students are eligible for related health services in schools, others are not. Because the insurance benefit plans of students who are insured vary a great deal, negotiation and conflict management skills are also essential as is teamwork with the interdisciplinary staff at school and in community agencies. Making the link between school, family, and community agencies is frequently a challenge.

Perhaps the best overall indicator of the impact of the evidence-based practice of SNPs, as reflected in Figure 8.1, is the developmental progress of the students academically, psychologically, socially, and physically. While problem-resolution rates and documentation of the cost-effectiveness of this role have special appeal to policy makers, what really matters in the end is whether children and youth grow and develop into healthy, well-adjusted adults.

School nurse practitioners need a variety of data-based assessment and intervention tools to operationalize the framework presented in Figure 8.1. Health history techniques for youth, who view such activities as interrogations, need to be designed to increase the reliability of the informant. Validated stress-management services for students who frequently seek assistance from SNPs are also needed. Even the centuries-old problem of head lice continues to consume an enormous amount of time, and benchmarking best practice must be done. Strategies to address nonadherence with care plans also deserve a great deal more attention.

HEALTH EDUCATION AND SCHOOL NURSE PRACTITIONERS

Health education in schools is a major component of school health programming. Although nurse practitioners could be taught classroom teaching skills, it seemed unlikely that they would be free from clinic responsibilities for this type of health teaching. Furthermore, their school nurse colleagues, in many instances, have already been well prepared and are working closely with school health educators and teachers to manage the classroom-based health education component of school health. Therefore, a new consumer health education program was designed in the 1970s for SNPs and other primary care providers at school to fill an existing void in the health education curriculum for schools. Known as HealthPACT, the consumer health education lessons taught by primary care providers focus on the development of a more participatory and informed consumer role beginning in early childhood (Igoe, 1991). Specifically, students, their families, teachers, and community health providers are introduced to a new set of social skills or norms for students to strengthen and enhance their consumer behavior during visits for health care. An acronym for this skill set, TLADD, helps them to remember and use the code: talk, listen and learn, ask, decide, do. Subsequently other HealthPACT lessons help students learn developmentally appropriate self-help measures. Finally, the topic "What is the health system and how does it work?" is being introduced into social studies classes at the elementary and middle school grade levels and into consumer studies in secondary schools.

THE FUTURE OF SCHOOL NURSE PRACTITIONERS

From the late 1980s to the present, numerous pediatric and family nurse practitioner programs have incorporated student learning experiences in the school setting, including school-based student health centers. Questions have been raised as to whether the content areas and supervised practice guidelines listed in Tables 8.1 and 8.2 have actually been integrated into these programs. Today, instruction time is limited and there is pressure to limit rather than expand the course work in graduate nurse practitioner programs. Therefore, postgraduate certificate programs for primary care providers who wish to subspecialize is a sensible option.

The complexity of student health problems has intensified. The design and operation of school-based health centers, including the linkage of data management systems between the community health system and the school for case management purposes, have also become more complicated. In addition, chronic health conditions such as asthma, diabetes, and eating disorders and complex problems like substance abuse, adolescent pregnancy, and depression demand additional skill from nurse practitioners.

Consequently, nurse practitioners working in school-based centers who lack experience in school health, primary health care, and educational systems and who need more advanced knowledge and skills in mental health, neurodevelopment, adolescent health, consumer health education, and care of students with special health care needs face many barriers in achieving results. Postmaster's education is one strategy for dealing with these challenges.

Following an invitational conference on school nursing roles sponsored by the Centers for Disease Control and Prevention, Division of Adolescent and School Health; the publication of an Institute of Medicine report on school health; and the availability of national health and safety guidelines for schools from the American Academy of Pediatrics and the National Association of School Nurses, it is clear that the delivery of primary care in schools will continue.

SCHOOL-BASED STUDENT HEALTH CENTERS

School-based student health centers (SBHCs) have grown rapidly in the United States since the first centers appeared in 1970. In the fall of 1994, 623 sites were reported, operating in middle schools and high schools. In 1997, 900 sites were in existence, and by 2000 there were 1,380 in 45 states and the District of Columbia (Making the Grade, 2000). School-based health centers still reach only a small fraction of U.S. students; however, the contributions of the primary care providers who work in these centers need more visibility within traditional school health organizations such as the American School Health Association, the National Association of School Nurses, and the National Assembly of School Based Student Health Centers. Indeed, the National Nurses Coalition for School Health, which represents all of these organizations, may be the nursing group to assume this responsibility.

Typically located in low-income communities underserved by other health providers, school-based student health centers offer a wide range of free or minimum-cost services, including treatment/referral for acute illnesses, injuries, pregnancy, and sexually transmitted diseases; routine screenings (vision, hearing); preventive care (physical examinations, immunizations); birth control services (prescribing/dispensing contraceptives); management of chronic diseases and disorders; and care, consultation, and referral for psychosocial problems (Kisker & Brown, 1996).

Elementary schools provide a setting to address the health needs of children before they develop unhealthy habits in nutrition, fitness, sexuality, and substance use. SBHCs are structured to serve an important function in teaching prevention and health education (National Health and Education Consortium, 1995). Staffing for SBHCs varies, depending on the facility. Typically, the full-time staff consists of a nurse practitioner or physician assistant, a school nurse or licensed practical nurse, a medical aide, and a receptionist. Part-time staff may include a physician, a licensed clinical social worker, nutrition and drug abuse specialists, and a health educator (Kisker & Brown, 1996).

The Clinton Administration looked to SBHCs in 1994 as one vehicle of health care reform, through which an improved system of personal health services for children and adolescents could be delivered on a national scale. Although federal health care reform legislation was never enacted, the Federal Bureau of Primary Care and the Maternal Child Health (MCH) Bureau of the Health Resources and Services Administration (HRSA) joined together in 1994 to provide the first direct federal funding, $11.9 million, for 27 SBHC demonstration projects (Santelli, Kouzis, & Newcomer, 1996; Santelli, Morreale, Wigton, & Grayson, 1996).

Community Support for SBHCs

Most school-based health centers encounter community scrutiny during the planning and implementation phases and, if they are established, have strong community backing, but with varying degrees of support for provision of reproductive health services. Goals stated for most school clinics are to improve child and adolescent access to primary care, including the reduction of teenage pregnancy. Most decisions about the scope of clinic services are made on the local level, although several states have passed laws limiting school-based reproductive health care (Santelli, Alexander, et al., 1992). Of the 45 states and the District of Columbia that have SBHCs, 24 states have created a governmental unit explicitly charged "to develop and support" the centers. The fastest growth of SBHCs has been in the Southwest and Rocky Mountain regions. Since these regions are generally more politically conservative, this development suggests a continued migration of SBHCs into the mainstream (Lear et al., 1999).

Working effectively in a coordinated fashion with a broad array of community stakeholders will be key to the success of each SBHC. Staff at the Edison SBHC in Kalamazoo, Michigan, faced challenges that forced them to embrace an encompassing systemic perspective and demonstrated that health services must be defined in relationship to all stakeholders in the student health care context (Cousins, Jackson, & Till, 1997). The SBHC served by the University of Rochester Community Nursing Center (CNC) is known in its community as a "center without walls." All students are eligible to participate with written parental permission. The major barrier is getting parents to complete the consent forms and provide insurance information. Lessons for other SBHCs from the CNC include its reputation for building true partnerships rather than simply "using" the community for research and education. The CNC also learned that it takes time to gain input and approval from community members, state personnel, county health department staff, and local school systems (Walker, Baker, & Civerton, 1997).

Finally, Denver's 1990 pilot project to once again prepare school nurses as school nurse practitioners was an effort to provide a school health workforce better designed to serve students in an environment of managed care and to meet the overlapping health and social needs of disadvantaged students. Although local physicians questioned the adequacy of the training that nurses received, stakeholder response was largely positive among school personnel and students. Community parents, in particular, were pleased with the convenience of Denver's program (Brindis et al., 1998). Currently, the challenge for Denver and other metropolitan areas in which SBHCs are located in schools, but are managed by local health departments, community health centers, or public hospitals, is to provide a seamless set of services through collaboration and cooperation with the rest of the school health team (school physicians, nurses, psychologists, counselors, social workers, etc.), who are employed by the school districts.

Access to Care

Many researchers and government studies have confirmed that school-based health centers have improved students' access to primary care health services, especially for low-income, medically underserved, and high-risk students (Santelli, Morreale, et al., 1996). Barriers to health care for adolescents include lack of health insurance; lack of providers who accept Medicaid; inability to obtain care on their own because of their age and limited financial resources; confidentiality concerns; lack of transportation to doctors' facilities; and school schedules that conflict with doctors' hours. SBHCs remove these barriers by offering free health care on the school premises, where most youth spend a significant portion of their day (Kisker & Brown, 1996). However, other barriers remain. Regional social conservatism and politically active religious organizations such as the Christian Coalition impede clinic success (Rienzo, Button, & Wald, 2000). Parental notification rules required of many clinics are also a barrier to providing reproductive and other health services (Fothergill & Feijoo, 2000).

A study of 24 Robert Wood Johnson Foundation-funded SBHCs found that for a small but significant number of students, the student health center became their usual place for receiving health care. These students were those with less access to other health care providers and those with greater health care needs (Kisker & Brown, 1996). School programs are increasingly perceived as key structures in the delivery of health care to our nation's youth, particularly youth from underserved populations (Parker & Logan, 2000). In fact, as one principal noted about the SBHC, "a lot of Hispanic kids and their families have access to human services for the first time in my school" (Dryfoos, 1998).

New Mexico's youth face some of the nation's highest rates of poverty, substance abuse, suicide, and school dropout. The state has pushed to increase access to SBHCs as an important intervention toward reducing youth homelessness, pregnancy, mental health problems, domestic violence, and entry into the juvenile justice system (Adelsheim, 1999).

While the number of SBHCs has grown extensively and some have expanded services, others have barely survived or even closed. Measures of clinic success and increased access include operating budget, average number of working hours, number of health services provided, and average number of hours open over the summer. Part of the reason student health centers have not become the usual place for student care lies in the fact that SBHCs do not provide 24-hour or weekend/holiday service. Tight budgets and lack of staff and resources limit most centers to operation only during school hours. Most centers must also limit their services to only their student population and not to adolescents in the broader community or to children of students or other members of a student's family. These limitations may be reduced if SBHCs become integrated into community systems of care (Santelli, Morreale, et al., 1996). The other option would be to increase the number of states that provide Medicaid reimbursement for school-based student health services and to maximize other existing reimbursements.

Student Usage Patterns

Studies of student enrollment and use of SBHCs correlate with several factors, including race, gender, insurance coverage, and existing health problems.

In a 1992 study of nine Baltimore schools with SBHCs, Santelli, Alexander, et al. found SBHC enrollees more likely than nonenrollees to be African American, female, attending one or more special education classes, or to have Medicaid. Enrollee percentages, however, were influenced by the fact that these nine schools had an overall higher proportion of Blacks and females. Other predictors of enrollment were one or more self-reported health problems, enrollment of close peers, and membership in a school club, sports team, or church organization. The most common reason for not enrolling was satisfaction with the current health provider (Santelli, Kouzis, & Newcomer, 1996).

In a West Virginia study assessing the ability of SBHCs to provide health care access to rural youth, it was found that youth who are uninsured or who receive public assistance made proportionately greater use of the SBHC than their counterparts (Crespo & Shaler, 2000). Another study showed that students with no health insurance coverage were 5% more likely to visit their SBHC than were students with private insurance or health maintenance organization coverage (Kisker & Brown, 1996).

Student use of a health center presumably increases as trust is developed through positive experiences. The enrollees in the nine Baltimore schools discussed above said they would be most supportive of using their SBHC for first aid, treatment for colds, and sports physical examinations and least supportive of using it for counseling services. Studies of SBHC use, however, show heavy use of counseling services, much of which may come from frequent SBHC users (Santelli, Kouzis, & Newcomer, 1996). In the nine schools, the students who reported the most favorable attitudes and trust were those who used their health centers the most. The researchers concluded that "treatment for minor problems probably increases adolescent willingness to use the health center for more serious problems" (Santelli, Kouzis, & Newcomer, 1996).

Twenty-four SBHCs located in major U.S. cities, funded by the Robert Wood Johnson Foundation, showed the following overall usage patterns in 1991–1992: 29% of student visits were for acute illness or injury; 18% for mental health problems; 18% for immunizations, nutrition counseling, and dental care; 15% for physical examinations; 10% for reproductive health, sexually transmitted diseases, and family planning; 6% for chronic disease management; and 4% for skin problems (Santelli, Morreale, et al., 1996).

In a study to assess adolescent use of services in a community health network (CHN) and an SBHC, users were predominately female (61%), Hispanic (67%), or African American (16.2%), and not on Medicaid (76%). The mean age of users at their first contact was 16.2 years of age. Out of 1,953 visits to both facilities, 64% were for medical and 36% were for mental health services. Mental health and substance abuse diagnoses were 20 times more likely to be generated at the SBHC than the CHN (Juszczak, 1999).

Further evidence of the need for mental health services at SBHCs is noted in a study of an urban high school SBHC. Of students surveyed, 31% had depression problems, 5% used alcohol daily, 10% had a history of a suicide attempt, and 50% knew someone who had been murdered (Pastore, Juszczak, Fisher, & Friedman, 1998). As noted by Jepson, Juszczak, and Fisher (1998), adolescents are less likely to seek services in an unfamiliar setting. Therefore, obtaining mental health services at an SBHC would be more likely since the setting is familiar and usage does not require extensive planning.

Evaluation of SBHC Outcomes

The outcomes produced by school-based health centers have yet to be thoroughly evaluated (Santelli, Morreale, et al., 1996). School-based health centers have diverse functions, including primary medical care, mental health care, counseling, and other social services; health education; health promotion interventions; and delinquency prevention. Because of this, researchers have had difficulty designing research models that will reveal the real effects of school-based health centers (Santelli, Morreale, et al., 1996).

Studies that have focused on a particular population or condition have had some concrete results. A school-based asthma clinic pilot program staffed by a nurse practitioner was limited by a small sample size but resulted in measurable improvement in asthma symptoms and functional status (Meng, 2000). In another study, a school wide asthma detection and treatment program in an inner-city elementary school health center resulted in significantly decreased hospitalization rates and increased outpatient care visits and visits to asthma specialists (Lurie, Bauer, & Brady, 2001).

Health Outcomes

Generally speaking, the health outcomes that could be expected of school-based health centers would include improvement of student overall health status, increase in health knowledge, increase in student preventive health practices, and reduction in risk-taking behaviors (Kisker & Brown, 1996). Some studies have showed SBHCs have positively influenced immunization administration rates and compliance (Sanford, 2001), as well as reductions in alcohol consumption, smoking, sexual activity, and pregnancy, but findings have been inconsistent (Santelli, Morreale, et al., 1996).

A study of 24 SBHCs, begun in 1989 by Kisker and Brown, followed students from their 9th or 10th grade in school through graduation age. Findings indicated that school-based health centers can increase students' access to health care and their health knowledge, particularly for homeless and low-income children, but that centers may not significantly reduce risk-taking behaviors, such as smoking, use of alcohol, and unprotected sexual activity. The researchers recommended that student health centers institute more intense, consistent interventions earlier, before students engage in risk-taking behavior.

Shuler (2000) recommended that a holistic approach to evaluating services and examining care utilization may yield better results in reducing risky behaviors. In the holistic approach, a multidisciplinary team coordinated by the nurse practitioner addresses students' health in the context of their physical, social, psychological, environmental, and other needs. Using similar logic, Simeonsson and Simeonsson (1999) concluded that the potential for a positive impact on health status increases when a population is viewed as a whole or as a set of subpopulations with specific health risks to be reduced or prevented.

School Performance Outcomes

Because good health is essential to effective learning, school performance outcomes occur after one or more health outcomes are observed. These could be expected to include consistent attendance, involvement in school activities, positive feelings about school and self, adequate progress in school, and high school graduation. The influence of the student health center in student education outcomes may be even more indirect, as the research described below seems to indicate.

McCord, Klein, Foy, and Fothergill (1993) studied student use of a school-based clinic and student absence, suspension, withdrawal, and grade promotion/graduation status over one academic year. Study subjects were high-risk adolescents attending an alternative high school in Greensboro, North Carolina. On average, the student body attended school only 56% of the time, 24% were suspended, and 26% were promoted. Researchers found that the students who used the school health clinic (49% of the student body) were just as likely to miss school or be suspended as were students not enrolled in the clinic; however, clinic users were twice as likely to stay in school and graduate or be promoted than nonclinic students. The greater the students' exposure to the clinic, the stronger the relationship between clinic use and graduation or promotion became. The research concluded that clinic personnel had provided students with positive role models and social support, which helped students identify with these role models and function better in school.

Another study compared students in 19 regular high schools, who were enrolled in their school health center, against a national sample of urban youths. In that study, the levels of absences because of illness were not significantly different between the two groups, but the percentage of students who progressed through school at the expected pace was slightly higher for the health center students than for the national urban sample. The difference was small but statistically significant: 78% vs. 75% (Kisker & Brown, 1996).

As many as 70% to 80% of children and youth who use mental health services receive that care only at school. A study of psychosocial functioning performed at a public high school SBHC with a large immigrant population concluded that adolescents identified by the screening tool who were referred to mental health services significantly reduced their rates of absence and tardiness (Gall, Pagano, Desmond, Perrin, & Murphy, 2000).

COLLABORATION

SBHCs can benefit from partnerships with community organizations and hospitals to maintain viability, attract funding, and share resources. In the most effective SBHC collaborations with business, political, and nonprofit organizations, benefits are shared equally. These benefits may include enhancing an organization's image; increasing access to services, populations, and resources; and increasing community acceptance (Juszczak, Moody, & Vega-Matos, 1998). Hospital sponsorship of SBHCs may improve a hospital's capacity to address its community and charity care mission and increase market share, efficiency, and quality. The benefits to the SBHC may include more clinical expertise, billing and fund-raising support, assistance in developing quality improvement programs, and increased credibility in negotiations with managed care organizations (VHA Health Foundation, 1999).

The Milwaukee Public Schools School-Based/School-Linked Health Centers' (SB/SLHCs) collaborative program increased access for children of working poor families by mobilizing resources among local leaders and the statewide health system. The program's efforts have included assessing needs, sharing data, seeking funds, prioritizing facilities, and establishing more than 30 SB/SLHCs (Willis, 2000).

In a study by Scheuring, Hanna, and D'Aquila-Lloyd (2000), a school of nursing and an SBHC staff joined together to meet each other's missions more effectively and to provide a broader safety net for a healthy student population. Some of their jointly planned services included screenings, a health fair, training, and mentoring. In Connecticut, advocacy groups for child and adolescent mental health were instrumental in convincing legislatures to enact safeguards to maintain SBHCs as providers of health and mental care under managed care (Armbruster, Andrews, Couenhoven, & Blau, 1999). Collaboration and communication with business, political, and other allied forces demonstrate how health care systems can effectively advocate for and impact local services for students, especially those in high-risk groups (Willis, 2000).

FINANCING SBHCs

The viability of SBHCs serving uninsured and Medicaid-insured children and youth increasingly depends on contracts with managed care organizations. Since enactment of the State Child Health Insurance Program (SCHIP), partnering with managed care has become a near necessity for most SBHCs. With congressional authorization of $40 billion for states to purchase health insurance for low-income, uninsured children, SCHIP has become the largest federal investment in child health since Medicaid.

Connecticut's Department of Public Health credits the continuing success of its SBHC program under SCHIP to ongoing communication between the public health and social services departments during the contracting process and to state threats of sanctions on health plans and SBHCs that would not contract. In Colorado, there was officially no problem in selling managed care plans on working with SBHCs because the centers are recognized as great locales for enrollment. School-based health centers also assist managed care organizations in meeting their National Center for Quality Assurance (NCQA) access standards. As these states exemplify, SBHCs can continue successfully under managed care if all partners share in the commitment to providing quality health care to the community (Koppelman & Lear, 1998).

Although there has been some stagnation in state funding of SBHCs (Lear et al., 1999), more than 30 states provide some financial support. Some states are also providing technical assistance and facilitating managed care partnerships (Rienzo et al., 2000). In addition, the overall growth of centers across the nation suggests that SBHCs have increasingly found significant avenues of support such as third-party payments and funding from private institutions. For instance, community and teaching hospitals such as the Duke Medical Center and the Henry Ford Hospital are funding SBHCs in order to receive tax incentives for investing in "community benefit" activities (Lear et al., 1999).

FUTURE OF SBHCs AND PRIMARY CARE IN SCHOOLS

The enormous influence of managed care requires that nurse practitioners invest in educating themselves on the managed care goals of disease prevention and case management. They need to be familiar with Medicaid managed care and waivers in their states and must be willing to become credentialed providers in as many managed care organizations as possible. They need to use and articulate research findings to support the benefits that nurse practitioners bring to managed care goals related to patient satisfaction, practice style, case management, and outreach (Cohen & Juszczak, 1997).

Interest in SBHCs continues not only because of the potential of SBHCs to improve youth and adolescent health in general, but also because of their potential to improve the country's social and economic conditions. For example, if school-based health centers were to become effective in reducing teen pregnancy and high school dropout rates, there could be a corresponding reduction in the multiple health problems associated with teen pregnancy and the unemployment, welfare dependency, and homelessness for which adolescents who do not finish high school are at increased risk (McCord et al., 1993).

The Assembly for School-Based Health Centers has developed standards and guidelines for primary care centers in schools (Brellochs & Fothergill, 1995), which should be very useful for health and education planners who want to establish school-based student health centers.

SUMMARY

Primary care providers in school settings and school-based student health centers are effective in their efforts to improve student health. Schools as nontraditional health settings are newcomers to the primary care delivery system. Therefore, it will be important in the years to come to recognize and take into account certain dilemmas that are somewhat unique to schools and to intensify our efforts to investigate these issues.

For example, the majority of America's school systems (79%)—urban, suburban, and rural—have total enrollments of 2,500 students or less. Hence, a challenge arises in terms of effective and economical staffing arrangements. Should there be a school-based student health center in all 15,000 school districts?

As school nurse supervisors struggle to design safe and sensible staffing arrangements, the issue of differentiated practice will also have to be addressed. A large number of paraprofessionals are now engaged in health-related activities in schools in addition to an estimated 57,954 school nurses (Spratley, Johnson, Sochalski, Fritz, & Spencer, 2000). What relationships need to exist among these individuals to ensure that the health services provided at school are of the highest quality? Certainly, the work of nurse practitioners in school-based student health centers and school nurses would be enhanced with more collaboration.

Finally, for some community organizations, school-based student health centers represent too much of a competitive threat because the student body is a captive audience. Others worry about the type of services being delivered and whether parental rights are being ignored. The point here is that advanced practice nurses have a great deal of knowledge and skill to contribute to these discussions. This author believes that, in the decades to come, school health will rise or fall depending upon the talent, creativity, and leadership of the nurses on its team. This chapter has provided an historical perspective of the SNP role, educational guidelines, and a conceptual framework for practice. Some of the key literature concerning school-based student health centers was also reviewed. Certification as an SNP (not available at present) might be a future possibility if the idea of

SNP postmaster's programs sparks interest. It is hoped that readers will be stimulated by this information to explore the opportunities and challenges the field of school health has to offer.

REFERENCES AND BIBLIOGRAPHY

Adams, E., Shannon, A., & Dworkin, P. (1996). The ready-to-learn program: A school-based model of nurse practitioner participation in evaluating school failure. *Journal of School Health, 66,* 242–246.

Adelsheim, S. (1999). School mental health in New Mexico. In A. H. Esman (Ed.), *Annals of the American society for adolescent psychiatry* (pp. 101–107). Hillsdale, NJ: Analytic Press.

American Nurses Association, American School Health Association, National Education Association, Department of School Nurses. (1978). Guidelines on educational preparation and competencies of school nurse practitioners: A joint statement. *Journal of School Health, 48,* 265–266.

Armbruster, P., Andrews, E., Couenhoven J., & Blau, G. (1999). Collision or collaboration? School-based health services meet managed care. *Clinical Psychology Review, 19,* 221–237.

Berlin, L. E., Stennett, J., & Bednash, G. D. (2002). *2001–2002 Enrollment and graduations in baccalaureate and graduate programs in nursing.* Washington, DC: American Association of Colleges of Nursing.

Brellochs, C., & Fothergill, K. (1995). *Ingredients for success: Comprehensive school based centers. A special report on the 1993 national work group meetings.* Bronx, NY: School Health Policy Initiative, Montefiore Medical Center, Albert Einstein College of Medicine.

Brindis, C. D., Sanghvi, R., Melinkovich, P., Kaplan, D. W., Ahlstrand, K. R., & Phibbs, S. L. (1998). Redesigning a school-health workforce for a new health care environment: Training school nurses as nurse practitioners. *Journal of School Health, 68,* 179–183.

CCD State Nonfiscal Survey of Public Elementary and Secondary Education: School Year 1999–2000. (2001). National Center for Education Statistics. Retrieved April 25, 2003 from http://nces.ed.gov/americaschildren/

Centers for Disease Control and Prevention. (2000, March). *The registered nurse population.* Washington, DC: U.S. Department of Health and Human Services Health Resources and Service Administration Bureau of Health Professions.

Cohen, S. S., & Juszczak, L. (1997). Promoting the nurse practitioner role in managed care. *Journal of Pediatric Health Care, 11,* 3–11.

Cousins, L. H., Jackson, K., & Till, M. (1997). Portrait of a school-based health center: An ecosystemic perspective. *Social Work in Education, 19,* 189–202.

Crespo, R. D., & Shaler, G. A. (2000). Assessment of school-based health centers in a rural state: The West Virginia experience. *Journal of Adolescent Health, 26,* 187–193.

Dryfoos, J. G. (1998). School-based health centers in the context of education reform. *Journal of School Health, 68,* 404–408.

Fothergill, K., & Feijoo, A. (2000). Family planning services at school-based health centers: Findings from a national survey. *Journal of Adolescent Health, 27,* 166–169.

Gall, G., Pagano, M. E., Desmond, M. S., Perrin, J. M., & Murphy, J. M. (2000). Utility of psychosocial screening at a school-based health center. *Journal of School Health, 70,* 292–298.

Goodwin, L. D. (1981). The effectiveness of nurse practitioners: A review of the literature. *Journal of School Health, 51,* 623–624.

Hacker, K., & Wessel, G. (1998). School-based health centers and school nurses: Cementing the collaboration. *Journal of School Health, 68,* 409–414.

Hinton, P., & Chiverton, P. (1997). The University of Rochester experience. *Nursing Management, 28,* 29–31.

Igoe, J. B. (1991). Empowerment of children and youth for consumer self-care. *American Journal of Health Promotion, 6,* 55–64.

Igoe, J. (2000). School nursing today: A search for new cheese. *Journal of School Nursing, 16,* 9–15.

Institute of Medicine. (1997). *Schools and health: Our nation's investment.* Washington, DC: National Academy Press.

Iverson, C. J., & Harp, B. (1994). School nursing in the 21st century: Prediction and readiness. *Journal of School Nursing, 10,* 19–24.

Jepson, L., Juszczak, L., & Fisher, M. (1998). Mental health care in a high school based health service. *Adolescence, 33,* 1–15.

Jones, M. E., & Clark, D. (1997). Increasing access to health care: A study of pediatric nurse practitioner outcomes in a school based clinic. *Journal of Nursing Quality Care, 11,* 53.

Juszczak, L. (1999). Use of health and mental health services by adolescents across multiple delivery sites. *Dissertation Abstracts International, 60,* 2639B.

Juszczak, L., Moody, J., & Vega-Matos, C. (1998). Business and faith: Key community partnerships for school-based health centers. *Journal of School Health, 68,* 429–433.

Kaplan, D., Calonge, N., Guernsey, B., & Hanrahan, M. (1998). Managed care and school-based health centers. *Archives of Pediatric and Adolescent Medicine, 152,* 25–33.

Key National Indicators of Well-Being. (2002). *Federal Interagency Forum on Child and Family Statistics.* Retrieved April 25, 2002 from http:childStats.gov/

Kisker, E. E., & Brown, R. S. (1996). Do school-based health centers improve adolescents' access to health care, health status, & risk-taking behavior? *Journal of Adolescent Health, 18,* 335–343.

Koppelman, J., & Lear, J. G. (1998). The new child health insurance expansions: How will school-based health centers fit in? *Journal of School Health, 68,* 441–446.

Lear, J. G., Eichner, N., & Koppelman, J. (1999). The growth of school based health centers and the role of state policies. *Archives of Pediatric and Adolescent Medicine, 153,* 1177–1180.

Lewis, C., & Lewis, M. A. (1989). Educational outcomes and illness behaviors of participants in a child-initiated care system: A 12-year follow-up study. *Pediatrics, 84*, 845–850.

Lurie, N., Bauer E. J., & Brady, C. (2001). Asthma outcomes at an inner city school-based health center. *Journal of School Health, 71*, 9–16.

Making the Grade. (2000). *School-based health centers: Results from a 50-state survey, school year 1999–2000.* Washington, DC: Center for Health and Health Care in Schools. Retrieved from http://www.healthinschools.org

McCord, M. T., Klein, J .D., Foy, J. M., & Fothergill, K. (1993). School-based clinic use and school performance. *Journal of Adolescent Health, 14*, 91–98.

Meeker, R. J., DeAngelis, C., Berman, B., Freeman, H. E., & Oda, D. (1986). A comprehensive school health initiative. *Image: Journal of Nursing Scholarship, 18*, 86–91.

Meng, A. (2000). A school-based asthma clinic: A partnership model for managing childhood asthma. *Nurse Practitioner Forum, 11*, 38–47.

National Health and Education Consortium. (1995). *Where the kids are: How to work with schools to create elementary school-based health centers.* Washington, DC: National Health and Education Consortium: An initiative of the Institute for Educational Leadership.

Oros, M. T., Perry, L. A., & Heller, B. R. (2000). School-based health services: An essential component of neighborhood transformation. *Family and Community Health, 23*, 31–35.

Parker, V. G., & Logan, B. N. (2000). Students', parents', and teachers' perceptions of health needs of school-age children: Implications for nurse practitioners. *Family and Community Health, 23*, 62–71.

Passarelli, C. (1993). *School nursing: Trends for the future.* Washington, DC: National Health and Education Consortium.

Pastore, D. R., Juszczak, L., Fisher, M. M., & Friedman, S. B. (1998). School-based health center utilization: A survey of users and non-users. *Archives of Pediatrics and Adolescent Medicine, 152*, 763–767.

Rienzo, B. A., Button, J. W., & Wald, K. D. (2000). Politics and the success of school based health centers. *Journal of School Health, 70*, 331–337.

Rosner, A. (1973). Cooperation and change in child health care. *Journal of School Health, 43*, 83–84.

Sanford, C. C. (2001). Delivering health care to children on their turf: An elementary school-based wellness center. *Journal of Pediatric Health Care, 15*, 132–137.

Santelli, J., Alexander, M., Farmer, M., Papa, P., Johnson, T., Rosenthal, B., & Hotra, D. (1992). Bringing parents into school clinics: Parent attitudes toward school clinics and contraception. *Journal of Adolescent Health, 13*, 269–274.

Santelli, J., Kouzis, A., & Newcomer, S. (1996). Students' attitudes toward school-based health centers. *Journal of Adolescent Health, 18*, 339–346.

Santelli, J., Morreale, M., Wigton, A., & Grayson, H. (1996, May). School health centers and primary care for adolescents: A review of the literature. *Journal of Adolescent Health, 17*, 68–76.

Sass, P., Cooper, K., & Robertson, V. (1996). School-based tuberculosis testing and treatment program: Comparing directly observed preventative therapy with preventative therapy. *Journal of Public Health Management and Practice, 2,* 32–40.

Scheuring, S., Hanna, S., & D'Aquila-Lloyd, E. (2000). Strengthening the safety net for adolescent health: Partners in creating realities out of opportunity. *Family and Community Health, 23,* 45–53.

Schwab, N. C., & Gelfman, M. H. B. (Eds.). (2001). *Legal issues in school health services.* North Branch, MN: Sunrise River Press.

Shuler, P. A. (2000). Evaluating student services provided by school-based health centers: Applying the Shuler nurse practitioner practice model. *Journal of School Health, 70,* 348–352.

Simeonsson, R. J., & Simeonsson N. E. (1999). Designing community-based school health services for at risk students. *Journal of Educational and Psychological Consultation, 10,* 215–228.

Spratley, E., Johnson, A., Sochalski, J., Fritz, M., & Spencer, W. (2000). *The registered nurse population: Findings from the National Sample Survey of Registered Nurses.* Rockville, MD: Health Resources and Services Administration, Bureau of Health Professions.

Tyson, H. (1999). A load off the teacher's backs: Coordinated school health programs. *Phi Delta Kappan, 80,* K1–K8.

U.S. Department of Health and Human Services. (2000). *Healthy people 2010: Understanding and improving health* (2nd ed.). Washington, DC: U.S. Government Printing Office.

VHA Health Foundation Inc. (1999). *Making the healthy connection: Establishing and sustaining the hospital sponsored school-based health center.* Irving, TX: Author.

Walker, P. H., Baker, J. J., & Civerton, P. (1997). Costs of interdisciplinary practice in a school-based health center. *Outcomes Management for Nursing Practice, 2,* 37–44.

Willis, E. (2000). School-based/school-linked health centers expanding points of access. *Wisconsin Medical Journal, 99,* 4–7.

Wold, S. (1981). *Assessing and promoting adaptation in school populations in school nursing: A framework for practice* (pp. 72–82). North Branch, MN: Sunrise River Press.

Chapter 9

MEETING THE NEEDS OF OLDER ADULTS FOR PRIMARY HEALTH CARE

Diane Stillman, Neville E. Strumpf, and Geraldine Paier

As they have for the past two decades, primary health care services in the United States continue to undergo rapid change. Professionals and consumers alike remain uneasy about the chaotic business of health care with its closures and consolidations, pressures imposed by managed care, and blurred lines between traditional nonprofit, community-based health care and for-profit, national corporations. These changes are driven by multiple factors, including demands for cost containment from both public and private sectors, the demographic imperative of a burgeoning population of elders, morbidity and mortality increasingly caused by chronic disease and lifestyle factors, and continuing advances in health and communication technologies.

Many decry the movement to managed care as a loss of autonomy for both practitioner and patient, and note its negative effects on the delivery of comprehensive and compassionate care. Others envision the positive potential of an environment focused on health outcomes and disease management with opportunities to provide integrated primary care. Restructuring of primary health care from traditional fee-for-service to managed care affects virtually everyone, but older Americans, because they experience more health problems and concomitant functional losses with aging, are more vulnerable to cost-cutting measures. Primary care providers and older adults are inevitably caught in a complex balancing act of tradeoffs between quality and cost.

The purposes of this chapter are to review the factors that influence the delivery of primary health care services to older Americans, to discuss the impact of managed care on older people, to articulate the evidence-based principles of comprehensive geriatric assessment, to describe the health promotion and disease prevention strategies that are the foundation of primary care, to note the importance of developing palliative care programs to serve older adults with life-limiting illnesses, and to describe the central role played by gerontologic advanced practice nurses in current and emergent models of primary care.

DEMOGRAPHICS, COST, AND HEALTH SERVICES UTILIZATION

Demographic features are well known to gerontologists and providers of care, but bear repetition as we examine the impact of older individuals on national needs for primary care now and in the future. Over the next 50 years, the United States will undergo a profound transformation, becoming a mature nation where 1 in 5 citizens is 65 or older (Older Americans 2000, n.d.). In 1900, persons over the age of 65 constituted only 4% of the total population, and in 2000, 13% (Bureau of the Census, 2000). The most dramatic increase will occur among the "oldest-old", those 85 years of age and over. Between 1960 and 1994, this latter group increased by 274% (Bureau of the Census, 1995). In 2000, the oldest-old were estimated to be 2% of the total population. It is expected that the oldest-old will soar to 19 million in 2050, or 24% of elderly Americans and 5% of all Americans (Bureau of the Census, 2000). Aging is now a worldwide phenomenon, resulting in a global society that is by far the oldest in human history (Butler, 2002).

Three out of four noninstitutionalized persons aged 65 to 74 consider their health to be good. Two in three aged 75 or older report similar feelings of good health (Bureau of the Census, 1995). Nevertheless, age increases the risk of poor health and dependency. For example, in the year 2000, 1.1% of those aged 65 to 74, as compared to nearly 20% of those aged 85 or older, lived in nursing homes. Among the community-dwelling population in 1990, 5% aged 65 to 74 years, but 22% aged 85 or older, needed assistance with everyday activities such as bathing, moving about, and preparing meals (Bureau of the Census, 1995).

Older Americans utilize acute health care services extensively, accounting for 28% of all hospital and 20% of all physician payments (Butler, 2002). Rates of hospitalization and lengths of stay are greater for the elderly than for younger persons. The average length of a hospital stay was 6.0 days for older persons, compared with 4.1 days for people under age 65. Average annual health care costs per person rise substantially with age, from $5,864 for individuals aged 65 to 74 years to $16,465 for those 85 and above (Health Care Financing Administration [HCFA], 2000a).

In addition to experiencing acute illness requiring primary care, older Americans suffer from many chronic conditions that require long-term care either at home or in nursing homes. While Medicare and private insurance cover primary care costs (excluding medications, etc.) they do not cover the long-term costs of home care or nursing home placement to any significant extent. Instead, older adults must rely on personal resources and, when these are exhausted, turn to Medicaid (Weiner & Illiston, 1994). At an average of more than $38,000 a year for nursing home care, with additional expenditures for prescription drugs, long-term care is the leading cause of out-of-pocket catastrophic health care costs among the older population (Bureau of the Census, 2000; Liu, Perozek, & Manton, 1993; Super, 2002). In the case of the nursing home, high costs are no guarantee of satisfactory care. It is thus not surprising that home health care is the alternative preferred by most older people and their families. The home care industry more than doubled its revenues from 1990 to 1995 from $13.1 billion to $28.6 billion, respectively (National Center for Health Statistics, 2001; The World of Home Care, 1997). In 1998, with the institution of the prospective payment system mandated by the Balanced Budget Act of 1997, claims dropped from eight visits per Medicare enrollee to five visits per enrollee. This is still an increase over the 1990 level of two visits per enrollee (HCFA, 2000a).

These demographics frame the significant challenges before us as we enter the 21st century. At a minimum, we must emphasize the efficiency of models shaped by a philosophy of primary health care, ones in which health promotion and disease prevention strategies are thoroughly understood and integrated, principles of interdisciplinary comprehensive geriatric assessment and collaborative practice are incorporated, and quality of life is emphasized. This requires achievement of the essential components and ideals of primary care—comprehensiveness, continuity, and accessibility. Although the current health care system remains in a state of flux, opportunities exist in evolving systems of care to achieve a fuller realization of a more seamless array of primary health care services for older people.

PRIMARY CARE AND EMERGENT MANAGED CARE SYSTEMS

The Institute of Medicine defines primary care as "the provision of integrated accessible health care services by clinicians who are accountable for addressing a large majority of personal health care needs, developing a sustained partnership with patients, and practicing in the context of family and community" (Vaneslow, Donaldson, & Yurdy, 1995, p. 8192). In a similar vein, the American Academy of Nursing states, "Nurse practitioners are primary care providers . . . they provide nursing and medical services to individuals, families, and groups . . . emphasis is placed on health promotion and disease prevention as well as diagnosis and management of acute and chronic diseases . . . Teaching and counseling are a major part of nurse practitioners' activities" (American Academy of Nursing, 1993, p. 1). In many ways, primary care exemplifies a nursing model where success is determined by physical, mental, and social function, with the focus on holistic approaches and participatory roles for patients and families (American Nurses Association, 1995). The realization of effective primary care for older people can be achieved by gerontologic advanced practice nurses who, by philosophy and education, are best suited to the role. In contrast to the long-standing domination of fee-for-service-based health care, a transition to the best elements of a managed care model could mean "the assumption of responsibility and accountability for the health of a defined population, and the simultaneous acceptance of the financial risks inherent in assuming that responsibility" (Pew Health Professions Commission, 1995, p. 4).

While managed care already plays a large role in the health care of older Americans, its future is uncertain. In 1999, more than 6 million older people were enrolled in health maintenance organizations (HMOs) and other competitive medical plans, and that number is expected to grow (HCFA, 1999). More recently, a crisis is occurring as private insurers contracting to administer Medicare HMO plans are drastically increasing premiums or dropping services to entire areas, citing the skyrocketing costs of prescription drugs as the reason (Pear, 2001). Debate over prescription drug coverage continues in Congress, and the future of Medicare HMOs remains unclear. While it is questionable whether managed care systems will ever achieve a true model of primary care for older adults, these systems nevertheless have several advantages. They often include the extensive use of gerontologic advanced practice nurses as primary care providers, they focus care on health promotion and disease prevention, and they manage both acute and chronic illnesses.

COMPREHENSIVE GERIATRIC ASSESSMENT, HEALTH PROMOTION, AND DISEASE PREVENTION

Healthy aging has been the major goal of health policy in the United States since the publication of *Healthy People: The Surgeon General's Report on Health Promotion and Disease Prevention* (U.S. Department of Health, Education, and Welfare, 1979). The role of healthy aging was further emphasized with the release of *Healthy People 2000: National Health Promotion and Disease Prevention Objectives* (U.S. Department of Health and Human Services, 1990) and *Healthy People 2010: National Health Promotion and Disease Prevention Objectives* (U.S. Department of Health and Human Services, 2000). Healthy People 2010 lists two goals to be achieved by the year 2010: (1) increase the span of healthy life and (2) reduce health disparities.

The provision of primary care for older adults is essential to the accomplishment of these goals. Central to primary care is the concept of comprehensive geriatric assessment (CGA). CGA was defined by the National Institutes of Health Consensus Development Panel (1987) as a "multidisciplinary evaluation in which the multiple problems of older persons are uncovered, described, and explained, if possible, and in which the resources and strengths of the person are catalogued, need for services assessed, and a coordinated care plan developed to focus interventions on the person's problems" (p. 342). Basic elements include physical and mental health, social and economic status, environmental characteristics, and functional status. The principles were first applied as part of the National Health Service in the United Kingdom more than 50 years ago (Barker, 1987).

In the United States, CGA is found mainly in academic health centers or in a growing number of managed care networks that use it for risk assessment of older clients. Findings from studies of CGA have thus far been inconsistent and inconclusive, particularly with regard to outcomes associated with geriatric consultation teams and outpatient geriatric evaluation. Nevertheless, the existing research does suggest that the effectiveness of CGA can be enhanced by targeting patients who are at greatest risk for poor outcomes and thus could benefit from a program of geriatric assessment aimed at modifying patient care and tailoring interventions in a systematic and ongoing manner (Cohen et al., 2002; Nikolaus, Specht-Leible, Bach, Oster, & Schlierf, 199; Reuben, Frank, Hirsch, McGuigan, & Maly, 1999; Rockwood et al., 2000). CGA may indeed prove extremely useful in managed care.

Health promotion is the second principle of primary care and the first phase of primary prevention (Lauzon, 1977). Broadly defined, health promotion is "any combination of health education and related organizational, political, and economic interventions designed to facilitate behavioral and environmental changes conducive to health" (Green, 1980, p. 7). At a systems level, it may involve increasing the problem-solving capacity of older persons or the community, providing a comprehensive continuum of community and social services, and helping to meet personal health objectives (Minkler & Pasick, 1986). Activities are aimed at persons without evidence of overt disease; emphasis is on facilitation or reinforcement of healthful living. In assessing the needs for health, the focus should be on determining practices that not only contribute to existing health but also could significantly delay or deter future problems.

Haber (1994) identifies health-related problems associated with aging and amenable to health promotion as nutrition, smoking, stress control, misuse of alcohol and drugs, accident prevention, and exercise and fitness. Prevailing notions that health promotion isn't "worth it" for older people are gradually disappearing. In the case of smoking cessation, for example, it has been demonstrated that within 5 years of smoking cessation, the relative risk of mortality declines in a population of community-dwelling adults 65 years of age or older (Scheitel, Fleming, Chutka, & Evans, 1996). Likewise, exercise and nutrition are positively associated with improved function (Cohen et al., 2002; Duffy & MacDonald, 1990; Schoenfelder, 2000; Sullivan, 1995). These findings clearly demonstrate the effectiveness of health promotion activities, and they underscore as well the need to support it in practice, policy decisions, allocation of resources, ongoing research, and education of providers and the public. Success of health promotion efforts will depend greatly on the ability to entice those most in need of services to participate: older individuals who are smokers, sedentary, isolated, heavily medicated, depressed, economically vulnerable, and suffering from sensory impairment (Omenn, 1990).

In contrast to health promotion, disease prevention is aimed at early detection of risk factors such as genetic history, age, weight, certain health habits, or environmental exposure, any of which could influence the onset of acute illness or the worsening of a chronic disease. Inconsistent screening recommendations, debate concerning the clinical effectiveness of screenings, and lack of reimbursement for preventive services hamper widespread use in practice (Haber, 1994).

The U.S. Preventive Services Taskforce, which was reconvened in the mid-1990s and published the second edition of the *Guide to Clinical Preventive Services* (U.S. Preventive Services Taskforce [USPS Taskforce], 1996), lists more than 80 diseases and conditions amenable to primary, secondary, and tertiary prevention. Primary prevention focuses on asymptomatic persons who may benefit from strategies such as counseling about behavioral risk factors, immunizations, and chemoprophylaxis. Secondary prevention targets individuals who are asymptomatic but also have identifiable health risks. Blood pressure, cholesterol, and diabetic screenings are the most widely implemented forms of secondary prevention. Tertiary prevention takes place after a disease or disability becomes symptomatic and focuses on the restoration or maintenance of function through rehabilitation. The taskforce recommends that practitioners discuss guidelines with patients and individualize recommendations based on health and risk factors.

Health screenings are important tools for disease prevention but must be carefully tailored, rather than routinely applied to entire populations (USPS Taskforce, 1996; Walter & Covinsky, 2001). "The most promising role for prevention in current medical practice may lie in changing the personal health behaviors of patients long before clinical disease develops" (USPS Taskforce, 1996). The health needs of people encompass lifestyle adjustments, health education, and self-care, elements that are both definitive characteristics of primary care and congruent with the expertise of advanced practice nurses.

DEVELOPMENT OF SPECIALIZED PRACTICE IN GERONTOLOGIC NURSING

Nursing has a long history of providing primary care for older people in a variety of settings. A 1925 editorial in the *American Journal of Nursing* alerted nurses to the growing need for care of older adults (Care of the Aged, 1925), but the first text in geriatric nursing was not published until 1950 (Newton, 1950). It described in detail the care of older persons, including constructive health practices and prevention of disease. Geriatric practice was established as one of five divisions of the American Nurses Association (ANA) in 1966. The first Standards for Geriatric Nursing Practice were published in 1970; the latest evolution of these initial guidelines appeared in 1995 as *Standards and Scope of Gerontological Nursing Practice* (American Nurses Association, 1995). The current standards are congruent with the basic tenets of primary health care, with particular emphasis on data collection, planning, continuity of care, and interdisciplinary collaboration.

Paralleling similar developments in advanced practice nursing in the United States, gerontologic clinical specialists and nurse practitioners emerged in the late 1960s. Advanced practice nurses now can be found in most care settings serving older populations; however, the present percentage of those with master's preparation in gerontology and skill in primary care covers a fraction of the actual need. In 1999, there were 4,081 gerontologic advanced practice nurses certified by the American Nurses Credentialing Center (ANA) as either nurse practitioners or clinical nurse specialists (Belza & Baker, 2000).

Practice characteristics of gerontologic advanced practice nurses (GAPNs) in ambulatory care, home care, acute care, and nursing homes embody the principles of primary care as identified by the ANA. Ruiz, Tabloski, and Frazier (1995) identified objectives in GAPN practice that incorporate improvement of functional ability of older persons, an emphasis on diagnosis and treatment of human responses to health and illness, patient and family education and interaction, and interdisciplinary collaboration to ensure quality of care. Positive patient outcomes are associated with primary care by GAPNs and include increased physical activity, decreased psychoactive drug use, and fewer hospital days for frail community-dwelling older adults (Leville et al., 1998), as well as maintenance of overall function and health in ambulatory care settings (Rubenstein, Bernabel, & Weiland, 1994). Improved illness prevention and disease management decrease hospitalization rates for nursing home residents (Haefmeyer, Convery, & von Sternberg, 2000; Kane et al., 1991; Wieland, Rubenstein, & Ouslander, 1986). Finally, attention to primary care needs and clinical management during and following hospitalization results in fewer readmissions to the hospital (Naylor, Brooten, Campbell, et al., 1999). The impact of interventions carried out by GANPs provides the clearest support for more widespread implementation of models of primary care.

MODELS OF PRIMARY CARE OF OLDER ADULTS

Innovative models for delivery of primary health care services to older adults have been proposed in all settings, from care in the community—including adult day care, day hospitals, hospice, geriatric evaluation programs, nurse-managed community centers, home care, and continuing care retirement communities—to care in hospitals and nursing homes. Central to the provision of high-quality, cost-effective care in these settings is utilization of the clinical expertise of gerontologic advanced practice nurses. Unfortunately, nontraditional models are rare, and many initiatives are discontinued as soon as funding disappears. A search of the current health care literature revealed few new models of primary care for older adults. In many cases, initiatives begin with specially designed funding sources and then fail when services fall outside customary reimbursement mechanisms.

Community-Based Primary Care

Cost-containment initiatives continue to shift care from hospitals to the community. It is increasingly unclear exactly who will be available to deliver community-based care to older adults (Super, 2002). Several successful programs have been described over the years, including the multistate National Long-Term Care Demonstration and the Program of All-Inclusive Care for the Elderly (PACE) pioneered by On Lok Senior Health Services Community Organization for Older Adults in San Francisco. Although outcomes vary across sites, Wieland et al. (2000) reported that overall short-term hospitalization was low compared to other older disabled populations. Additionally, in a report to HCFA, hospital and nursing home admissions were decreased, along with decreased hospital lengths of stay and functional decline. Furthermore, the model increased the use of ambulatory care and improved life satisfaction, socialization, and overall survival (Chatterji, Burnstein, Kidder, & White, 1998).

Another model, the Community Nursing Organization (CNO), utilizes advanced practice nurses to provide health promotion, screening, and early intervention to patients in the community. Four demonstration practice sites were funded by HCFA: the Visiting Nurse Service of New York (VNSNY), serving 4 boroughs of New York City and constituting the largest nonprofit Medicare-certified home health agency in the city; Carle Clinic Association in Urbana, Illinois, a multispecialty physician group practice; Carondelet Health Services in Tucson, Arizona, a health system using nurse-managed clinics as a primary component; and the Living Home/Block Nurse program in St. Paul, Minnesota, a community-based program of health care and supportive services to older persons at home, delivered primarily by volunteers (Daley & Mitchell, 1996).

The CNO uses a model of community-focused nursing that includes patient services and identification of aggregate needs, planning, and intervention. Nursing practice integrates family, environment, and community. CNO practice sites include senior centers and clubs, churches, apartment complexes, storefront offices, and homes. The nurses provide assessments and screening, ongoing monitoring of acute and chronic conditions, patient education, and education concerning health promotion and illness prevention to groups of CNO members (Daley & Mitchell, 1996; Ethridge, 1997; Schraeder & Britt, 1997; Strorfjell, Mitchell, & Daly, 1997).

The Collaborative Assessment and Rehabilitation for Elders (CARE) program, established by the School of Nursing at the University of Pennsylvania in Philadelphia, utilized the British Day Hospital model to provide a comprehensive approach to care of frail older adults, bridging the gap between acute home-based and institutional long-term care. With a gerontologic nurse practitioner as care manager, clients received an intensive, individualized, time-limited program of nursing, rehabilitation, mental health, social, and medical services in one setting several times a week. The targeted population of frail older persons had complex medical problems and lived at home. Individuals needed to qualify for multiple services, including at least one rehabilitation therapy, and were deemed unsuitable for inpatient rehabilitation. Preliminary data supported the beneficial effects, and economic feasibility of this approach (Evans, Yorkow, & Siegler, 1995). Unfortunately, this program was discontinued with Medicare changes in reimbursement in 1997–1998 for comprehensive outpatient rehabilitation.

The Veterans Integrated Service Network (VISN) is currently developing a program of nurse-managed primary care clinics led by gerontologic advanced practice nurses (see chapter 14). The clinics emphasize health promotion and disease prevention and focus on appropriate use of health care services. The program will be evaluated for customer satisfaction, quality outcomes, resource utilization, and functional status (Robinson, 2000).

These evolving models of primary care in the community demonstrate the positive impact of gerontologic nursing expertise and advanced practice nursing, and also show the effectiveness of home health services in decreasing mortality and admissions to nursing homes (Elkan et al., 2001). Except for very sick patients requiring highly complex care, or those with serious disabilities or with rehabilitative and subacute care needs, older adults receive care in outpatient, home, and community-based settings. GAPNs will thus be an essential element in the design and implementation of any future programs to meet the needs for quality, community-based care.

Hospital-Based Primary Care

Models of nursing care for hospitalized older adults have evolved over the last 20 years. These models now include geriatric consultation teams, geriatric evaluation and management (GEM) units, a program for transitional care, the Hospital Elder Life program (HELP), and initiatives that fall under the umbrella of NICHE: Nurses Improving Care to Health Systems Elders (Fulmer et al., 2002).

Geriatric consultation teams usually consist of specialists from nursing, medicine, social work, and psychiatry. Providers function in a variety of ways, such as evaluation of all hospital patients above a certain age, response to specific consultation requests, follow-up of all patients admitted from other geriatric services in the system (i.e., home care or ambulatory geriatric clinic), or care of patients in a dedicated GEM unit.

Typically, a consultation team focuses on problems related to functional status, mental status, drug therapy, potential for rehabilitation, and discharge planning (Strumpf, 1994). Improved outcomes for hospitalized patients receiving geriatric consultation have been reported, including better utilization of resources (Germain, Knoeffel, Weiland, & Rubenstein, 1995); reduced medications (Boult et al., 2001); slowed decline or improved physical and mental status (Boult et al., 2001; McVey, Becker, Saltz, Feussner, & Cohen, 1989; Wanich, Sullivan-Marx, Gottlieb, & Johnson, 1992); improved well-being and life satisfaction (Burns, Nichols, Martindale-Adams, & Graney, 2000); and higher survival rates (Applegate et al., 1990; Cohen et al., 2002; Hogan & Fox, 1990; Rubenstein et al., 1994). The best results have been documented in combination with geriatric assessment and rehabilitation, or on inpatient units focused on individuals with potential for improved function. Assessment and rehabilitation without adequate post-discharge follow-up may be of little benefit (Epstein et al., 1990; Stuck, Siu, Weiland, Adams, & Rubenstein, 1993). The use of GEMs peaked in the mid-1980s and, due to difficulty with funding, only a few remain (Miller, 2000).

The transitional care model, tested at the University of Pennsylvania, incorporates a protocol in which patients are enrolled within 24 to 48 hours of admission. Geriatric advanced practice nurse specialists assess both the patient and the caregiver, make interim hospital visits at least every 48 hours until discharge, and maintain contact with the patient for 2 weeks after discharge with follow-up telephone calls. Patients receiving the transitional care protocol had fewer readmissions, fewer rehospitalization days, lower readmission charges, and lower charges for health care services after discharge (Naylor, Brooten, Campbell, et al., 1999; Naylor, Brooten, Jones et al., 1994; Naylor & McCauley, 1999). A wide-scale replication of this model is being planned.

The Hospital Elder Life Program (HELP), developed at Yale-New Haven Hospital, is based on both the GEM and ACE models of care. It differs, however, in that it provides skilled staff to carry out interventions throughout the hospital and focuses on targeted evidence-based interventions to prevent functional decline, particularly delirium (Inouye, Bogardus, Baker, Leo-Summers, & Cooney, 2000). An interdisciplinary team, including a geriatric nurse specialist, specially trained elder life specialists, and trained volunteers are responsible for older adults who are screened as positive for risk factors associated with functional decline. The HELP program significantly reduced new cases of delirium in a controlled clinical trial (Inouye, Bogardus, Charpentier, et al., 1999). Further analysis of the program suggests that it may decrease functional decline as well as inappropriate use of sleep-inducing sedative drugs (Inouye, Bogardus, Baker, et al., 2000).

Nurses Improving Care to Health Systems Elders (NICHE) is a model developed to improve geriatric care that focuses primarily on nursing care. Evolving from the John A. Hartford Foundation's Hospital Outcomes Project for the Elderly (HOPE) (Fulmer & Mezey, 1999; Inouye, Armpra, et al., 1993), NICHE provides nursing models and tools to help hospitals achieve a system change in how they deliver care to older patients. NICHE models include the geriatric resource nurse (GRN), acute care of the elderly (ACE) unit, and the Disease Specific Model (Finch-Guthrie, Edinger, & Schumacher, 2002; Fulmer & Mezey, 1999; Fulmer et al., 2002; Margitic et al., 1993; Miller, 2000; Swauger & Tomlin, 2002).

The NICHE GRN model uses unit-based geriatric resource nurses to provide care and to guide other nurses' care of older patients with complex clinical needs, such as incontinence, functional and mental status changes, delirium, and pressure ulcers. Gerontologic advanced practice nurses (GAPNs) act as consultants, teachers, and role models to the GRNs. In addition, an interdisciplinary team collaborates on complex issues of patient care. Several reports have documented improved patient outcomes associated with implementation of the GRN model (Francis, Fletcher, & Simon, 1998; Fulmer & Mezey, 1999; Lee & Fletcher, 2002; Pfaff, 2002). Barriers to implementation include the difficulty of sustaining a GRN program due to staff turnover and a changing managed care environment.

Acute care of the elderly (ACE) units are dedicated to care of targeted groups of acutely ill older patients (Barrick, Karuza, & Levitt, 1999; Palmer, Counsell, & Landfeld, 1998; Siegler, Glick, & Lee, 2002). The roles played by geriatric specialists from nursing and medicine are significant, and the team bases care on mutually agreed-upon clinical protocols. In addition, the physical environment of ACE units is designed to meet the functional needs of older patients, including low beds, an activity room, reclining chairs, and levered doors (Strumpf, 1994). ACE units appear to be cost-effective and to reduce functional decline in hospitalized elders (Kresevic et al., 1998; Landefeld, Palmer, Kresevic, Fortinsky, & Kowal, 1995). The number of hospitals with ACE units nationwide is unknown, although one study reports on staffing ratios for these units in 33 hospitals (Siegler et al., 2002).

The disease-specific model that is part of NICHE focuses on helping hospitals address a specific condition throughout the facility. Issues that hospitals participating in NICHE have addressed include recognition and management of delirium, limiting the use of physical restraints, and improved management of pressure ulcers (Foreman, Fletcher, Mion, & Simon, 1996; Guthrie, Edinger, & Schumacher, 2002; Swauger & Tomlin, 2002).

The majority of these models of hospital-based care emphasize the importance of GAPNs in the attainment of positive outcomes for older adults. Indeed, many of these innovative approaches arose from nurses who recognized that the complexities of acute care often complicate or diminish overall functional status and contribute to loss of independence for older adults.

Nursing Home Care

Although provision of adequate health care for older people must be considered from the standpoint of a continuum of services from home to hospital to long-stay institutions, nursing homes dominate and symbolize the problems and dilemmas of long-term care (Wunderlich & Kohler, 2001). Earlier hospital discharge to long-term care settings has substantially increased the needs and acuity of residents in nursing homes. A persistent lack of funds continues to affect quality of care and the ability to attract and pay professional staff. Despite recommendations for higher staffing ratios (Harrington et al., 2000), federal regulations continue to require only 8 hours of coverage by a registered nurse per day for all nursing homes, regardless of size (Omnibus Budget Reconciliation Act, 1987). A recent report to Congress found that care suffered when registered nurse coverage fell below 0.45 hours per resident per day (HCFA, 2000b). Here lies the greatest challenge of all: getting primary care services to these vulnerable older adults.

A significant effort toward improving nursing home care was undertaken through the Robert Wood Johnson Foundation Teaching Nursing Home Program (Mezey & Lynaugh, 1991; Mezey, Mitty, & Bottrell, 1997; Shaughnessy, Kramer, Hittle, & Steiner, 1995). This experiment in social change was conceived as a model for restructuring and enhancing clinical care. Its purposes were to upgrade care of residents using a cadre of nurse specialists, to create an environment supportive of education, and to promote research. The 5-year national demonstration project involved 11 schools of nursing and 12 nursing homes with established joint appointments.

Along with the findings from the Teaching Nursing Home Program, the literature clearly supports the effectiveness of GAPNs as primary care providers in nursing homes (Burl, Bonner, & Rao, 1994; R. A. Kane et al., 1988; R. L. Kane, Flood, Keckhafer, & Rockwood, 2001; Kane, Garrard, Buchanon, et al., 1991; Kane, Garrard, Skay, et al., 1989; Reinhard & Stone, 2001). In collaboration with physicians, GAPNs respond to changes in resident status, conduct assessments, monitor medication, provide direct care or supervision for complex problems, and counsel patients and their families.

With attention to primary care, hospitalization rates of nursing home residents are lowered (Burl et al., 1994; Shaugnessy et al., 1995). Residents have better functional outcomes, fewer urinary catheters, less incontinence, fewer nosocomial infections, better attention to behavioral symptoms with more appropriate use of medications, and limited use of physical restraints. Presence of a GAPN ensures the transmittal of timely and accurate information to physicians and reduces unnecessary transfers to the hospital emergency department (Shaugnessy et al., 1995).

Although past evaluations to date support a significant role for GAPNs in nursing homes without significant additional costs (Buchanon et al., 1990), little incentive exists for advanced practice in nursing homes, other than the EverCare Program. EverCare, a HCFA demonstration project started by two gerontologic nurse practitioners, is now an established national program of nurse-physician collaboration to provide ongoing assessment and management of acute and chronic health problems for nursing home residents (R. L. Kane, Flood, et al., 2001; Ryan, 1999). The effectiveness of GAPNs is clearly established in nursing homes; what remains is to make this presence as widespread as possible.

Palliative Care

Palliative care embodies the principles of primary care, having relevance at many stages of serious illness, as well as when death is approaching (Tuch & Strumpf, 2002). Palliative care is defined as "the study and management of patients with active, progressive, far advanced disease for whom the prognosis is limited and the focus of care is on the quality of life" (Doyle, Hanks, & MacDonald, 1998). Alternatively, the World Health Organization defines it as "active, total care of patients whose disease is no longer responsive to curative treatment" (World Health Organization, 1990). Cassel and Foley (1999) delineated core principles for end-of-life care that have been widely adopted, which include assurance of effective symptom management, respect for the wishes of patients and families, and attention to psychological and spiritual concerns.

By the year 2020, 2.5 million older adults will die each year, and roughly 40% of these deaths will occur in nursing homes (Brock & Foley, 1998). Among older adults, most deaths occur after a long, progressive chronic illness such as congestive heart failure or Alzheimer's disease. Until recently, interest was minimal in the end-of-life experiences of older people. The landmark SUPPORT study, which followed more than 9,000 severely ill patients, found them likely to die in pain, in intensive care units, on ventilators, and with little physician awareness of their advance directives

(SUPPORT Principal Investigators, 1995). While the study focused on those dying in the hospital, recent research on death in nursing homes suggests that many residents die without advance directives (Levin et al., 1997; Teno et al., 1997), in pain (Fries, Simon, Morris, Hodstrom, & Bookstein, 2001; Won et al., 1999), and with inadequate psychosocial support (Baer & Hanson, 2000; Murphy, Hanrahan, & Luchins, 1997).

During the past three years, with funding from the Robert Wood Johnson Foundation through an initiative called, "Promoting Excellence in End of Life Care," a palliative care program was carried out as a collaboration between the University of Pennsylvania School of Nursing and Genesis ElderCare. The program specifically addressed advance care planning, pain and symptom management, and psychosocial support, and introduced an integrated palliative care delivery process. An expert nurse clinician acted as a palliative care consultant and role model at the participating homes. The staff at participating homes felt that the clinician's expertise and guidance was crucial to the successful integration of palliative care principles into nursing home care (Tuch et al., 2003).

Palliative care, as a multidisciplinary, patient-centered approach, fits well with current models of geriatric nursing care (Tuch & Strumpf, 2002). As models are developed to better meet the needs of older adults at the end-of-life across settings, advanced practice nurses will be called on to provide support, education, and expert palliative care to older adults and their families.

CONCLUSIONS

Elder care has benefited from "an impressive array of innovative gerontologic practices using nurses, nursing interventions, and the interdisciplinary care team in a variety of settings and across the continuum of care" (Strumpf, 1994, p. 523). Nursing must continue in its efforts to redefine how America cares for older adults, utilizing its expertise in coordinated, comprehensive approaches that maintain the health, well-being, and independent living of older adults.

In its current transitional phase, it is difficult to determine the effects of managed care on primary care services for older adults. Regardless, the 21st century will require individualized approaches for large numbers of older persons and their families, and the move to community-based primary and long-term care will accelerate. Models of primary care practice incorporating gerontologic advanced practice nurses will best serve the needs of older persons and their families, as well as contribute to patient outcomes. As the shape of heath care services continues to unfold in the United States, nursing must continue to argue convincingly for its beneficial and cost-effective role, using outcomes-based research as an essential point in the quest for quality care. This argument must address not only the direct provision of care, but also the preparation of a workforce capable of providing this care (Kovner, Jones, Zhan, Gergen, & Basu, 2002; Mezey, Fulmer, & Fairchild, 2000, Reinhard, Barber, Mezey, Mitty, & Peed, 2002). Nursing must remain faithful to its historical and most fundamental mission—to advocate the best care for patients and families in all health care settings. Only then can the components of care articulated in this chapter be practiced by all providers and offered with satisfaction and confidence to every older American.

REFERENCES

American Academy of Nursing. (1993). *Managed care and national health reform: Nurses can make it work.* Washington DC: American Academy of Nursing.

American Nurses Association. (1995). *Standards and scope of gerontological nursing practice.* Kansas City, MO: Author.

Applegate, W. B., Miller, S. T., Graney, M. J., Elam, J. T., Burns, R., & Atkins, D. E. (1990). A randomized controlled trial of a geriatric assessment unit in a community rehabilitation hospital. *New England Journal of Medicine, 322,* 1572–1578.

Baer, W. M., & Hanson, L. (2000). Families' perceptions of the added value of hospice in the nursing home. *Journal of the American Geriatrics Society, 48,* 879–882.

Barker, W. H. (1987). *Adding life to years: Organized geriatric services in Great Britain and implications for the United States.* Baltimore: Johns Hopkins University Press.

Barrick, C., Karuza, J., & Levitt, J. (1999). Impacting quality: Assessment of a hospital-based geriatric acute care unit. *American Journal of Medical Quality, 14,* 133–137.

Belza, B., & Baker, M. W. (2000). Maintaining health in older adults: Initiatives for schools of nursing and The John A. Hartford Foundation for the 21st century. *Journal of Gerontologic Nursing, 26*(7), 8–17.

Boult, C., Boult, L. B., Morishita, L., Dowd, B., Kane, R. L., & Urdangarin, C. F. (2001). A randomized clinical trial of geriatric evaluation management. *Journal of the American Geriatrics Society, 49,* 317–319.

Brock, D. B., & Foley, D. J. (1998). Demography and epidemiology of dying in the U.S. with emphasis on deaths of older persons. In J. K. Harrold & J. Lynn (Eds.), A good dying: Shaping health care for the last months of life. *Hospice Journal, 13,* 49–60.

Buchanon, J. L., Bell, R. M., Arnold, S. B., Witsberger, C., Kane, R. L., & Garrard, J. (1990). Assessing cost effects of nursing home based geriatric nurse practitioners. *Health Care Financing Review, 11*(3), 67–78.

Bureau of the Census. (1995). Sixty-five plus in the United States. *Statistical brief.* Issued May 1995 by U.S. Dept. of Commerce.

Bureau of the Census. (2000). Retrieved from http://factfinder.census.gov/

Burl, J. B., Bonner, A., & Rao, M. (1994). Demonstration of the cost-effectiveness of a nurse practitioner/physician team in long-term care facilities. *HMO Practice, 8,* 157–161.

Burns, R., Nichols, L. O., Martindale-Adams, J., & Graney, M. J. (2000). Interdisciplinary geriatric primary care evaluation and management: Two-year outcomes. *Journal of the American Geriatrics Society, 48*(1), 8–13.

Butler, R. (2002). *A national crisis: The need for geriatrics faculty training and development.* Washington, DC: Alliance for Aging Research.

Care of the aged. (Editorial). (1925). *American Journal of Nursing, 25*(5), 394.

Cassel, C. K., & Foley, K. M. (1999). *Principles for care of patients at the end-of-life: An emerging consensus among the specialties of medicine.* New York: Milbank Memorial Fund.

Chatterji, P., Burnstein, N. R., Kidder, D., & White, A. (1998). Evaluation of all-inclusive care for elderly (PACE) demonstration: The impact of PACE on patient outcomes. HCFA Contract # 500-96-0003/T04.

Cohen, H. J., Feussner, J. R., Weinberger, M., Carnes, M., Hamdy, R. C., Hsieh, F., Phibbs, C., Courtney, D., Lyles, K. W., May, C., McMurtry, C., Pennypacker, L., Smith, D. M., Ainslie, N., Hornick, T., Brodkin, K., & Lavori, P. (2002). A controlled trial of inpatient and outpatient geriatric evaluation and management. *New England Journal of Medicine, 346,* 906–912.

Daley, G. M., & Mitchell, R. D. (1996). Case management in the community setting. *Nursing Clinics of North America, 31*(3), 527–534.

Doyle, D., Hanks, G., & McDonald, N. (1998). *Oxford textbook of palliative medicine* (2nd ed.). Oxford: Oxford University Press.

Duffy, M., & MacDonald, E. (1990). Determinants of the functional health of older persons. *Gerontologist, 30*(4), 503–509.

Elkan, R., Kendrick, D., Dewey, M., Hewitt, M., Robinson, J., Blair, M., Williams, D., & Brummell K. (2001). Effectiveness of home based support for older people: Systematic review and meta-analysis. *British Medical Journal, 323,* 719–725.

Epstein, A., Hall, J., Fretwell, M., Feldstein, M., DiCiantis, M., Tognetti, J., Cutler, C., Constantine, M., Besdine, R., Rowe, J., & McNeil, B. (1990). Consultative geriatric assessment for ambulatory patients. *Journal of the American Medical Association, 263,* 538–544.

Ethridge, P. (1997). The Carondelet experience. *Nursing Management, 28*(3), 26–27.

Evans, L. K., Yurkow, J., & Siegler, E. L. (1995). The CARE program: A nurse-managed collaborative outpatient program to improve function of frail older people. *Journal of the American Geriatrics Society, 43,* 1155–1160.

Finch-Guthrie, P., Edinger, G., & Schumacher, S. (2002). TWICE: A NICHE Program at North Memorial Health Care. *Geriatric Nursing, 32,* 133–139.

Foreman, M. D., Fletcher, K., Mion, L. C., & Simon, L. (1996). Assessing cognitive function. *Geriatric Nursing, 17,* 228–232.

Francis, D., Fletcher, K., & Simon, L. K. (1998). The geriatric resource nurse model of care: A vision for the future. *Nursing Clinics of North America, 33,* 481–496.

Fries, B. E., Simon, S. E., Morris, J. N., Flodstrom, C., & Bookstein, F. L. (2001). Pain in U.S. nursing homes: Validating a pain scale for the minimum data set. *Gerontologist, 41,* 173–179.

Fulmer, T., & Mezey, M. (1993). *Report of hospital outcomes project for the elderly.* New York: The John Hartford Foundation.

Fulmer, T., & Mezey, M. (1999). Contemporary geriatric nursing. In W. R. Hazzard, J. P. Blass, W. H. Ettinger, Jr., J. B. Halter, & J. G. Ouslander (Eds.), *Principles of geriatric medicine and gerontology* (4th ed., pp. 355–363). New York: McGraw-Hill.

Fulmer, T., Mezey, M., Bottrell, M., Abraham, I., Sazant, J., Grossman, S., & Grisham, E. (2002). Nurses Improving Care for Healthsystem Elders (NICHE): Using outcomes and benchmarks for evidenced-based practice. *Geriatric Nursing, 23,* 121–127.

Germain, M., Knoeffel, F., Weiland, D., & Rubenstein, L. Z. (1995). A geriatric assessment and intervention team for hospital inpatients awaiting transfer to a geriatric unit: A randomized trial. *Aging, 7*(1), 55–60.

Green, L. W. (1980). *Health education planning: A diagnostic approach.* Palo Alto, CA: Mayfield.

Guthrie, P. F., Edinger, G., & Schumacher, S. (2002). TWICE: A NICHE program at North Memorial Health Care. *Geriatric Nursing, 23,* 133–138.

Haber, D. (1994). *Health promotion and aging.* New York: Springer Publishing.

Haefmeyer, J. W., Convery, L., Manninen, R. P., & von Sternberg, T. (2000). The Minnesota Model of sunacute care. *Clinics in Geriatric Medicine, 16,* 725–734.

Harrington, C., Kovner, C., Mezey, M., Kayser-Jones, J., Burger, S., Mohler, M., Burke, R., & Zimmerman, D. (2000). Experts recommend minimum nurse staffing standards for nursing facilities in the United States. *Gerontologist, 40*(1), 5–16.

Health Care Financing Administration. (1999). *Managed care and Medicare. Fact sheet.* Baltimore MD: Centers for Medicare and Medicaid Services.

Health Care Financing Administration (2000a). Retrieved from http://www.hcfa.gov/stats

Health Care Financing Administration (2000b). Retrieved from http://www.hcfa.gov/medicaid/reports/rp700hmp.htm

Hogan, D. B., & Fox, R. A. (1990). A prospective controlled trial of a geriatric consultation team in an acute care hospital. *Age and Ageing, 19,* 107–113.

Inouye, S., Armpra, D., Miller, R., Fulmer, T., Hurst, L., & Cooney, L. (1993). The Yale Geriatric Care Program: A model of care to prevent functional decline in hospitalized elderly patients. *Journal of the American Geriatrics Society, 41,* 1345–1352.

Inouye, S. K., Bogardus, S. T., Baker, D. I., Leo-Summers, L., & Cooney, L. M. (2000). The Hospital Elder Life Program: A model of care to prevent cognitive and functional decline in older hospitalized patients. *Journal of the American Geriatrics Society, 48,* 1697–1706.

Inouye, S. K., Bogardus, S. T., Charpentier, P. A., Leo-Summers, L., Acampora, D., Holford, T. R., & Cooney, L. M. (1999). A multicomponent intervention to prevent delirium in hospitalized older patients. *New England Journal of Medicine, 340,* 669–676.

Kane, R. A., Kane, R. L., Arnold, S., Garrard, J., McDermott, S., & Kepferle, L. (1988). Geriatric nurse practitioners as nursing home employees: Implementing the role. *Gerontologist, 28,* 469–477.

Kane, R. L., Flood, S., Keckhafer, G., & Rockwood, T. (2001). How EverCare nurse practitioners spend their time. *Journal of the American Geriatrics Society, 49,* 1530–1534.

Kane, R. L., Garrard, J., Buchanon, J. L., Rosenfeld, A., Skay, C., & McDermott, S. (1991). Improving primary care in nursing homes. *Journal of the American Geriatrics Society, 39,* 359–367.

Kane, R. L., Garrard, J., Skay, C., Radosevich, D. M., Buchanon, J. L., McDermott, S. M., Arnold, S. B., & Kepferle, L. (1989). Effects of a geriatric nurse practitioner on process and outcome of nursing home care. *American Journal of Public Health, 79,* 1271–1277.

Kovner, C., Jones, C., Zhan, C., Gergen, P. J., & Basu, J. (2002). Nurse staffing and postsurgical adverse events: An analysis of administrative data from a sample of U.S. hospitals, 1990–1996. *Health Services Research, 37,* 611–629.

Kresevic, D. M., Counsell, S. R., Covinsky, K., Palmer, R., Landefeld, C. S., Holder, C., & Beeler, J. (1998). A patient-centered model of acute care for elders. *Nursing Clinics of North America, 33,* 515–527.

Landefeld, C. S., Palmer, R. M., Kresevic, D. M., Fortinsky, R. H., & Kowal, J. (1995). A randomized trial of care in a hospital medical unit especially designed to improve the functional outcomes of acutely ill older patients. *New England Journal of Medicine, 332,* 1338–1344.

Lauzon, R. J. (1977). An epidemiological approach to health promotion. *Canadian Journal of Public Health, 68,* 311–317.

Lee, V. K., & Fletcher, K. R. (2002). Sustaining the geriatric resource nurse model. *Geriatric Nursing, 23,* 128–132.

Leville, S. G., Wagner, E. H., Davis, C., Grothaus, L., Wallace, J., LoGerfo, M., & Kent, D. (1998). *Journal of the American Geriatrics Society, 46,* 1191–1198.

Levin, J. R., Wenger, N. S., Ouslander, J. G., Zellman, G., Schnelle, J. F., Buchanan, J., Hirsch, S. H., & Reuben, D. B. (1997). Life-sustaining treatment decisions for nursing home residents: Who discusses, who decides, and what is decided? *Journal of the American Geriatrics Society, 47*(1), 82–87.

Liu, K., Perozek, M., & Manton, K. G., (1993). Catastrophic acute and long-term care costs: Risks faced by disabled elderly persons. *Gerontologist, 33,* 299–307.

Margitic, M., Inouye, S., Thomas, J., Cassel, C., Regenstreif, D., & Kowal, J. (1993). Hospital Outcomes Project for the Elderly (HOPE): Rationale and design for a prospective pooled analysis. *Journal of the American Geriatrics Society, 41,* 258–267.

McVey, L. J., Becker, P. M., Saltz, C. C., Feussner, J. R., & Cohen, H. J. (1989). Effect of a geriatric consultation team on functional status of elderly hospitalized patients. *Annals of Internal Medicine, 110*(1), 79–84.

Mezey, M., & Lynaugh, J. (1991). Teaching Nursing Home Program: A lesson in quality. *Geriatric Nursing, 12*(2), 76–77.

Mezey, M., Fulmer, T., & Fairchild, S. (2000). Enhancing geriatric nursing scholarship: Specialization versus generalization. *Journal of Gerontological Nursing, 27*(7), 28–35.

Mezey, M., Mitty, E., & Bottrell, M. (1997). The Teaching Nursing Home Program: Enduring educational outcomes. *Nursing Outlook, 45,* 133–140.

Miller, D. K. (2000). Effectiveness of acute rehabilitation services in geriatric evaluation and management units. *Clinics in Geriatric Medicine, 16,* 775–782.

Minkler, M., & Pasick, R. J. (1986). Health promotion and the elderly: A critical perspective on past and future. In K. Dychtwald (Ed.), *Wellness and health promotion for the elderly* (pp. 39–54). Rockville, MD: Aspen.

Murphy, K., Hanrahan, P., & Luchins, D. (1997). A survey of grief and bereavement in nursing homes: The importance of hospice grief and bereavement for end stage Alzheimer's disease patient and family. *Journal of the American Geriatrics Society, 45,* 1104–1107.

National Center for Health Statistics. (2001). *Health, United States, 2001, with urban and rural health chartbook,* Pub. No. (PHS) 01-1232. Hyattsville, MD: U.S. Department of Health and Human Services.

National Institutes of Health Consensus Development Panel. (1987). National Institutes of Health Consensus Development Conference Statement: Geriatric assessment methods for decision making. *Journal of the American Geriatrics Society, 36*(4), 342–347.

Naylor, M. D., Brooten, D., Campbell, R., Jacobsen, B. S., Mezey, M. D., Pauly, M. V., & Schwartz, J. S. (1999). Comprehensive discharge planning and home follow-up of hospitalized elders: A randomized clinical trial. *Journal of the American Medical Association, 281,* 613–620.

Naylor, M., Brooten, D., Jones, R., Lavizzo-Mourey, R., Mezey, M., & Pauley, M. (1994). Comprehensive discharge planning for the hospitalized elderly: A randomized clinical trial. *Annals of Internal Medicine, 120,* 999–1006.

Naylor, M. D., & McCauley, K. M. (1999). The effects of a discharge planning and home follow-up intervention on elders hospitalized with common medical and surgical cardiac conditions. *Journal of Cardiovascular Nursing, 14*(1), 44–54.

Newton, K. (1950). *Geriatric nursing.* St. Louis, MO: Mosby.

Nikolaus, T., Specht-Leible, N., Bach, M., Oster, P., & Schlierf, G. (1999). A randomized trial of comprehensive geriatric assessment and home intervention in the care of hospitalized patients. *Age and Ageing, 28:* 543–550.

Older Americans 2000. (n.d.). Retrieved from http://www.agingstats.gov/chartbook/2000/population.html

Omenn, G. S. (1990). Prevention and the elderly. *Health Affairs, 9*(2), 80–93.

Omnibus Budget Reconciliation Act of 1987, Nursing Home Reform Amendments, 42 U.S.C. §1819.

Palmer, R. M., Counsell, S., & Landfeld, C. S. (1998). Clinical intervention trials. The ACE unit. *Clinical Geriatric Medicine, 14,* 831–839.

Pear, R. (2001, December, 4). H.M.O.s flee Medicare despite rise in payments. *New York Times,* p. 16.

Pew Health Professions Commission. (1995, August). *Health professionals' education and managed care: Challenges and necessary responses* (pp. 1–34). San Francisco: Author.

Pfaff, J. (2002). The Geriatric Resource Nurse Model: A culture change. *Geriatric Nursing, 23,* 140–144.

Reinhard, S., & Stone, R. (2001). *Promoting quality in nursing homes: The Wellspring Model.* (Publication No. 432). New York: The Commonwealth Fund.

Reinhard, S. C., Barber, P. M., Mezey, M., Mitty, E., & Peed, J. A. (2002). *Initiatives to promote the nursing workforce in geriatrics.* Washington, DC: Institute for the Future of Aging Services.

Reuben, D. B., Frank, J. C., Hirsch, S. H., McGuigan, K. A., & Maly, R. C. (1999). A randomized trial of comprehensive geriatric assessment and home intervention in the care of hospitalized patients. *Journal of the American Geriatrics Society, 47,* 269–276.

Robinson, K. R. (2000). Nurse-managed primary care delivery clinics. *Nursing Clinics of North America, 35,* 471–479.

Rockwood, K., Stadnyk, K., Carver, D., MacPherson, K. M., Beanlands, H. E., Powell, C., Stolee, P., Thomas, V. S., & Tonks, R. S. (2000). A clinimetric evaluation of specialized geriatric care for rural dwelling frail older people. *Journal of the American Geriatrics Society, 48:* 1080–1085.

Rubenstein, L. Z., Bernabel, R., & Weiland, D. (1994). Comprehensive geriatric assessment into the breach. *Aging, 6*(1), 1–3.

Ruiz, B. A., Tabloski, P. A., & Frazier, S. M. (1995). The role of gerontological advanced practice nurses in geriatric care. *Journal of the American Geriatrics Society, 43,* 1061–1064.

Ryan, J. W. (1999). An innovative approach to the medical management of the nursing home resident: The EverCare experience. *Nurse Practitioner Forum, 10*(1), 27–32.

Scheitel, S. M., Fleming, K. C., Chutka, D. S., & Evans, J. M. (1996). Geriatric health maintenance. *Mayo Clinic Proceedings, 71,* 289–302.

Schoenfelder, D. P. (2000). A fall prevention program for elderly individuals: Exercise in long-term care settings. *Journal of Gerontological Nursing, 26*(3), 43–51.

Schraeder, C., & Britt, T. (1997). The Carle Clinic. *Nursing Management, 28*(3), 32–34.

Shaughnessy, P. W., Kramer, A. M., Hittle, D. F., & Steiner, J. F. (1995). Quality of care in teaching nursing homes: Findings and implications. *Health Care Financing Review, 16*(4), 55–83.

Siegler, E. L., Glick, D., & Lee, J. (2002). Optimal staffing for acute care of the elderly (ACE) units. *Geriatric Nursing, 32,* 152–155.

Storfjell, J. L., Mitchell, R., & Daly, G. M. (1997). Nurse-managed health clinics: New York's community nursing organizations. *Journal of Nursing Administration,* 27(10), 21–27.

Strumpf, N. E. (1994). Innovative gerontological practices as models for health care delivery. *Nursing and Health Care, 15,* 522–527.

Stuck, A. E., Siu, A. L., Weiland, G. D., Adams, J., & Rubenstein, L. Z. (1993). Comprehensive geriatric assessment: A meta-analysis of controlled trials. *Lancet, 342,* 1032–1036.

Sullivan, D. H. (1995). Impact of nutritional status on health outcomes of nursing home residents. *Journal of the American Geriatrics Society, 43,* 195–196.

Super, N. (2002, January 23). Who will be there to care for the growing gap between caregiver supply and demand? *National Health Policy Forum Background Paper.* Washington, DC: The George Washington University.

SUPPORT Principal Investigators. (1995). A controlled trial to improve care for seriously ill hospitalized patients. The Study to Understand Prognoses and Preferences for Outcomes and Risks of Treatments (SUPPORT). *Journal of the American Medical Association, 274,* 1591–1598.

Swauger, K., & Tomlin, C. (2002). Best care for the elderly at Forsyth Medical Center. *Geriatric Nursing, 23,* 145–150.

Teno, J. M., Branco, K. J., Mor, V., Phillips, C. D., Hawes, C., Morris, J., & Fries, B. E. (1997). Changes in advance care planning in nursing homes before and after the Patient Self-Determination Act: A report of a 10-state survey. *Journal of the American Geriatrics Society, 45,* 939–944.

Tuch, H., & Strumpf, N. E. (2002). Palliative care. In V. T. Cotter & N. E. Strumpf (Eds.), *Advanced practice nursing with older adults* (pp. 361–371). New York: McGraw-Hill.

Tuch, H., Strumpf, N. E., Stillman, D., Parrish, P., Morrison, N., & Parmelee, P. (2003). *Developing and integrating palliative care programs in community nursing homes.* Manuscript submitted for publication.

U.S. Department of Health, Education, and Welfare. (1979). *Healthy people: The surgeon general's report on health promotion and prevention.* DHEW (PHS) Publication No. 79-55071. Washington, DC: U.S. Government Printing Office.

U.S. Department of Health and Human Services. (1990). *Healthy people 2000: National health promotion and disease prevention objectives.* Washington, DC: U.S. Government Printing Office.

U.S. Department of Health and Human Services. (2000). *Healthy people 2010: National health promotion and disease prevention objectives.* Washington, DC: U.S. Government Printing Office.

U.S. Preventive Services Taskforce (1996). *Guide to clinical preventive services* (2nd ed.). Baltimore, MD: Williams and Wilkins.

Walter, L. C., & Covinsky, K. E. (2001). Cancer screening in elderly patients: A framework for individualized decision-making. *Journal of the American Medical Association, 285,* 2750–2756.

Wanich, C., Sullivan-Marx, E., Gottlieb, G., & Johnson, J. (1992). Functional status outcomes of a nursing intervention in hospitalized elderly. *Image: Journal of Nursing Scholarship, 24,* 201–207.

Wieland, D., Rubenstein, L. Z., & Ouslander, J. G. (1986). Organizing an academic nursing home. Impacts on institutionalized elderly. *Journal of the American Medical Association, 255,* 2622–2627.

Weiner, J. M., & Illiston, L. H. (1994). Health care reform in the 1990s: Where does long-term care fit in? *Gerontologist, 34,* 402–408.

Won, A., Lapane, K., Gambessi, G., Bernabei, R., Mor, V., & Lipsitz, L. A. (1999). Correlates and management of non-malignant pain in the nursing home. *Journal of the American Geriatrics Society, 47,* 936–942.

World Health Organization. (1990). *Cancer pain relief and palliative care.* (Technical Report Series 804). Geneva: Author.

The world of home care. (1997, May). *Provider,* 33–48.

Wunderlich, G. S., & Kohler, P. (Eds.). (2001). *Improving the quality of long-term care.* Washington DC: National Academy Press.

Chapter 10

ADVANCED PRACTICE PSYCHIATRIC–MENTAL HEALTH NURSING

Madeline A. Naegle

Nursing has traditionally used an interpersonal context to address a broad spectrum of health care needs of clients and their families. Hildegard Peplau operationalized this context in the 1950s in an interpersonal relations paradigm (Sills, 1993, p. 201). Peplau focused on "what goes on between nurse and patient . . . needs, expectations, dynamics of the interaction." Awareness and understanding of these components allow for the transformation of the interaction into a therapeutic relationship.

In the primary mental health care model, the advanced practice primary mental health nurse (APN-PMH) delivers broad-based care while addressing psychotherapeutic needs. The model's value rests on the consolidation of care delivery by one provider, thereby decreasing the fragmentation associated with many relationships and enhancing patient trust, and consequently, patient adherence to therapeutic regimens. This chapter discusses the unique benefits of this nursing role, which are demonstrated in the nursing management of illnesses characterized by complex psychophysiologic relationships. It also discusses how the traditional psychotherapeutic relationship is enhanced when elements of primary care expand services delivered by one provider. Complex psychophysiologic conditions are evidenced in both dysfunctional behavior and physiologic changes; sensory deprivation and alcoholism are examples. The chapter articulates how APN-PMH interventions are designed for different levels of health and illness, incorporating the concepts of primary care delivery, coordination of care providers, and advocacy behaviors within a variety of community and health care delivery systems. The chapter concludes by using the alcoholic client as an exemplar for APN-PMH practice.

EVOLUTION TO CONTEMPORARY ROLES

Three levels of primary mental health care frame the role functions of the APN-PMH: (1) primary mental health activities that focus on at-risk groups to enhance function and mental health (prevention activities are included in this category); (2) primary mental health services that address management and treatment interventions by identifying mental health problems as early as possible, reducing the time that mental health problems exist, and halting the progression of severity and limiting the coexistence of other mental health problems; and (3) primary mental health interventions that decrease the likelihood of relapse (Haber & Billings, 1995). A final level added by Murphy and Moller (1993) addresses maintenance interventions that decrease disability, enhance prevention of relapse, and promote optimal functional status and quality of life.

A bio-psychosocial perspective supports psychiatric-mental health nursing practice. The bio-psychosocial approach recognizes the biological, cultural, environmental, psychological, and sociological determinants of mental health, as well as mental illness, and supports a broad base for nursing practice. This broad base expands the nurse's role to include assessment and treatment of basic heath (as well as mental health) problems, and requires master's-level preparation in pathophysiology, pharmacotherapeutics, and physical assessment.

Primary mental health care conforms to the Institute of Medicine (1996, p. 5) definition of primary care: "the provision of integrated, accessible health care services by clinicians who are accountable for addressing the majority of personal healthcare needs, developing a sustained partnership with patients, and practicing in the context of family and community." The components of this definition were seen in the earliest nursing models of contracts between the independently practicing nurse and the client and/or client's family and included (1) a sustained partnership, including the assumption of primary and long-term responsibility for the patient regardless of the presence or absence of disease, (2) the community context manifested in the formation and coordination of networks of resources and care providers within the health care system and/or the community, and (3) accessibility and consistent contact with other health care providers.

Today, the mental health-primary care components come together in the primary mental health nurse's role, as described by Haber and Billings (1995). In identifying the primary care components of the mental health specialty, they described the expansion of nursing interventions in the majority of personal health care needs through assessment, direct care, and referral. They noted that the primary care components of the psychiatric-mental health nursing role have been less frequently emphasized than specialized practice, which employs theories of human behavior and purposeful use of self as its art. This role finds support in earlier mandates calling for the lowering of the incidence of mental disorders as a primary care activity (Leininger, 1973), and psycho-education on stress and mental health risks (Christman, 1987).

Primary mental health care interventions fall within the scope of practice of both generalist nurses and mental health nurse specialists. Universal preventive measures, for example, deemed desirable for everyone in a given population, are implemented to enhance functioning and mental health (Mrazek & Haggerty, 1994). Examples of these include culturally congruent parenting education and promotion of self-esteem. Selective preventive interventions are also used for at-risk populations and include elder support groups, respite for caregivers, and bereavement counseling. An excellent example is health teaching on prescribed and over-the-counter medication use by the elderly. Of prescriptions written in the United States, the largest number are written for persons over 65 (Solomon, Manepalli, Freland, & Mahon, 1993), leading to polypharmacy, which manifests in the misuse of medications by the consumer and high incidences of drug interactions with negative outcomes. Drug properties may produce mood changes, drug interactions may change pharmacotherapeutic outcomes, and side effects of drugs may cause undesirable effects in emotional, sexual, and digestive systems (Agency for Health Care Policy and Research, 1993). Health teaching of the "well" elderly who are, or may soon be using multiple medications can prevent adverse outcomes.

The renewed emphasis on biological science as central to mental health has important implications for the APN-PMH nursing role. Recent research has elucidated new biological factors influencing mental-emotional illness, and consumer groups now demand definitions of psychiatric illnesses as brain disorders. Neuroscientific research supports brain dysfunction as central to both the diagnosis and treatment of psychiatric disorders and is now central to psychiatric nursing education. Psychiatric nurse leaders (McBride,

1996; McEnany, 1991) have stressed the need for integration of neurological and psychiatric mental health knowledge and urged expanding the biologic bases for practice if nursing interventions are to be effective. Such knowledge is now required and a foundation to the curricula for advanced practice psychiatric-mental health nurses for prescribing and monitoring medication, teaching clients and families about treatment, and understanding the implications of coexisting medical conditions.

Clinical nurse specialists have long been recognized for expert psychiatric-mental health nursing knowledge used in direct care of acutely ill patients/clients, families, and groups. Nurses in this role provide education, consultation, and research perspectives on care provision for colleagues, consumers, and organizations. Psychiatric nurse practitioners share this expert knowledge and their role also includes education on the specialty, consultation, and research, but they conduct more primary care activities, including medical management and medication prescribing. In 2001, the American Nurses' Credentialing Center (ANCC) recognized both roles by creating a credential designating all advanced practice nurses. ANCC now credentials many advanced practice nurses as APRN-BC, advanced practice nurse, board certified.

A forerunner of primary mental health nursing emerged in the 1970s in community mental health centers. Psychiatric-mental health clinical nurse specialists in these centers worked primarily in ambulatory care; were highly autonomous; delivered treatment in modalities traditionally reserved for psychiatrists, social workers, and others; and provided mental health teaching, education, and consultation to schools, social agencies, and service centers. Shaped by the needs of the health care delivery system and recent research on psychiatric illness, the education, competencies, and role functions of psychiatric-mental health nurse clinical specialists and psychiatric nurse practitioners today are increasingly similar. The master's degree is the accepted requirement for both roles, and both share the same core competencies of expert knowledge and specialist skills on consultation, research, and education roles. Preparation includes courses in pathophysiology, pharmacotherapeutics, and advanced physical assessment, which are foundations for identifying basic health problems and preparing the nurse for primary care and prescribing. Skills derived from Peplau's (1987) interpersonal and psychosocial model continue to be central to role implementation. Master's preparation provides a foundation to assess clients' basic health needs and to assess and treat mental health concerns.

Nursing approaches represent a marked shift away from the medical model because they place heavy emphasis on a comprehensive, sociopsychological assessment of client and family as well as basic health assessments

(Cotroneo, Outlaw, King, & Brince, 1997). For example, cognitive changes, diminished sensory and learning capacities, and social losses make older individuals especially vulnerable to the confusion caused by fragmentation in the health care delivery system. When care is comprehensive and coordinated by the APN-PMH, brief superficial contacts with an array of health care personnel can be decreased.

Talley and Caverly (1994) offer excellent examples of primary mental health care provided by advanced practice psychiatric-mental health nurses. These services include (1) maintenance of the medical health care record in the mental health treatment record; (2) provision of selected health screening and health education in mental health settings (e.g., blood pressure, cholesterol screening, weight checks, and education); (3) evaluation of health care risks and problems secondary to psychiatric illnesses or psychopharmacologic interventions; and (4) monitoring before and during drug treatment, and at the time of drug discontinuation, with special monitoring of laboratory and medical procedures needed to ensure safe psychopharmacological interventions. In Peplau's paradigm, these activities performed conjointly with psychotherapy provide openings to "find the ways to come to know a person as a human being in difficulty" (Peplau, 1987, p. 204).

The psychiatric-mental health nurse's role includes the interventions described above as well as (1) client advocacy, (2) accountability, and (3) collaborative activities with nurses and members of other disciplines. Psychiatric nurses in primary care practice adhere to the Scope and Standards of Psychiatric Mental Health Clinical Nursing Practice (American Nurses Association, American Psychiatric Nurses Association, & International Society of Psychiatric-Mental Health Nurses,, 2000). Typically, the advanced practice psychiatric nurse will have prescribing privileges in accordance with state nurse practitioner statutes and collaborative physician and institutional agreements. Consistent with the practice of all advanced practice nurses, psychiatric nurses in primary care practice use knowledge about culturally diverse traditions and variations among racial and ethnic groups to understand health and illness, differences in sexual preference and lifestyles, and the social realities experienced by patients and families.

ROLE RECOGNITION AND REIMBURSEMENT

Only recently have psychiatric nurses been employed as direct care providers in community-based clinics or private practice. Social agencies have begun to employ APN-PMHs. Nevertheless, because of the newness of the role of psychiatric nurses as primary providers, there are many unanswered questions about, and challenges to, APN-PMH activities. The role has been most effectively delineated by identifying billable services that the APN-PMH delivers in private practice, in clinics, at home, or in correctional facilities.

As with all other APNs, APN-PMH nurses benefit from the successful lobbying by national and specialty nursing organizations that has produced legislation supporting the advanced practice role, generally (see chapter 23). The Balanced Budget Act of 1997 enables advanced practice nurses to be directly reimbursed under Medicare Part B. Health care agencies tend to delineate the role of advanced practice nurse around billable services, even though this may be more restrictive than the professional role for which the nurse is prepared. For APN-PMH nurses, for example, numerous social agencies define the role as that of physician substitute and delineate APN-PMH activities primarily as medication prescribing and monitoring.

Initial and continuing education for APN-PMHs should include content on the definitions and scope of practice and on reimbursement, specifically, on coding terms since reimbursement is compromised by inaccurate billing. The APN-PMH nurse may see a patient briefly for medication adjustment and cannot bill for a full 45- or 50-minute psychotherapy session. When discussion with the patient encompasses more than 50% of the encounter time, the nurse may bill for counseling, describing the nature of the discussion and noting the amount of time (Rapsilber & Anderson, 2000). (See chapters 15 and 22).

Ability to use the *Diagnostic and Statistical Manual,* fourth edition, text revision (American Psychiatric Association, 2000) is also a required competency for the APN-PMH. Clinical judgment and experience reinforce the use of diagnostic codes and enrich the clinician's understanding of the behavior. Agency policy and billing procedures require all axes diagnoses applicable to the patient and generally ask for a numerical measure of the patient's rank on the Global Assessment of Functioning scale (GAF scale). In addition to providing evidence for the APN-PMH nurse's financial productivity, guidelines have helped concretize nursing functions, particularly in relation to prescribing, medical diagnoses, and assessment. Guidelines may be issued as consensus statements by expert panels, managed behavioral care companies, or the federal government, such as guidelines for the delivery of culturally competent care through Medicaid managed care.

In many of the settings where the APN-PMH role has been introduced, services are fragmented, resulting in discreet interventions being performed by several providers. One cause for this fragmentation is overlapping roles among health care providers: the provision of psychotherapy or drug and alcohol counseling by one set of providers (a social worker or substance abuse counselor) and prescribing and monitoring of medication by a nurse. Another cause for fragmentation is state regulations that may restrict the role of APN-PMH nurses, for example, specific provisions in state regulations that allow APN-PMH nurses to conduct secondary but not initial psychiatric assessments. In New York state, for example, nurses may not authorize involuntary psychiatric hospitalization for observed treatment under Kendra's Law (NYS OMH, 2000).

In summary, the evolution of the role in the marketplace is influenced by legislation, state regulation, customs and traditions of hospitals and social agencies, and the competencies demonstrated by the APN-PMH (Naegle & Krainovich-Miller, 2001). Nurses can influence these factors by supporting the activities of professional nursing specialty or state organizations that seek to change existing regulations and through community-level action on health policy. Through education, the advanced practice nurse is well equipped to implement or support change agent roles and assumes leadership responsibility in collaboration with intra- and interdisciplinary colleagues.

PRACTICE SETTINGS AND ROLES OF APN-PMH NURSES

Professional trends support greater autonomy in practice for APN-PMH nurses. Brief inpatient stays and more outpatient programs, such as partial hospitalization and observation units, provide job opportunities away from the institution. At the same time, mental health is now emphasized rather than the earlier focus on psychiatric pathology. Optimally, the APN-PMH provides continuous care for the client in need of primary mental health or psychiatric care through interventions that address mental health needs on a continuum from preventive counseling to grief counseling to psychopharmacologic management. These APN-PMH activities would include reviewing and monitoring of health care provided by other practitioners, as well as symptom assessment. APN-PMH roles include those of direct care provider, case manager, consultant, collaborator, interdisciplinary team member, researcher, and educator. These roles can be implemented in hospitals, community agencies, clinics, and long-term care. Roles in psychiatric-liaison consultation also present institution-based options to blend primary and specialist care.

Direct Care Provider

In the climate of managed care, psychiatric hospitalization is reserved for individuals who are in acute illness states, have complex diagnostic profiles, require pharmacologic management, or are a danger to themselves or others. APN-PMHs perform activities congruent with the Peplau interpersonal framework that include counseling, psychoeducation, and psychotherapy in an inpatient therapeutic milieau. In a therapeutic milieu, nurses, according to early nurse leaders, create and maintain a proper psychological atmosphere (Johns & Pfefferkorn, 1934), "manipulate environmental factors" (Render, 1947), and create an environment conducive to recovery. The APN-PMH actively participates in defining processes of a therapeutic milieu. In many inpatient units, APN-PMHs now perform the intake admission histories and physicals and the initial comprehensive mental status assessment. As direct providers, their scope of practice includes mental and basic health assessments; psychiatric diagnoses; nursing diagnoses; treatment interventions, including medication prescription and monitoring; counseling and psychotherapy; and psychoeducation (Naegle & Krainovich-Miller, 2001). They may address immediate, short-term needs for medication prescription and administration. APN-PMHs are expected to be knowledgeable of and alert to physiologic symptoms and conditions as well.

Most clients/patients receiving secondary and tertiary psychiatric care live in the community in group homes, halfway houses, or subsidized housing or single-room occupancies. These clients benefit substantially from care by nurses who are competent to address both their physical and psychological needs. Homelessness can be a frequent problem, depending on geographic location and resources. Undomiciled clients with severe and persistent mental illness and dual diagnoses seek care sporadically in general and psychiatric settings. Many can be maintained in community settings through crises and require hospitalization only during acute exacerbation of illness. Comorbidity may be high in these populations and may include HIV-AIDS, hepatitis, diabetes, and hypertension, which require monitoring by the APN-PMH as well as interdisciplinary team management.

The APN-PMH cares for these complex patients in individual, group, and family sessions. The nurse is accountable for treating and evaluating treatment outcomes of a caseload of clients/patients (case management) in collaboration with members of other disciplines. Examples of treatment settings that employ mental health nurses in the direct provider role include psychiatric emergency departments, mental health and substance abuse agencies that are expanding services to include primary care, group homes for the severely and persistently mentally ill and developmentally disabled, day care settings, nursing homes, and centers for vocational rehabilitation counseling and client services.

Case Manager

The case manager role in psychiatric nursing may include elements of the direct provider role or may be limited to case management functions. Case management focuses on meeting treatment outcomes related to an illness episode, in a given period of time. As a case manager, the psychiatric-mental health nurse is responsible for coordinating care delivered to an assigned group of patients or to clients/patients in his or her own caseload. Care is provided according to guidelines for diagnostic groups and standard-based protocols developed between the nurse and a collaborating physician or nurse colleague. It includes some health teaching and health maintenance activities (Cohen & Cesta, 1994). In addition to the direct provider functions, the nurse oversees the use of resources by determining the eligibility and reimbursement potential for a client in a specific program. The nurse case manager engages in follow-up and review of the case and the patient's progress. Psychiatric nurses are increasingly being employed in this role in drug and alcohol treatment facilities, by managed care companies, and by acute-care psychiatric facilities.

Consultant

This role is well described in *Scope and Standards of Psychiatric-Mental Health Nursing Practice* (ANA et al., 2000). Some excellent examples are the use of APN-PMHs in community-based clinics that treat individuals in the criminal justice system, using a drug court model. Men and women arraigned in the community and evaluated for alternatives to incarceration have a high prevalence of substance-related and/or mental health problems. On site, nurses assess and screen for basic health problems and mental/emotional illness within the plan of action ordered by the court, that is, detoxification, community service with mental health follow-up, or psychiatric hospitalization. A comprehensive plan of action involves collaboration with adult health nurse practitioners, physicians, and/or social workers or counselor coworkers. In primary care settings where individuals with mental health problems are often seen but remain undiagnosed or misdiagnosed, the APN-PMH provides consultation for the provision of effective and appropriate mental health care. An exemplar is the use of an APN-PMH as consultant to nurse care managers in a new role supporting the treatment of depression by practitioners in primary care.

Psychiatric-Consultation Liaison Nurse

Psychiatric-consultation liaison nurses have opportunities to implement an APN-PMH model as they seek to increase the accessibility of mental health services for patients/clients served in settings not specific to mental health or substance abuse. These nurses are institution-based and respond to nursing and medical staff requests for psychiatric and psychosocial evaluation of clients/patients. Following an assessment and diagnosis, nurses assist staff caring for the patient in designing interventions tailored to the client's mental health and medical illness-related needs. These nurses may assist in developing interventions ranging from health promotion to crisis intervention to illness rehabilitation. They provide services in psychiatric and substance abuse treatment settings, general hospital units, primary care clinics, and emergency departments.

Interdisciplinary Team Member

The APN-PMH is uniquely prepared to function as a member of multidisciplinary and interdisciplinary teams in all health care settings. Expert knowledge and skills in communication, conflict resolution, leadership, and group dynamics, as well as interpersonal skills, increase the efficiency of teams in their goals to improve organizational functions and provide optimal patient care (McGivern, 1993). Knowledge of human behavior and experience in solving problems related to mental health and human behavior equip the nurse with skills for collaboration, maintenance of a positive work environment, and tolerance for the ambiguity and role diffusion that often characterize team development and function.

Roles in Education and Research

The APN-PMH continues his or her own education, participates in educating others, and engages in and collaborates with others in the research process (ANA, 2000). With the emergence of newer models of care and an emphasis on primary mental health care, APN-PMHs increasingly design and develop psychoeducation. Behavioral change, the desired outcome of psychoeducation, requires tailoring the education to meet the learner's need to develop life skills and coping strategies that must be integrated into behavior. Nurses delivering psychoeducation must understand behavioral change processes. With a renewed emphasis on consumer education and empowering clients and families for self-care and disease prevention, this role presents new challenges for the nurse.

Similarly, the APN-PMH launches evidence-based interventions, evaluating outcomes of care, and formulating questions for further investigation. Effective interventions with measurable outcomes are central to achieving cost-effective use of resources. Interventions often take the form of protocols developed according to standards of psychiatric nursing care and standardized mental health approaches used in related disciplines. The implementation and evaluation of protocols are shaping the directions for new models of care delivery and new nursing role functions.

THE ALCOHOLIC CLIENT: AN EXEMPLAR OF APN-PMH PRACTICE

Alcoholism is a multidimensional disorder, highly prevalent in the population at large. Most individuals with this disorder rarely receive comprehensive care, that is, primary care and care of specific co-occurring psychiatric syndromes. In addition, other problems, such as anxiety disorders, depression, and substance abuse are commonly misdiagnosed categories in primary care practice (National Institutes of Health Consensus Development Panel, 1992), resulting in large numbers of individuals who are not treated for the disorders that trouble them most (National Institute of Mental Health, 2002). Broad-based APN-PMH functions in treating alcoholism: (1) address the majority of personal health needs; (2) develop a sustained partnership; and (3) support practice of one's role in the context of family and community (IOM, 1996).

As many as 6 million individuals meet DMS-IV criteria for alcohol dependence (SAMHSA, 1995), and another 11 million are heavy drinkers (SAMHSA, 1997). Most are not treated because signs are not recognized by primary care providers, because drinkers are unlikely to seek help, and because symptoms of heavy consumption, like fatigue, headaches, and low-back pain are presented as only physical in origin. The client often denies excessive consumption and does not report the links between consumption and symptoms; providers often do not solicit adequate histories. Alcohol-related problems occur on a continuum from use to early problem drinking to frank alcoholism. Nursing interventions must assess the beginning level for severity, evaluate the intermediate stages, and detect progression in an entrenched pattern of alcoholism where the client fluctuates between degrees of health and illness. The APN-PMH who understands both primary care and primary mental health is in a unique position to assist the client during phases of sobriety as well as during preliminary stages of recovery and periods of relapse.

Prevention takes the form of dealing with stressful situations early, avoiding heavy alcohol consumption and over-reliance on prescription drugs, and use of positive coping strategies to deal with daily hassles and problems. Primary prevention and basic health care are supported by "sensible" drinking or a drug-free lifestyle and by use of health education to promote physical and mental well-being. The APN-PMH emphasizes health promotion at all stages of health and illness, recognizing changes in the signs and symptoms of alcohol-related problems.

In the role of direct provider, the APN-PMH develops a comprehensive self-care plan with the client. Alcohol use, often in combination with use of other drugs, persists for long periods, and clients often neglect exercise, dental hygiene, and good nutrition. The nurse imparts important information on these topics and interprets their value in the context of positive self-regard and support for sobriety.

The biologic components of alcohol abuse and dependence figure prominently in meeting health care needs and require a biopsychosocial approach. The APN-PMH develops a database beginning with a comprehensive history and physical assessment. The alcohol and other drug history, in combination with physical signs and laboratory data, are central to nursing and medical diagnoses. Since defensiveness and denial of excessive drinking may result in under-reporting, other sources of data, such as collateral reports from family and friends, must be considered in relation to national standards of sensible drinking to establish a diagnosis of a drinking problem. Screening tools used in primary care and specialty practice help identify the individual whose drinking places him or her at risk for health problems. The two that have been found to be helpful in primary care settings are the CAGE questionnaire (Ewing, 1984) and the WHO (World Health Organization) AUDIT (Saunders, Aasland, Babor, de la Fuente, & Grant, 1993). In addition, the nurse reviews the physical examination and laboratory findings for indicators of heavy consumption and signs of other drug use, such as tracks from injecting drugs or obliteration of structures in nasal passages, indicating cocaine use. The mental status exam (MSE) identifies mental health problems, such as anxiety disorders or depression, and the associated signs of affective and cognitive changes that contribute to alcohol consumption. The APN-PMH may choose to use a brief intervention, which has been found to reduce consumption significantly in persons drinking alcohol in amounts that result in serious health, legal, or occupational problems. A brief intervention consists of a counseling interview in which the clinician reviews the current and potential outcomes of alcohol use for the individual (Miller & Rollnick, 2002).

The APN-PMH will find primary care components essential for alcohol-dependent clients who require detoxification on an inpatient or ambulatory basis. Careful pharmacological and nursing management are key to the restoration of health and to motivating the client to deal with the addiction. Basic assessment, nutritional guidance, nursing care, and counseling skills are components of comprehensive nursing care provided by the APN-PMH. In stages of illness that follow detoxification, the nurse may use pharmacotherapy in conjunction with other treatment approaches.

Partnership with Patients

A trusting, therapeutic nurse-patient relationship is the essential framework for APN-PMH care delivery, and time is needed to build this trust and a secure, credible relationship. A chronic illness like alcoholism may necessitate hospitalizations and contacts with numerous agencies and providers. For trust to continue, a relationship of continuity must be maintained over time and through many communication channels. Outreach efforts, essential in the delivery of broad-based care, include a willingness to visit the client at home and to assess factors such as family or caretaker interaction with the client and the safety and stability of the home and community.

The APN-PMH facilitates trust when the working relationship reflects both accessibility and commitment. Since "slips" and relapses occur in all phases of the chronic disease of alcoholism, the nurse must establish a contract with the client about a plan. Depending on the nature of the illness, the plan may be for controlled drinking or abstinence. An open agreement and the assurance that the nurse will not abandon the patient should relapse occur will encourage honest reporting and diminish expectations about punishment or rejection. A long-term working relationship, characterized by support for basic and psychological health care, increases opportunities to achieve personal growth as well as sobriety.

Contexts of Family and Community

For the APN-PMH, direct primary care interventions include family and community as well as the individual. The alcoholic's family system is often diminished in size and spirit by death, separation, and other losses consequent to many years of alcohol-induced abusive behavior. The APN-PMH uses family counseling and/or psychotherapy to facilitate problem solving and decision making. Adult children of alcoholics report many life problems, and a significant number of them develop dependencies on alcohol and other drugs. By assessing family systems, the APN-PMH can develop strategies for health education, support, and counseling needs for families with alcoholic members.

Tertiary prevention consists of relapse counseling and health maintenance and requires that the client acquire new learning in the psychotherapeutic relationship. Relapse prevention assists the client in learning strategies to recognize and deal with high-risk situations, including skills training for coping, cognitive reframing, and lifestyle balance (Marlatt & Gordon, 1998).

Because alcoholism and other drug dependencies have wide ramifications for the lives of client and family, the APN-PMH is key in interpreting the availability and appropriate use of reliable community resources. The focus of the psychotherapeutic work is the client's drug use and central psychological problems. Support and learning opportunities that move the individual toward a new view of self are particularly important. The nurse facilitates appropriate referrals to legal, vocational, and health agencies, as well as to other care providers and self-help groups, such as Alcoholics Anonymous, Smart Recovery, Rational Recovery, and Women for Sobriety, that can provide guidance and information to the recovering alcoholic.

SUMMARY

APN-PMH practice integrates a level of primary care into mental health care to provide a holistic care model for vulnerable clients whose ability to attend to their own physical and mental health needs is compromised (Talley & Caverly, 1994). Major changes in health care delivery support the greater use of psychiatric nurses in advanced practice roles generally, and the primary mental health care provider role in particular. Aided by managed care approaches, access to third-party payment, and federally funded programs, APN-PMHs are responding to the growing need for community-based mental health for individuals and families with human immunodeficiency virus, the frail elderly, addicts, the severely and persistently mentally ill, the developmentally disabled, and those housed in correctional facilities. In these settings, APN-PMHs are cost-effective because they address health in a comprehensive way while providing psychiatric care at primary, secondary, and tertiary levels.

Primary care as a health care delivery model presents challenging opportunities. Skills in addressing both basic and mental health problems while formulating evidence-based interventions, addressing client/family problems, organizing environmental patterns in support of treatment approaches, and facilitating circumstances to influence the client's ability to attain optimum wellness support the potential for a broad range of role functions and responsibilities.

REFERENCES AND BIBLIOGRAPHY

Agency for Health Care Policy and Research. (1993). *Depression in primary care, Volume I: Detection and diagnosis, Volume II: Treatment of major depression.* Rockville, MD: U.S. Department of Health and Human Services.

Aiken, L., & Sage, W. M. (1993). Staffing national health care reform: A role for advanced practice nurses. *Akron Law Review, 26,* 1–30.

Alexopolous, G. S. (1996). Geriatric depression in primary care. *International Journal of Psychiatry, 11,* 397–400.

Alexopoulos, G. S., Katz, I. R., Reynolds, C. F., Carpenter, D., & Docherty, J. P. (2001). *Pharmacotherapy of depressive disorders in older patients: The expert consensus guideline series.* Minneapolis, MN: McGraw-Hill Healthcare Information Programs.

American Nurses' Association, American Psychiatric Nurses' Association, & International Society of Psychiatric-Mental Health Nurses. (2000). *Scope and standards of psychiatric-mental health nursing practice.* Washington, DC: American Nurses' Association.

American Psychiatric Association. (1994). *Diagnostic and statistical manual of mental disorders* (4th ed., text revision). Washington, DC: Author.

American Psychiatric Association. (1995). *Practice guidelines for substance-related disorders.* Washington, DC: Author.

Astrom, M., Adolfsson, R., & Asplund, K. (1993). Major depression in stroke patients. *Stroke, 24,* 976–982.

Beyer, J., & Marshall, J. (1981). The interpersonal dimension of collegiality. *Nursing Outlook, 29,* 662.

Christman, L. (1987). Psychiatric nurses and the practice of psychotherapy: Current status and future possibilities. *American Journal of Psychotherapy, 41,* 384–390.

Cohen, E., & Cesta, T. (1994). Case management in the acute care setting: A model for health care reform. *Journal of Case Management, 3*(3), 83–87.

Conwell, Y., Duberstein, P. R., Cox, P. R., Hermann, J. H., Forbes, N. T., & Caine, E. D. (1996). Relationships of age and axis I diagnoses in victims of completed suicide: A psychological autopsy study. *American Journal of Psychiatry, 153,* 1001–1008.

Cotroneo, M., Outlaw, F. H., King, J., & Brince, J. (1997). Advanced practice psychiatric-mental health nursing in a community-based nurse-managed primary care program. *Journal of Psychosocial Nursing Mental Health Services, 35*(11), 18–25.

Courage, M. M., Gobdey, K. L., Ingram, D. L., & Schramm, L. L. (1993). Suicide in the elderly: Staying in control. *Journal of Psychosocial Nursing & Mental Health Services, 31*(7), 26–31.

Diagnosis and treatment of depression in late life: Results of the NIH Consensus Development Conference. (1992). Washington, DC: American Psychiatric Press, 9–19.

Dongier, M., Hill, J., Kealy, S., & Lawrence, J. (1994). Screening for alcoholism in general hospitals. *Canadian Journal of Psychiatric Care, 39*(1), 12–20.

Ebersole, P. (1998). *Caring for the psychogeriatric client.* New York: Springer Publishing.

Ells, M. A. (1991). Family therapy. In G. E. Bennett & D. Woolf (Eds.), *Substance abuse* (pp. 267–279). Albany, NY: Delmar.

Ewing, J. A. (1984). Detecting alcoholism: The CAGE questionnaire. *Journal of the American Medical Association, 252,* 1905–1907.

Haber, J., & Billings, C. (1995). Primary mental health care: A model for psychiatric-mental health nursing. *Journal of the American Psychiatric Nurses Association, 1,* 5.

Institute of Medicine. (1996). *Primary care: America's health in a new era.* Washington, DC: National Academy Press.

Johns, E., & Pfefferkorn, B. (1934). *An activity analysis of nursing.* New York: Committee on the Grading of Nursing Schools.

Jenike, M. A. (1996). Psychiatric illnesses in the elderly: A review. *Journal of Geriatric Psychiatry and Neurology, 9,* 57.

Leininger, M. (1973). *Contemporary issues in mental health nursing.* Boston: Little, Brown.

Liskow, B., Campbell, J., Nickel, E. J., & Powell, B. J. (1995). Validity of the CAGE Questionnaire in screening for alcohol dependence in a walk-in (triage) clinic. *Journal of Studies on Alcohol, 56*(3), 277–281.

Marlatt, G. A., & Gordon, J. R. (Eds.). (1998). *Harm reduction: Pragmatic strategies for managing high risk behaviors.* New York: Guilford Press.

McBride, A. B. (1996). Psychiatric nursing in the twenty-first century. In A. B. McBride & J. K. Austin (Eds.), *Psychiatric-mental health nursing: Integrating the behavioral and biological sciences* (pp. 1–10). Philadelphia: W.B. Saunders.

McEnany, G. W. (1991, October). Psychobiology and psychiatric nursing: A philosophical matrix. *Archives of Psychiatric Nursing, V,* 5.

McGivern, D. (1993). The role of the nurse on the interdisciplinary treatment team. In M. A. Naegle (Ed.), *Substance abuse education in nursing, Vol. III* (pp. 183–210). New York: National League for Nursing.

Miller, W., & Rollnick, S. (2002). *Motivational interviewing.* New York: Guilford Press.

Moller, M. D., & Haber, J. (1996). Advanced practice psychiatric nursing: The need for a blended role. *Online Journal of Issues in Nursing, 14*(41), 16–24.

Morris, D. L. (2001). Geriatric mental health: An overview. *Journal of the American Psychiatric Nurses Association, 7*(6), S2–S7.

Morris, J. A. (1995). Alcohol and other drug treatment: A proposal for integration with primary care. *Alcohol Treatment Quarterly, 13*, 45–56.

Murphy, M. F., & Moller, M. D. (1993). Relapse management in neurobiological disorders. The Moller-Murphy Symptom Management Assessment Tool. *Archives of Psychiatric Nursing, 7*, 226–235.

Mrazek, P. J., & Haggerty, R. J. (1994). *Reducing risks for mental disorders.* Washington, DC: National Academy Press.

Naegle, M. (1983). The role of psychotherapist within the primary health care model. In L. Breslan & M. Hang (Eds.), *Depression and aging* (pp. 156–167). New York: Springer Publishing.

Naegle, M. A., & Krainovich-Miller, B. (2001). Shaping the advance practice psychiatric-mental-health nursing role: A futuristic model. *Issues in Mental Health Nursing, 2*, 461–482

National Institute of Mental Health (NIMH). (2002). Retrieved May 15, 2002, from http://www/nimh.nih.gov

New York State Office of Mental Health. (1999). Kendra's law: New York's assisted outpatient treatment. *OMH Quarterly, 5*(3), 3–8.

Peplau, H. (1987). Interpersonal constructs for nursing practice. *Nurse Education Today, 1*, 201–208.

Rapsilber, L. M., & Anderson, E. H. (2000). Understanding the reimbursement process. *Nurse Practitioner, 25*(5), 36–56.

Render, H. W. (1947). Nurse–patient relationships in psychiatry. New York: McGraw-Hill.

SAMSHA. (1995). *Substance abuse and mental health statistics sourcebook.* B. A., Rouse (Ed.). Rockville, MD: U.S. Department of Health and Human Services.

SAMHSA. (1997). *Preliminary results from the 1996 National Household Survey on Drug Abuse.* Rockville, M.D: U.S Department of Health and Human Services.

Saunders, J. B. Aasland, T. F., Babor, T. F., de la Fuente, C., & Grant, M. (1993). Development of the Alcohol Use Disorders Identification Test (AUDIT): WHO collaborative project on early detection of persons with harmful alcohol consumption. *Addiction, 88*, 791–804.

Schuckit, M. A. (1989). *Drug and alcohol abuse: A clinical guide to diagnosis and treatment* . New York: Plenum.

Shiffinan, S., & Balabaris, M. (1996). Do drinking and smoking go together? *Alcohol Health and Research World, 20*, 107–110.

Sills, G. (1993). Foreword. In A. W. O'Toole, & S. F. Welt (Eds.), *Interpersonal theory in nursing practice: Selected works of Hildegard E. Peplau* (pp. ix–xi). New York: Springer Publishing.

Solomon, K., Manepalli, J., Freland, G. A., & Mahon, G. M. (1993). Alcoholism and prescription drug abuse in the elderly: St. Louis University Grand Rounds. *Journal of the American Geriatrics Society, 41*(1), 57–69.

Talley, S., & Brooke, P. (1992). Prescriptive authority for psychiatric clinical specialists: Framing the issues. *Archives of Psychiatric Nursing, 6*(2), 71–82.

Talley, S., & Caverly, S. (1994). Advanced practice psychiatric nursing and health care reform. *Hospital and Community Psychiatry, 45,* 545–547.

World Health Organization Study Group. (1996). A cross-national trial of brief interventions with heavy drinkers. *American Journal of Public Health, 86*(7), 948–955.

U.S. Department of Health and Human Services. (1999). *Mental health: A report to the surgeon general.* Rockville, MD: U.S. Department of Health and Human Services.

Chapter 11

ADVANCED PRACTICE IN HOLISTIC NURSING

Carla Mariano

Holistic health care emphasizes the fundamental wholeness and integrity of the individual and views the body, mind, and spirit as inseparable and interdependent. All behaviors, including health and illness, are manifestations of the life process of the whole person (Quinn, 1995). Health can be described as a condition of wholeness, balance, and harmony of the body, mind, emotions, and spirit. It is not a goal or a state to be achieved—it is a life process of growth and change toward one's potential and a feeling of being alive. Additional assumptions that underlie holistic practice are cited by Fontaine (2000).

> Even Hippocrates, the father of Western medicine, espoused a holistic orientation when he taught doctors to observe their patients' life circumstances and emotional states. Socrates agreed, declaring "Curing the soul; that is the first thing." In alternative medicine, symptoms are believed to be an expression of the body's wisdom as it reacts to cure its own imbalance or disease. Other threads or concepts common to most forms of alternative medicine include the following:
>
> - An internal self-healing process exists within each person.
> - People are responsible for making their own decisions regarding their health care.
> - Nature, time, and patience are the great healers.

Einstein said that matter is energy, energy and matter are interchangeable, and all matter is connected at the subatomic level. No single entity could be affected without all connecting parts being affected. In this view, the universe is a living web. The human body is animated by an integrated energy called the life force. The life force sustains the physical body but is also a spiritual entity that is linked to a higher being or infinite source of energy. When the life force flows freely throughout the body, a person experiences optimal health and vitality. When the life force is blocked or weakened, organs, tissues, and cells are deprived of the energy they need to function at their full potential, and illness or disease results (p. 6).

The word *heal* comes from the Greek word *halos* and the Anglo-Saxon word *haelan*, which means "to be or to become whole." The word *holy* also comes from the same source. *Healing* means "making whole"—or restoring balance and harmony. It is movement toward a sense of wholeness and completion. *Healing* in this context is defined as:

the return toward the natural state of integrity and wholeness of an individual; the process of bringing together aspects of one's self, body-mind-spirit, at a deep level of inner knowing in a way that leads toward integration and balance and integration, with each aspect having equal importance and value; can lead to more complex levels of personal understanding and meaning; may be synchronous but is not synonymous with curing (Dossey & Guzetta, 2000, p. 6).

When the focus is on healing, a successful outcome is not dependent on whether the person lives. "Curing may or may not be possible, but healing is always possible" (Quinn, 2000). Through healing, people appreciate what they already are and move toward a greater sense of the meaning of their lives and their experiences. Even when little can be done physically to change the course of illness or disease, much can be done to make the human experience more meaningful and understandable (Fontaine, 2000; Quinn, 2000).

Contemporary authors describe nursing as central to the paradigm shift occurring in health and illness care (Bright, 2001; Watson, 1999). Burkhardt (2001) described this shift as one from an "illness oriented, biomedically dominated" system to a "model that encompasses health, quality of life and the recognition of the primacy of relationship and or 'interbeing' among all living things" (p. vi). Bright (2001) emphasized that nurses who have integrated a holistic paradigm "hold the vision of health that will continue to transform client care, the means with which to restore wholeness to our beleaguered ecosystem, and the faith that healing possibilities are infinite" (p. 44). Nurses, particularly those educated in the holistic paradigm, carry the hopeful stance that is needed now more than ever to consider and to plan for the future health care delivery system.

Nursing is especially suited to holistic practices because its tradition is based on a philosophy of humanness, compassion, and viewing the individual as an integrated whole within a culture and an environment. Within that philosophy, nurses strive to support people in transition achieving the most comfortable and/or best outcome for the person. This may not be the cure that is commonly the goal of medicine, but rather a more transformative and integrative *healing* of body-mind-spirit.

The treatment of the body alone during illness does not take into account the profound effect the mind has on disease states. Advanced practice holistic nurses integrate complementary therapies into clinical practice to treat patients' physiological, psychological, and spiritual needs. Doing so does not negate the validity of conventional medical therapies but serves to complement, broaden, and enrich the scope of nursing practice and to help patients access their greatest healing potential.

Fontaine (2000) emphasized that this stance places nurses with a foot in each camp—biomedicine and complementary alternative approaches. Currently most experts in the field, as well as the National Center for Complementary and Alternative Medicine (NCCAM), advocate integration rather than separation. Holistic nursing education and practice restores those traditions of seeking healing, restoration, and growth through comfort-enhancing measures such as touch and relaxation-imagery approaches, and by helping the client be in the best situation for healing through such measures as nutritional support, health counseling, and environmental management. Nurses with advanced education in holistic practice are also needed to participate more effectively as partners in the much-needed research into the efficacy and safety of complementary alternative medicine (CAM) modalities. They have a valuable role to play in the expanding world of holistic health care.

COMPLEMENTARY/INTEGRATIVE HEALTH CARE

Kim Jobst (1998), editor in chief of *The Journal of Alternative Medicine,* states that public and professional demand for, and interest in, complementary and alternative therapies and holistic systems of health is part of a profound change taking place in health care that no country can afford to ignore, either economically or socially. We need a rigorous and coordinated commitment to evaluation of these modalities and systems for appropriate integration into health care practice and policy. Western medicine is proving wholly, or partially, ineffective for a significant proportion of the common chronic diseases. Furthermore, highly technological health care is too expensive to be universally affordable.

Many conventional health care institutions are developing programs such as stress management, energy therapies, healers in the operating rooms, and acupuncture. Programs such as Reiki or therapeutic touch for chronic pain, support groups using imagery for breast cancer, and groups espousing meditation for health and wellness are commonly advertised across the United States. These programs are led by both lay and professional people, some of whom are skilled and experienced while others are novice. Similarly, local pharmacies and health food stores are selling an array of supplements, herbs, homeopathic preparations, vitamins, hormones, and various combinations of these that were not considered marketable 5 years ago. The number of books, journals, and Web sites devoted to complementary, integrative, and holistic healing practices has also dramatically increased.

According to a survey published in the *Journal of the American Medical Association* (K. L. Eisenberg, 1993), one of every three Americans seeking medical help in 1991 received what would be considered unconventional treatment. D. M. Eisenberg et al.'s (1998) updated survey showed a sharp increase in use which he estimated will continue in the next 20–30 years (see Table 11.1).

According to D. M. Eisenberg et al. (1998), the estimated expenditures for alternative medicine professional services increased by 45.2% from 1990 to 1997 and the expenditure of 12.2 billion out-of-pocket dollars in 1997 exceeded the out-of-pocket expenditures for all U.S. hospitalizations. The total expenditure for 1997 was conservatively estimated at $27 billion, which compares with the projected total out-of-pocket expense for all physician services.

D. M. Eisenberg et al. (1998) includes various modalities that nurses are increasingly incorporating into their practices: massage therapy, biofeedback, relaxation techniques, guided imagery, spiritual healing, hypnosis, herbal remedies, and energy healing with touch, magnets, and other devices. Other studies (Boutin, Buchwald, Robinson, & Collier, 2000; Wolsko et al., 2000) indicate that the heavy use of these modalities spans all socioeconomic groups. These modalities may decrease overall use of standard methods of care, including costly emergency department visits, by enhancing comfort and helping individuals maintain quality of life with chronic illnesses. Although no controlled studies exist on the use of these modalities in poor and underserved populations, it is known that folk remedies

TABLE 11.1   Comparison of Eisenberg's Findings 1990/1997

Findings	1990	1997
Americans using alternative medicine	61 million	83 million
Visits to alternative practitioners	427 million	629 million
Visits to conventional practitioners	386 million	338 million
Use of at least one alternative modality	33.8% of sample	42.1% of sample
Probability of a person visiting an alternative practitioner	36.3%	46.3%

and modalities are often employed (McGuire, 1994). Kessler et al. (2001), in a survey of 2,005 respondents, found that the range of CAM modalities used increased over the respondents' life times. This study indicates that the use of these modalities is likely to continue to rise as the baby boomers age and develop more chronic illnesses.

Weil (2000) noted that a "major impetus for the integrative medicine movement is the large and growing gulf between what consumers want and what doctors [health care providers] are trained to do. Consumers want [those] who have the time to help them understand the nature of their medical problems; who will not propose drugs and surgery as the only treatment options; who are aware of nutritional influences on health and can answer questions about dietary supplements; who are sensitive to mind-body interactions and able to see patients as more than just physical bodies; and who will not laugh at them for bringing up topics like Chinese medicine and homeopathy" (p. 6).

The White House Commission on Complementary and Alternative Medicine Policy (WHCCAMP, 2001) report includes the testimony of 300 consumers. Consumer interest in and use of complementary modalities apparently has not changed since the landmark epidemiologic studies done by Eisenberg and associates (1993; 1998). Weeks (2001) outlined several trends in CAM that demonstrate how consumer use is influencing insurance coverage, education, and practice: (1) The majority of physicians support at least the use of one or more CAM, (2) Approximately two thirds of health maintenance organizations offered some coverage for CAM modalities, and that trend is increasing, (3) In 1999, The American Hospital Association developed a program to educate member institutions on how to offer CAM services, (4) Integrative clinics that include both CAM and conventional providers are increasing across the country. This driving force will propel mainstream health care increasingly in this direction, and nurses therefore need to be adequately prepared to meet this need.

ADVANCED PRACTICE HOLISTIC NURSING

The American Holistic Nurses Association (2002) described the graduate prepared holistic nurse (GPHN), a term used instead of advanced practice holistic nurse, and the master's or doctoral-level preparation needed for that role:

> Graduate preparation in [advanced practice] holistic nursing is aimed at specialization in an holistic approach to care. . . . [It] emphasizes critical thinking based on advanced thinking based on advanced assessment skills, advanced knowledge of physiology, psychoneuroimmunology, psychology, pharmacology, and in-depth understanding of health care policy, financing, and organization as well as advanced clinical and ethical decision making based on holistic philosophy, theory and a broad understanding of human diversity and complex social issues and health promotion and disease prevention. Graduate preparation for the holistic nurse emphasizes a holistic perspective and expert enactment of the roles of advanced practice including clinician and facilitator of healing, consultant and collaborator, educator and guide, administrator, leader, change agent, researcher and advocate.
>
> Graduate prepared holistic nurses model a wellness lifestyle and value lifelong learning, all ways of knowing, and interconnectedness. They are aware of their assets and limitations and their effect on others and work to contribute to the well-being of individuals, families, groups, communities, and the earth. [They] recognize themselves as integral to a larger universe consciousness and endeavor to contribute in a positive and meaningful way to the larger reality. . . . [They] facilitate the healing process by using themselves as instruments of healing through the integration of advanced holistic nursing knowledge with the core values of holistic nursing. (p. 9)

The American Holistic Nurses' Association (AHNA) *Standards of Advanced Holistic Nursing Practice for Graduate Prepared Nurses* (2002) define and establish the scope of holistic practice, serve as a guide to practice, and describe the care expected from an advanced practice holistic nurse. The Standards are grouped under five core values: holistic philosophy, theory, and ethics; holistic education and research; holistic nurse self-care; holistic communication, therapeutic environment, and cultural diversity; and holistic caring process. The standards are quite specific and, therefore, will be used here as the basis for identifying the role and responsibilities of the GPHN.

Core Value I: Holistic Philosophy, Theory, and Ethics

Graduate prepared holistic nurses subscribe to a philosophy that values healing as the desired outcome of the practice of caring and the human health experience as a complicated, dynamic relationship of health, illness, and wellness. Their practice is based on scientific foundations; however, nursing is truly valued as an art. It is relationship-centered, aesthetic, and culturally, socially, and ecologically sensitive. The holistic philosophy further recognizes that the client is the authority on his or her own health experience, and honors that ethic. Client narratives, whether they arise from individuals, families, or communities, provide the context of the experience and are used as an important focus in understanding the client situation. GPHNs hold the belief that they are not the healer but the guide and facilitator of the client's own healing.

Philosophically, there are differences between allopathic and holistic models of care, and this strongly affects the practice of the graduate prepared holistic nurse. Table 11.2 lists the differences.

Graduate prepared holistic nurses hold to a professional ethic of caring and healing that seeks to preserve wholeness and dignity of self and others in all practice settings. GPHNs support human dignity by advocating and adhering to the patient's bill of rights. The components of traditional ethics (its morals, values, and cultural ideals) are not excluded from holistic ethics; indeed, they serve as the foundation.

The view of holistic ethics encompasses traditional ethical principles and also emphasizes the unity of the self and the universe. According to Keegan (2000), holistic ethics is a particular theory of ethics emphasizing the "unity and integral wholeness of all people and of all nature that is identified and pursued by finding unity and wholeness within the self and within humanity" (p. 162).

In the belief that all things are connected, the holistic perspective espouses the belief that an individual's actions have a ripple effect throughout humanity. Holism places the greatest worth on individuals' developing higher levels of human awareness. This, in turn, elevates the whole of humanity. Keegan (2000) stated that "unethical acts are those that degrade or brutalize the individual who performs the act and detract from his or her conscious evolution . . . the unethical act dissolves unity . . . and takes away wholeness. Holistic ethics is a process of developing an attitude of the sacredness of ourselves and of all nature . . . our inner self and the collective greater self have stewardship not only over our bodies, mind and spirit, but also over our planet and the total universe" (p. 165). Holistic ethics is about relationship. It concerns itself with the meaning and quality of life deriving from a person's own character and from the person's relationship to the universe rather than imposed from without.

Kylea Taylor (1995) coined the term *holotrophic ethics,* which is the process of therapists, teachers, and caregivers moving themselves toward

TABLE 11.2 Conventional/Allopathic and Holistic Perspectives of Care

Conventional/Allopathic Perspective	Holistic Perspective
• Cure, symptom treatment, repair • Diagnosed by practitioner • Patient is dependent, passive • Effective for some, but not all people; cure may or may not be possible • Mechanistic; separation of body, mind, spirit • Specialization • Use of invasive treatments, e.g., drugs, surgery, radiation • Illness is interpreted as negative • Neutrality and objectivity	• Healing, growth, evolution • Meaning, understanding, insight, self-awareness • Person is autonomous, active partner • Healing is possible for all individuals even during death • Body-mind-spirit viewed as holistic, dynamic, inseparable, and interdependent • Integration • Integrative treatments that include diet, herbs, stress management, energy work, and reflection • Illness is viewed as a teacher • Human caring and connectedness; value oriented

Modified from Fontaine (2000) and Dossey & Keegan (2000).

and assisting clients to move toward mental, physical, psychological, and spiritual wholeness. Holotrophic ethics is the expanding of the caregiver's "ethical consciousness to include more and more integrity. Such an understanding of ethics goes beyond morals and ethical codes. Rather, morality and ethical behavior are in the service of our highest nature. They are at the same time a natural product of our growing attunement with our spiritual natures" (p. 4).

Core Value II: Holistic Education and Research

The entry level for advanced practice holistic nursing is a graduate degree. Presently there is only one holistic nurse practitioner program in the country (New York University) and three holistic clinical nurse specialist programs (College of New Rochelle; Beth-El College, University of Colorado; and Tennessee State University). Increasingly, graduate programs are incorporating courses or concentrations into their master's degree programs. The American Holistic Nurses Association's recently approved *Standards of Advanced Holistic Nursing Practice for Graduate Prepared Nurses (2002)* provides a guide for graduate curriculum design and will serve as the basis for the upcoming development of the advanced practice certification examination (presently, the generalist holistic nursing certification [HNC] examination is used to certify holistic nurses).

Graduate prepared holistic nurses participate in life-long learning and teach others in a manner that demonstrates a holistic philosophy and values all ways of knowing and learning. GPHNs believe that illness and adversity are our greatest teachers and that we have a great deal to learn from them if we take advantage of the opportunity to do so. Often clients need guidance in developing this perspective that is so helpful on the path to self-healing.

As the American public increasingly uses CAM therapies, more rigorous scientific research and information on the safety and efficacy of these modalities will be needed. To demonstrate the importance of research in this area, the appropriations to the National Center for CAM increased dramatically from $19.5 million in 1998 to $68.3 million in 2000, and the National Institute of Health, including the NCCAM, plan to fund more than $220 million for research and research training in fiscal year 2002 (WHCCAMP, 2001). The Commission noted that this research might be best served by collaborations between conventional and CAM researchers and clinicians.

The importance of GPHNs conducting and/or evaluating research in this area cannot be overstated. As they are often in a position to guide clients and families in their health care decisions, especially between conventional allopathic and complementary practices, they must be knowledgeable about the best evidence available. They develop evidence-based practices using research, practice guidelines, expertise, and client values. GPHN researchers need to attend to scholarly rigor, clinical significance, ethics, consultation when necessary, dissemination of findings, interdisciplinary discourse, and quality improvement generated by their research.

There is a question, however, about what method is most appropriate for the study of holistic phenomena. The scientific method or quantitative approach has been the most commonly used method of scientific inquiry to date in nursing. Qualitative methods may be better suited to capture the wholeness of one's experience rather than a part of it, and the fit between quantitative methods and holistic nursing practice may not always be ideal. It is therefore important for GPHNs to look at alternative philosophies of science and research methods that are compatible with investigations of humanistic and holistic occurrences. Also needed are studies exploring the context in which phenomena occur and the meaning of patterns that evolve.

With regard to quantitative studies, researchers must approach quantitative intervention studies more holistically by taking into consideration the interactive nature of the body, mind, and spirit. Rather than isolating the effects of one part of an intervention, more comprehensive interventions and more sensitive measurement instruments that measure the interactive nature of each client's biological, psychological, sociological, emotional, and spiritual patterns are needed. Comprehensive comparative outcome studies are needed to ascertain the usefulness of and indications and contraindications for integrative therapies. And researchers must also evaluate these interventions for their usefulness in promoting wellness as well as preventing illness (Mariano, 2001b).

As can be seen, both quantitative and qualitative approaches are needed in holistic research.

Core Value III: Holistic Nurse Self-Care

Self-care and personal awareness of being an instrument of healing are significant requirements for advanced practice holistic nurses. GPHNs value themselves and mobilize the necessary resources to care for themselves. "They integrate self-care into their lives and engage in self-management in ways that honor their unique patterns and the cycles of growth and development of the body, the psychological-social-cultural self, the intellectual self, and the spiritual self" (AHNA, 2002, p. 17). Nurses cannot facilitate healing unless they are in the process of healing themselves. It is a lifelong process.

The American Holistic Nurses' Association (1992) code of ethics for holistic nurses states "the nurse has a responsibility to model health behaviors. Holistic nurses strive to achieve harmony in their own lives and assist others to do the same" (p. 3). It is important for graduate prepared holistic nurses to create healing environments for themselves by attending to their own well-being, letting go of self-destructive behaviors and attitudes, practicing centering and stress reduction techniques, and keeping balance in their lives. Roach and Nieto (1997), in discussing the role of nurse healers, identified five self-care areas and questions that need to be explored:

1. Spiritual self-care—Is spirituality important in my life; what is my relationship with God or a higher power; why am I here and what is my purpose; what is my relationship to the universe?
2. Emotional self-care—Can I identify my emotions; how do I deal with them; am I usually in control; can I discuss my emotions; am I open to others and do I respect the feelings of others or do I jump to conclusions; when do my emotions get out of control?

3. Physical self-care—What areas of my lifestyle are unhealthy or do I have a healthy lifestyle; what can I do to improve my lifestyle?

4. Mental self-care—Am I knowledgeable and do I continually increase my knowledge; am I satisfied with the status quo or am I open to new ideas; what am I doing to stimulate my mind?

5. Relationships self-care—Am I open and honest with myself and others; do I have satisfying relationships with others; am I willing to accept the thoughts and feelings of others even though they are different from my own or am I judgmental; must I have all the control or can I share it; do I have a balance between work, home, and leisure? (pp. 171–175)

Graduate prepared holistic nurses realize that suffering, illness, and disease are natural components of the human condition that need attention and have the potential to teach us about ourselves, our relationships, and our universe. Every experience is valued for its uniqueness and its lesson. In addition, GPHNs honor creative expression as a way of knowing that assists them in finding meaning in experience. Creativity can be demonstrated through ingenuity in practice, teaching, management, and research. Honoring the creative self can add beauty to one's life and practice and further enhance the art of caring.

Core Value IV: Holistic Communication, Therapeutic Environment, and Cultural Diversity

How GPHNs communicate is a vital factor in their effectiveness as advanced practitioners. Their communication attempts to ensure that each individual experiences the presence of the nurse as authentic, caring, compassionate, and sincere; there is an atmosphere of shared humanness and interconnectedness. The importance of context in understanding the client's health experience is always recognized. Space and time are allowed for exploration. As each client's health encounter is unique and may be contrary to conventional knowledge and treatments, the GPHN must be comfortable with ambiguity, paradox, and uncertainty. Approaching the client with openness or a "beginner's mind" allows for mutual respect and reciprocal knowing. "Graduate prepared holistic nurses have an expanded knowledge base of the use and meanings of symbolic language. . . . [They] incorporate in their practices therapies based on symbolic language such as imagery, creation of sacred space and personal rituals, dream exploration, and the use of aesthetic therapies such as music, visual art and danced. . . . [They] encourage and support others in the use of prayer, meditation or other spiritual and symbolic practices for healing purposes" (AHNA, 2002, p. 20).

Graduate prepared holistic nurses have a particular obligation to create a therapeutic environment that values holism, caring, social support, and integration of conventional and CAM approaches to healing. They create environments where individuals, both clients and staff, feel connected, supported, and respected. Referring to a holistic environment, Mariano (2000) says it is essential that "the staff, the janitors, the elevator operator, the client—all have to be honored because they are integrally connected. This requires a different type of thinking. Holistic healing is a collaborative approach; you know that you're connected with each other. You honor the client's meaning of illness or treatment; the ego has no place in healing" (p. 186). The nurse, through his or her presence, provides an environment of support and caring by creating an environment to evoke the healing response. This environment is sacred—the nurse engages with clients in an authentic exchange of energy, truth, and communication in order to help them attune to their own healing capacities and their inner teacher and guide (McKivergin, 2000).

In keeping with this thinking, GPHNs also take an active role in trying to remove the political and financial barriers to the inclusion of holistic care in the health care system. In addition, GPHNs actively participate in building an ecosystem that sustains the well-being of all life. This includes raising the public's consciousness about environmental issues and stressors that affect not only the health of people but the health of the planet.

Culture, beliefs, and values are an inherent component of a holistic approach. Concepts of health and healing are based in culture and often influence people's actions to promote, maintain, and restore health. Culture also may provide an understanding of a person's concept of the illness or disease and appropriate treatment. GPHNs must be reflective practitioners, "getting in touch with their beliefs/values, with their preconceived ideas, with their spirituality and sense of wholeness, and with their views about life and about themselves. . . . The attempt is not to change [your] belief system but to appreciate and honor someone else's belief system and someone else's journey. . . . Holism is very culturally oriented, because you have to deal with that as an integral part of people's behavior and their health care beliefs" (Mariano, 2001a, p. 7). GPHNs possess knowledge and understanding of numerous cultural traditions and health care practices from various racial, ethnic, and social backgrounds. These understandings then are used to provide culturally competent care that corresponds with the beliefs and values, traditions, and health practices of clients.

Core Value V: Holistic Caring Process

Holistic caring is a process that involves six often simultaneously occurring steps: assessment; pattern/problem/need identification; therapeutic plan of care; implementation; outcomes; and evaluation. GPHNs apply the holistic caring process with individuals, families across the lifespan, population groups, and communities, and in all settings. Holistic nursing takes place wherever healing occurs.

Graduate prepared holistic nurses incorporate a variety of roles in their practice, including expert clinician and facilitator of healing; consultant and collaborator; educator and guide; administrator, leader, and change agent; researcher; and advocate (AHNA, 2002). GPHNs utilize empirical, ethical, aesthetic, intuitive, personal, and sociological ways of knowing while partnering with the client in the decision-making process. They accept and honor the supposition that behavior has meaning and intent has an integral role in the healing process.

Advanced holistic assessments include not only the physical, functional, psychosocial, mental, emotional, cultural, and sexual aspects, but also the spiritual, transpersonal, and energy field assessments of the whole person. Appropriate laboratory, screening, and other diagnostic tests are used, as indicated, when dealing with individual assessments. Holistic assessments of groups and communities include many of the same parameters described above and also include group and community energy field dynamics and patterns. Holistic assessment data are interpreted into "patterns/challenges/needs from which meaning and understanding of the health/disease experience can be mutually identified with the client" (AHNA, 2002, p. 25). GPHNs, using critical thinking and diagnostic reasoning, synthesize assessment data (both nursing and medical) to establish differential diagnoses and create a holistic diagnosis, including levels of acuity, severity, and complexity.

In their role as advanced practice nurses, GPHNs consult, collaborate, prescribe, and refer, as necessary, both to conventional allopathic providers and to other holistic practitioners. An important responsibility is that of helping the client to identify risk factors such as lifestyle, habits, personal and family health history, and age-related conditions that influence health and to recognize opportunities to increase well-being.

In healing, some outcomes may not be immediately apparent because of the nonlinear nature of the process. The GPHN and client together specify the expected outcomes of care and also appreciate evolving outcomes of healing. Therapeutic plans of care are created mutually with the client and present options and encourage choice. The plan respects the client's experience and the uniqueness of each healing journey. Therapeutic plans focus on health, growth, and wholeness. They value the beliefs, culture, traditions, and background of the client. A significant focus is on guiding clients to utilize their own inner strength and resources through the course of healing. Appropriate and evidence-based information (including current knowledge, practice, and research) regarding the health condition and various treatments and therapies and their side effects is consistently provided.

Interventions in holistic care always occur within the scope and standards of practice of advanced practice registered nursing and in accordance with state and federal laws and regulations. GPHNs prescribe and implement care based on client needs and the holistic assessment. This care is grounded in current knowledge, practice, and research. In addition to conventional advanced practice nursing interventions, GPHNs use a number of CAM approaches, which have been categorized by the National Center for Complementary and Alternative Medicine (2001–2005 *Five-Year Strategic Plan*). These include the following:

1. Alternative medical systems, such as Ayurveda, traditional oriental medicine, homeopathy, naturopathy, Native American practices, and Latin American practices).
2. Mind-body interventions, such as meditation, imagery, hypnosis, yoga, prayer, art and music therapies, mental healing, cognitive-behavioral therapy, therapeutic counseling, stress reduction).
3. Biologically based therapies, such as herbal therapies, diet therapies (e.g., Atkins, Ornish, Pritkin, and Weil diets, nutritional supplements, megadose vitamins, laetrile, bee pollen, chelation therapy, metabolic therapy).
4. Manipulative and body-based methods, such as chiropractic, massage therapy, osteopathy, Rolfing).
5. Energy therapies, such as therapeutic touch, Reiki, Qi gong, reflexology, accupressure, electromagnetic fields, biofield therapeutics.

GPHNs prescribe medications as legally authorized and instruct clients regarding drug, herbal, and homeopathic regimens as well as side effects and interactions. They provide information and counseling about alternative, complementary, integrative, and conventional health care practices; provide continuity of care; and facilitate negotiation of services as they guide individuals and families between these two systems. As in all aspects of the holistic caring process, GPHNs, in partnership with the client, evaluate if care is effective and if there are changes in the meaning of the health experience for the client.

Practice settings include free standing complementary and alternative care centers; integrative or complementary health or medicine departments in ambulatory or acute care facilities; private practitioners in primary care, specialty care, or complementary/integrative care; women's health centers; mental health centers; student and employee health; health maintenance organizations; specialty outpatient clinics (e.g., oncology, AIDS, cardiac, substance abuse); home care; rehabilitation centers; and schools, to name a few. As the public increasingly requests these services, advanced practice holistic nurses will be increasingly in demand and practice in a wider array of settings.

ISSUES IN HOLISTIC NURSING

A number of issues exist or will emerge in the future of advanced practice holistic nursing. They can be categorized into the areas of education, research, clinical practice, and policy. It is important to note that many of these issues face not only holistic nursing but other disciplines as well. Therefore, an interdisciplinary approach is imperative to the successful outcomes of a number of these questions.

At a May 2002 nursing summit in St. Paul, Minnesota, a group of holistic nursing leaders addressed the issue of nursing's leadership in the complementary/alternative/integrative health care movement ("Leading the Way," 2003). The purposes were to identify issues and strategies relating to the integration of complementary/alternative therapies into nursing education, research, and patient care, examine financial and legal implications, including scope of practice and reimbursement models; and develop a plan for strengthening nursing's presence and visibility within the field and for advancing this agenda.

The White House Commission on Complementary and Alternative Medicine Policy (WHCCAMP, 2000) recently completed its final report to the President through the Secretary of Health and Human Services. It contains legislative and administrative recommendations that will ensure the potential benefits of CAM to all citizens.

The Integrated Health Care Consortium—a multistakeholder ad hoc group represented by such diverse parties as educators from accredited conventional and CAM schools and professional organizations and representative of various disciplines, payers (e.g., Medicare, private insurance companies), natural health care product manufacturers, employers, consumer advocacy groups, and government agencies—developed a report that included recommendations on research, education, underserved and special-needs populations, regulation and access to CAM, clinical practice and quality of care, and public and community health.

The nursing summit, the White House Commission on Complementary and Alternative Medicine Policy, and the Integrated Health Care Consortium identified the following issues facing holistic nursing.

Education

There are several areas of educational challenge in the holistic arena. With increased use of complementary and alternative therapies by the American public, both students and faculty need knowledge and skill in their use. Of priority is the integration of complementary and alternative modalities into nursing curricula. Core content appropriate for advanced practice programs needs to be identified, and models for integration of both content and experiences into existing curricula are necessary. An elective course is not sufficient to imbue this knowledge to future practitioners of nursing because of the increasing number of patients and clients who are recipients of these modalities. Holistic nurses will need to work with the accrediting bodies of master's degree programs to ensure that this content is included in educational programs. There is a definitive need for increased scholarship and financial aid to support advanced training in this area. Faculty development programs also will be necessary to support faculty in teaching these therapies.

Licensure and credentialing provide another challenge for holistic nursing. As complementary/alternative medicine has gained national recognition, state boards of nursing began to attend to the regulation issues. In 2001, Captain Andrew Sparber of the U.S. Public Health Service undertook a study to ascertain the number of boards of nursing that had a formal policy, position, or inclusion of complementary therapies under the scope of practice (Sparber, 2001). He found that 25 states (47%) that permitted practice had statements or positions that included specific complementary therapies or examples of these practices, 7 (13%) were discussing the topic, and 21 (40%) had not formally addressed the topic but did not discourage these practices. It will be important in the future to monitor state boards of nursing for evidence of their recognition and support of integrative nursing practice and requirements that include CAM for nursing educational program approval. Finally, holistic nursing has the challenge of working with the state boards to incorporate this content into the National Council Licensure Examination thus ensuring the credibility of this practice knowledge.

Although certification at the generalist level exists for holistic nurses through the American Holistic Nurses Certification Corporation, there is a pressing need for certification of holistic nurses at the advanced practice level. Credentialing is necessary for credibility with the public, inside the profession, and with other disciplines, as well as for reimbursement. Both the American Holistic Nurses Association (AHNA) and the American Holistic Nurses Certification Corporation (AHNCC) have deemed this a priority, and an advanced practice exam for holistic nurses will be forthcoming.

To improve the competency of practitioners and the quality of services, CAM education and training needs to continue beyond basic and advanced academic education. Continuing education programs at national and regional specialty organizations and conferences may assist in this need. Working with practitioners in other areas of nursing to increase their understanding of the philosophical and theoretical foundations of holistic nursing practice (e.g., intention, presence, and centering) will also be a role of holistic nurses.

Research

Research in the area of holistic nursing will become increasing important in the future. There is a great need for an evidence base establishing the effectiveness and efficacy of complementary/alternative therapies. However, one of the formidable tasks for nurses will be to identify and describe outcomes of CAM therapies such as healing, well-being, and harmony to develop instruments to measure these outcomes. Presently, most outcome measures are based on physical or disease symptomatology. In Addition, methodologies need to be expanded to capture the wholeness of the client/patient experience because the philosophy of these therapies rests on a paradigm of wholeness.

Nurses need to address how to secure funding for their CAM research. They need to apply to other National Institutes of Health (NIH) centers and institutes than the National Institute of Nursing Research for funding of CAM research, particularly the National Center for Complementary and Alternative Medicine. But hand in hand with this is the need for nurses to be represented on study sections and review panels to educate and convince the biomedical/NIH community about the value of nursing research; the need for models of research focusing on health promotion and disease prevention, wellness, and self-care instead of just the disease model; and the importance of a variety of designs and research methodologies versus the randomized controlled trial alone.

Another area of responsibility for advanced practice holistic nurses will be the dissemination of their research findings to various media sources (e.g., television, newsprint) and at non-nursing, interdisciplinary conferences. Publishing in non-nursing journals and serving on editorial boards of non-nursing journals also broadens the appreciation of other disciplines for nursing's role in setting the agenda and conducting research in the area of CAM.

Clinical Practice

Clinical care models reflecting holistic assessment, treatment, health, healing, and caring are important in the development of CAM integration. Models (discussed earlier in the chapter) are an enormous challenge to operationalize in today's health care environment. Their acceptance will require a paradigm shift for many providers who subscribe to a disease model of care. Advanced practice holistic nurses with their education and experience are the logical leaders in integrative care and must advance that position.

Policy

Three major policy issues face holistic nursing in the future: reimbursement, regulation, and access.

Public or private policies regarding coverage of and reimbursement for health care services play a crucial role in shaping the health care system and will play a crucial role in deciding the future of CAM in the nation's health care system. Often CAM is offered as a supplemental benefit rather than as a core or basic benefit, and many third-party payers do not cover such services at all. Coverage of and reimbursement for most services depend on the provider's ability to furnish services legally within the scope of practice. The legal authority to practice is given by the state in which services are provided. Reimbursement of advanced practice nurses also depends on appropriate credentialing. Advanced practice holistic nurses will need to work with Medicare and other third-party payers, insurance groups, boards of nursing, health care policy makers, legislators, and other professional nursing organizations to ensure that holistic nurses are appropriately reimbursed for services rendered. Another issue regarding reimbursement is the fact that the effectiveness of CAM is influenced by the holistic focus and integrative skill of the provider. Consequently, reimbursement must be included for the process of integrating care, not just for providing the specific modality.

There are many barriers to the use of CAM therapies, providing yet another challenge for holistic nurses in the future. Although the number of users is growing, more than half of Americans did not use CAM therapies in 2001. Factors affecting use include lack of awareness of the therapies and their benefits, uncertainty about their effectiveness, inability to pay for them, and limited availability of qualified providers. Access is even more difficult for rural populations; uninsured or underinsured populations; special populations, such as racial and ethnic minorities; and vulnerable populations, such as the chronically and terminally ill (WHCCAMP, 2002). Advanced practice holistic nurses have a unique opportunity to educate the public more fully about complementary/alternative modalities and practitioners and to guide clients so that they can make informed choices among the array of health care alternatives and individual providers. Holistic nurses also must actively participate in the political arena as leaders in this movement to ensure an increased focus on wellness and access and affordability for all.

CONCLUSIONS

Advanced practice holistic nursing is an art and a science. It is also an integrative practice. As consumers continue to demand a holistic approach to their health care and the use of holistic modalities continues to expand, nurses' knowledge and use of these modalities in all areas of practice becomes increasingly important. Now the question is, "Who will provide this care?"

Advanced practice holistic nurses play a vital role by assessing, implementing, coordinating, and evaluating holistic care throughout wellness/illness, as well as counseling and educating patients, clients, and families and facilitating continuity of care between conventional biomedicine and complementary/alternative practices.

Advanced practice holistic nurses, by developing theoretical and empirical knowledge, will advance holistic nursing practice and education and contribute significantly to the formalization and credibility of this work. They will provide the leadership in the profession in research, the development of educational models, and the integration of a more holistic approach in nursing practice and health care.

ACKNOWLEDGMENT

The author wishes to acknowledge Rothlyn Zahourek, PhD, RN, CS, HNC for her input.

ADDITIONAL RESOURCES

American Holistic Nurses Association
P.O. Box 2130
Flagstaff, AZ 86003-2130
Phone: (800) 278-2462
Web site: http://www.ahna.org

National Center for Complementary and Alternative Medicine (NCCAM)
National Institutes of Health
P.O. Box 8218
Silver Spring, MD 20907-8218
Phone: (888) 644-6226
Fax: (301) 495-4957
Web site: http://nccam.nih.gov/

REFERENCES

American Holistic Nurses Association. (1992). *American Holistic Nurses Association position statement on holistic nursing ethics.* Flagstaff, AZ: Author.

American Holistic Nurses Association. (2002). *AHNA standards of advanced holistic nursing practice for graduate prepared nurses.* Flagstaff, AZ: Author.

Boutin, P. D., Buchwald, D., Robinson, L., & Collier, A. C. (2000). The use of and attitudes about alternative and complementary therapies among outpatients and physicians at a municipal hospital. *Journal of Alternative & Complementary Medicine, 6,* 335–343.

Bright, M. A. (2001). Health, healing and holistic nursing. In M. A. Bright (Ed.), *Holistic health and healing* (pp. 31–46). Philadelphia: F.A. Davis.

Burkhardt, P. (2001). Foreword. In M. A. Bright (Ed.), *Holistic health and healing* (pp. v–vi). Philadelphia: F.A. Davis.

Dossey, B., & Guzzetta, C. (2000). Holistic nursing practice. In B. Dossey, L. Keegan, & C. Guzzetta (Eds.), *Holistic nursing: A handbook for practice* (pp. 5–33). Gaithersburg, MD: Aspen.

Eisenberg, D. M., Davis, R. B., Ettner, S. L. Appel, S., Wilke, S., Van Rompay, M., & Kessler, R. C. (1998). Trends in alternative medicine use in the United States, 1990–1997. *Journal of the American Medical Association, 280,* 1569–1575.

Eisenberg, K. L. (1993). Unconventional medicine in the United States. *Journal of the American Medical Association, 328,* 246–252, 328.

Expanding horizons of health care. (2001–2005). National Center for Complementary & Alternative Medicine's Five-Year Strategic Plan. Bethesda, MD: National Institute of Health.

Fontaine, K. L. (2000). *Healing practice: Alternative therapies for nursing.* Upper Saddle River, NJ: Prentice Hall.

Jobst, K. A. (1998). Complementary and alternative medicine: Essential for the future of effective, affordable healthcare (Editorial). *Journal of Alternative & Complementary Medicine, 4,* 261–266.

Keegan, L. (2000). Holistic ethics. In B. Dossey, L. Keegan, & C. Guzzetta (Eds.), *Holistic nursing a handbook for practice* (pp. 159–169). Gaithersburg, MD: Aspen.

Kessler, R. C., Davis, R. B., Foster, D. F., Van Rompay, M. I., Walters, E. E, Woilkey, S. A., Kaptchuk, T. J., & Esienbery, D. M. (2001). Long-term trends in the use of complementary and alternative medical therapies in the United States. *Annals of Internal Medicine, 135,* 262-268.

Leading the Way: The Gillette Nursing Summit on Integrated Health & Healing. (2003). St. Paul Minnesota Report of Proceedings. *Health and Medicine* (Suppl.), *9,* 1A–10A.

Mariano C. (2000). Holistic ethics. *American Journal of Nursing, 101,* 24A–24C.

Mariano, C. (2001a). *Holistic ethics and holistic research in nursing.* Unpublished manuscript.

Mariano, C. (2001b). Incorporating holistic care into nursing practice. *NYU Nursing, 4*(2), 6–7.

McGuire, M. B. (1994). *Ritual healing in suburban America.* New Brunswick, NJ: Rutgers University Press.

McKinergin, M. (2000). The nurse as an instrument of healing. In B. Dossey, L. Keegan, & C. Guzzetta (Eds.), *Holistic nursing: A handbook for practice* (pp. 207–227). Gaithersburg, MD: Aspen.

National Policy Dialogue to Advance Integrated Health Care: Finding Common Ground. (2002). *Alternative Therapies in Health and Medicine* (Suppl.), *18*(3), S1–S16.

Quinn, J. (1995). The healing arts in modern health care. In D. Kunz (Ed.), *Spiritual healing* (pp. 116–124). New York: Theosophical Publishing.

Quinn, J. (2000). Transpersonal human caring and healing. In B. Dossey, L. Keegan, & C. Guzzetta (Eds.), *Holistic nursing: A handbook for practice* (pp. 37–48). Gaithersburg, MD: Aspen.

Roach, S., & Nieto, B. (1997). *Healing and the grief process.* New York: Delmar Publishing.

Sparber, A. (2001). State boards of nursing and scope of practice of registered nurses performing complementary therapies. *Online Journal of Issues in Nursing, 6*(3), Manuscript 10. Retrieved from http://www.nursingworld.org/ojin/topic15/tpc/15_6.htm

Taylor, K. (1995). *The ethics of caring.* Santa Cruz, CA: Hanford-Mead.

Watson, J. (1999). *Postmodern nursing and beyond.* Edinburgh: Churchill Livingston.

Weeks, J. (2001). Foreword. In L. W. Freeman & G. F. Lawlis (Eds.), *Mosby's complementary & alternative medicine: A research-based approach.* St. Louis: Mosby.

Weil, A. (2000). *Self healing* (newsletter). December 1, p. 6.

White House Commission on Complementary and Alternative Medicine Policy. (2001). Interim progress report. *Alternative Therapies in Health and Medicine, 7*(6), 32–40.

Wolsko, P., Ware, L., Kutner, J. Lin, C. T., Albertson, G., Cyran, L., Shilling, L., & Anderson, R. (2000). Alternative/complementary medicine: Wider usage than generally appreciated. *Journal of Alternative & Complementary Medicine, 6, 321–326.*

C h a p t e r **12**

NURSE-MIDWIFERY AND PRIMARY HEALTH CARE FOR WOMEN

Joyce E. Thompson

Primary health care for women in a community setting focuses on the promotion of health and support for the practice of healthy behaviors by women from menarche through the rest of their lives. Health care activities include health education and self-care instruction, health screening, and health supervision for women. The principal foci of primary health care services for women include wellness counseling; health promotion activities; conception and contraception planning; childbearing services; well-woman gynecology; including screening for reproductive cancers; and sexual and lifestyle counseling, including interventions targeted to reducing gender-based violence. The principal health care provider referred to in this chapter will be the American College of Nurse-Midwives Certification Council (ACC) certified nurse-midwife (CNM).

WOMEN AND HEALTH CARE

We live in a time when women are actively seeking to control their own destinies and are receiving increasing support in their efforts in both national and global arenas (Family Care International [FCI], 2000; J. E. Thompson, 2002; United Nations, 1996). Feelings of independence, self-control, and self-determination are fostered when women take an active role in decisions affecting their health care and assume responsibility for self-care activities. Until recently, society has accorded women low status and few opportunities for self-determination and control of their own lives (Craft, 1997; Potts & Walsh, 1999; Scully, 1980; J. B. Thompson & Thompson, 1981; J. E. Thompson & Thompson, 2001; United Nations, 1996; Woods, 1995). The beginning of the 21st century has brought increased attention to women's health and lives and using a human rights framework for approaching the health care needs of adolescent girls and women (J. E. Thompson & Thompson, 2001). This framework is based on treating women as human beings, and understanding that full rights accorded to adolescent girls and women will contribute to their health and well-being and their ability to be productive members of any society. It also recognizes the complex interaction of factors that affect the health and well-being of women (Tresolini & the Pew-Fetzer Task Force, 1994). Modern contraceptive means, although of some risk to the users, have given millions of women a choice in childbearing instead of almost certain motherhood (FCI, 2000; J. B. Thompson & Thompson, 1981). Though some think this choice wrong, for the majority of women, the freedom to choose whether and when to bear children has opened up opportunities for greater control over their lives, including wider options in career choice, improved health with the spacing of children, and improved education without interruption for childbearing (J. E. Thompson, 1996).

Self-care is a process of education and action in which an individual learns to provide effectively for his or her own health care needs. It also includes knowing when to seek professional care. Self-care skills are learned, and this learning can be self-initiated, group-taught, or learned through an organized educational program in a health care facility or community with the professionals as consultants. Today the types of self-care activities gaining in importance involve nutrition and weight management, exercise, self-medication (especially with natural remedies), how to deal with violence, and stress management. All of these and other self-care activities important to the health of women serve as a model for primary health care. The practice of primary health care by CNMs is based on a cooperative, educative, reflective, and supportive relationship with women as partners in health promotion and health care activities (American College of Nurse-Midwives [ACNM], 1997a; J. E. Thompson, Oakley, Burke, Jay, & Conklin, 1989; Tresolini & the Pew-Fetzer Task Force, 1994).

If one accepts the premises that women need health care services during and after their reproductive years in order to maintain or improve their health status, and that healthy women are needed for a healthy nation, it seems logical that provision of such services should be a national health priority, supported by lawmakers as well as by the people for whom the services are intended—women. Though our nation has written and monitored *Healthy People 2000* objectives and, more recently, 2010 objectives, there remains evidence that these objectives were and are not being met, especially among the most vulnerable populations of women (U.S. Department of Health and Human Services [USDHHS], 1991; 1996). *Healthy People 2010* goals (USDHHS, 2000) continue to emphasize promoting the health of women, focusing on physical activity, overweight and obesity, tobacco use, mental health, and injury and violence, to name a few of the leading health indicators. These indicators reflect that we as a nation still have much work to do to have healthy adolescent girls and women, as well as men. To be healthy, one needs to understand and be responsible for one's own personal habits as well as have access to cost-effective, quality primary health care services that help to make good health a reality.

THE NURSE-MIDWIFE AS A PRIMARY HEALTH CARE PROVIDER FOR WOMEN

The primary care nurse working most closely with healthy women of childbearing age and beyond is the certified nurse-midwife (CNM). The nurse-midwife is an individual educated in the two disciplines of nursing and midwifery within an American College of Nurse-Midwives-accredited or -preaccredited program (ACNM, 1997c). A CNM is a graduate nurse-midwife who has been certified for entry into practice by successfully completing a national examination administered by the ACNM Certification Corporation, Inc. (ACC). In 2002, there were approximately 5,700 CNMs practicing in the United States (ACNM, 2001b). Approximately 400 new nurse-midwives are certified annually (J. E. Thompson, 1997).

Nurse-midwifery practice, as defined by the ACNM (1997d), includes the autonomous management of the care of healthy newborns and women throughout the childbearing cycle and the primary care of women seeking contraceptive and/or gynecological services (ACNM, 1997a). Nurse-midwifery practice occurs within a health care system that provides for medical consultation and collaborative management or referral as needed, and is in accord with the *Standards for the Practice of Nurse-Midwifery* as defined by the ACNM (1993a; 1997b; Paine, Dower, & O'Neil, 1999).

The CNM utilizes written policies and protocols as guidelines for practice and works collaboratively with physicians when the health care needs of the woman require medical attention. The protocols delineate areas of care (antepartum, intrapartum, family planning, etc.); describe procedures used by the CNM (e.g., vaginal delivery, local anesthesia, intrauterine device [IUD] insertions, newborn examinations); medication that may be used in the treatment of specific conditions, such as anemia, vaginitis, or urinary tract infections; and the indications for referral to a physician, such as placenta previa, pregnancy-induced hypertension, and recurrent pelvic inflammatory disease (ACNM, 1994). Though practice protocols are helpful in providing primary care for women, the CNM must rely on current knowledge, clinical skills, and judgment (accountability) to know what to do at any given time and when to call for assistance from other professionals (ACNM, 1994; Paine et al., 1999).

Given the above definition of practice, the CNM is a *nurse and a midwife* who provides *health* care to women seeking *primary care* services. In addition, nurse-midwives practice according to a philosophy whose central themes are family- and woman-centered care, the woman's right to self-determination in her health care, and the CNM's support of client and family as "captains" of the health care team (ACNM, 1989; ACNM, 1993b; Paine et al., 1999). Self-determination in health care requires understandable information, fully informed consent, and responsibility for the outcomes of one's choices (J. B. Thompson & Thompson, 1981; J. E. Thompson, Oakley, et al., 1989), which in turn require learning and interest in self-care activities. Motivation for self-care is one of the primary goals of nurse-midwifery care.

EDUCATION OF NURSE-MIDWIVES FOR PRIMARY CARE

The education of nurse-midwives as providers of primary health care services was begun in the United States in 1932 at the Maternity Center Association in New York City, following the introduction of the nurse-midwife as a public health practitioner in 1925 at Frontier Nursing Service in Hyden, Kentucky. Standardization of curriculum has evolved along with a formal accreditation process administered by the ACNM since 1957, with its official recognition by the U.S. Department of Education as the accrediting agency for nurse-midwives since 1982. National certification by examination for entry into practice was begun by the ACNM in 1971, and is now administered by a sister corporation, the ACNM Certification Council, Inc. There are currently two routes to basic preparation as a nurse-midwife: the 9- to 12-month postbaccalaureate certificate and the 16- to 20-month master's degree programs (ACNM, 2001b). In 2002, there were 45 ACNM-accredited or -preaccredited programs preparing nurse-midwives.

Of these, 40 offer midwifery within a master's degree program, and 5 are post-baccalaureate certificate programs, including 1 direct-entry program (ACNM, 2002c; Roberts, 2001).

The core competencies in midwifery required in all ACNM-accredited programs include theory and clinical practice in the autonomous management of women's health care, focusing particularly on preconception care, pregnancy, childbirth, the postpartum period, care of the newborn, and the family planning and gynecological needs of well women (ACNM, 2003). Knowledge of common pathological conditions of pregnancy is required, although clinical practice with high-risk pregnant women is not. Both knowledge and clinical practice with common primary care conditions of women was reintroduced into the curriculum in the 1980s (original practice in rural Kentucky, New York City, and New Mexico included primary care as practiced by public health nurses). Emphasis throughout the program is placed on health promotion activities, client/family-centered care, and development of the woman's ability to care for herself and to know when she should seek professional care.

The nurse-midwifery curriculum in many educational programs is based on the health model of care because nurse-midwives believe in the natural mind-body-spirit phenomena of pregnancy, birth, and menopause (Paine et al., 1999) and direct their care efforts toward the attainment and maintenance of optimal health for the woman and for her fetus when pregnant. Perhaps nowhere else in the health care system is the truism of personal responsibility for health more obvious than during a normal pregnancy. As long as all is going well, only the pregnant woman can maintain that optimal health state through proper nutrition, exercise, sleep, and management of life's stresses. The role of the nurse-midwife is one of expectant observation, watchful screening (at times referred to as masterly inactivity or the art of doing nothing well [Kennedy, 2000]) teaching, support, and supervision (ACNM, 2003; J. E. Thompson, Fullerton, & Brogan, 2002; J. E. Thompson, Oakley, et al., 1989).

Health education constitutes approximately 90% of the clinical activities of nurse-midwives and includes teaching self-care skills, preparation for childbearing and childrearing, and knowledge of the anatomy and physiology of women throughout all phases of their lives. Based on a national study in 1996, 90% of all visits to a CNM were for primary, preventive health care, and 20% were for care outside the maternity cycle, including annual gynecological care and reproductive health visits (ACNM, 2001b; Clarke, Martin, & Taffel, 1997; Johnson, Oshia, Fisher, & Fullerton, 2001; Roberts, 2001; Scupholme, DeJoseph, Strobino, & Paine, 1993). These educational activities also provide women with knowledge of their minds and bodies, contraceptive choices, pregnancy progress, and general health care needs so that informed and active participation in health care decisions is facilitated. The theoretical framework of health education builds on the woman's perception of her state of health, her view of herself as a person and as a woman, her accepted roles in society, and her particular stage of growth and development (Bermosk & Porter, 1979; J. B. Thompson, 1980; J. E. Thompson, 1990; J. E. Thompson, Oakley, et al., 1989; J. E. Thompson & Thompson, 2001; Tresolini & the Pew-Fetzer Task Force, 1994).

A concrete example of the nurse-midwife's belief in and promotion of self-determination for women is her willingness to offer care options to childbearing families. Women were encouraged to make informed decisions about the frequency of prenatal visits long before the NIH/HHS Expert Panel on the Content of Prenatal Care suggested fewer visits for healthy women (1989). Women are also asked who their support people will be during childbirth and what their birth plan is (type of delivery, place of birth, procedures to avoid, etc.). Concurrent with the nurse-midwife's encouragement and support of women taking an active role in decisions about their health care is the education of women for the responsibilities inherent in self-determination. For example, if a woman plans a home birth, she must also be willing to maintain her body in optimum condition for labor; prepare herself and her family for the labor, delivery, and needs of a postpartum mother and newborn; and consent to prenatal supervision so that her appropriateness for home birth is reassessed at frequent intervals. The women-as-partners concept is often clearly delineated in the consent forms for nurse-midwifery care.

MODEL OF PRIMARY HEALTH CARE FOR WOMEN

Any model of primary health care must be based on knowledge of what determines health, what activities promote health, which type of health care provider can best support or carry out these health-promoting activities, and how that health care provider should be educated for such a crucial role in our national health care system. Each individual has a responsibility for adopting healthy behaviors and giving up careless, self-destructive habits. Blum (1974) noted that medical care and the provision of health services are relatively minor inputs into one's state of health. He placed greatest emphasis for the state of one's personal health on a broad range of environmental factors, including the fetal and physical environment, socioeconomic status, culture, and level of education and, secondly, on one's personal health habits, attitudes, and behaviors. For women, consideration of gender and status must enter the health equation because, in many areas of the world, being born female means certain ill health, beginning with poor nutrition and little education, and continuing with many forms of violence (J. E. Thompson, 1996). Healthy People 2010 Objectives (USDHHS, 2000) reinforced the fact that one of the main determinants of personal health is the way of life an individual chooses to follow, reinforcing the work of Blum (1974) and McKeown (1978).

If one's lifestyle is a principal determinant of one's state of health, what could be a more cost-effective health program than one that promotes self-care and a healthy lifestyle? A model of primary health care for women should be based on a holistic health concept fostering healthy behaviors and habits by the woman and her significant others, supported by knowledge of healthy lifestyles and how to adopt and maintain them.

Health is a continuum from most to least healthy, and most people along the "healthy" end, without major illness or disease. Health is a separate condition from disease, but health and illness are not necessarily opposites of one another, as explained recently by the work on relationship-centered care (Tresolini & the Pew-Fetzer Task Force, 1994).

Education for Self-Care

If health is principally determined by one's lifestyle and environment, it may be concluded that any cost-effective model of primary health care must focus on education: teaching individuals to know what constitutes health for them; explaining how it may be achieved or maintained through alterations in their lifestyles, if necessary; and preparing individuals to assume the responsibility for self-care, when appropriate. Education for self-care and assuming responsibility for one's own health are key components of the primary health care model described in this chapter, and they are the most difficult components of the model to teach and learn, primarily because most of us, whether consumer or provider, tend to hold on to some destructive habits. Perhaps we have all fallen into the mistaken notion, often promoted by the medical world, that any disease or infirmity can be treated and health regained no matter what we do to ourselves (McKeown, 1978; J. E. Thompson & Thompson, 1985).

Personalized, Caring Concern

A second important component of a primary health care model is a personalized, caring concern (relationship) exhibited at all times by health care providers for the whole person and for that person's significant others. This *caring* concern is not, however, equated with a *controlling* concern by the professional (Garrett & Garrett, 1982; J. E. Thompson, Oakley, et al., 1989; J. E. Thompson & Thompson, 2001). All people need exposure to health care providers who not only encourage them to assume health-promoting behaviors but are concerned enough to provide them with information and allow them the space to make informed decisions about their health and its supervision, so that they may maintain control over their own bodies and lives. Health professionals need to recognize the illogical nature of their demands that clients be "good," submissive patients and yet also become responsible adults in control of their health. Such dichotomous demands often leave patients with little choice but to distrust the "system" and go it alone. The health care professional must also be aware of and understand the client's desire to use natural remedies and therapies, such as herbs, acupuncture, meditation, Reiki, yoga, biofeedback, and faith healing. It may be difficult and unnecessary for the professional health care worker to provide all of these modalities, but it is important to know about them.

Part of the caring concern for women is knowing when to use a directive approach to health care, when to be supportive, and when mutual participation is indicated. Research (J. E. Thompson, 1980; J. E. Thompson, Oakley, et al., 1989) on the process of care used by nurse-midwives to supervise the health status of pregnant women concluded that even though some women responded very well to learning about pregnancy and took an active role in decisions about their care, other women seemed more responsive to being taken care of by the nurse-midwife. It seems impractical to expect all women or all people to want and be able to participate fully in working toward mutually agreed-upon health goals, although this type of interaction is an important goal to strive toward.

Health Screening and Supervision

The other two necessary components of any model for primary health care are the activities of health screening and health supervision. The health screening component for women includes such things as routine cancer smears; breast examination, tests for sexually transmitted diseases and vaginitis, screening for violence and abuse, screening for depression, and general physical fitness exams relative to nutrition, weight, exercise, sleep, and work patterns (ACNM, 1997f; ACNM 2002a; ACNM, 2002b). The health supervision component for women includes preconception, pregnancy, contraceptive, and well-woman gynecological care for women through menopause and beyond. An integral part of health supervision is the integration of counseling activities, consultation with and/or referral to other sources of care (e.g., dentist, safe homes, etc.), and ongoing health education activities.

Several models of primary health care have been proposed in the literature and used in practice (American Nurses Association [ANA], 1976, 1991; Bermosk & Porter, 1979; Choi, 1981; Fagin, 1992; Kennedy, 2000; Klima, 2001; Tresolini & the Pew-Fetzer Task Force, 1994; Welch, 1996; Young, 1993). They range from minor modifications of the medical model to include health screening activities to global ideas of holistic health care and feminist philosophy in which the provider needs expertise in science and natural remedies, as well as philosophy and women's ways of "knowing" (Belenky, Clinchy, Goldberger, & Tarule, 1997). The shortage of health care of the type needed by women, as described in this chapter, led to the development of the Thompson model over 15 years ago, and is reinforced by more current writings (Kennedy, 2000; Klima, 2001; Paine et al., 1999;).

The Thompson "Women's Primary Health Care Model"

The schematic representation of a women's primary health care model is illustrated in Figure 12.1. Most health care activities are the responsibility of the individual woman. Supervision and screening activities by the health care provider come after the woman makes her initial contact with the nurse-midwife and seeks out these activities. Health education is the foundation of all activities carried out by the CNM. The overlap of health activities between woman and CNM is illustrated by the appearance of certain action-needs above and below the level of interaction with the nurse-midwife, that is, the individual's point of entry into a health care system. Since there is little or no apparent need for the well woman to be taken care of by others, the health care provider (CNM) enters into the individual's mind-body-spirit system rather than providing an outside system that the woman must enter. This type of health care is represented by mutual participation/interaction providing an open system at the point of interaction with the CNM, should consultation or referral to a disease-illness system become necessary.

This model of health care also clearly indicates that it is the woman who is in control of her health and that the responsibility or decision to seek out a professional health worker is also hers. The model also attempts to portray the mind-body-spirit wholeness of the woman influenced by who she is, what she believes in and values, where she lives, and who her family, friends, and community are. All of these factors are brought to bear on

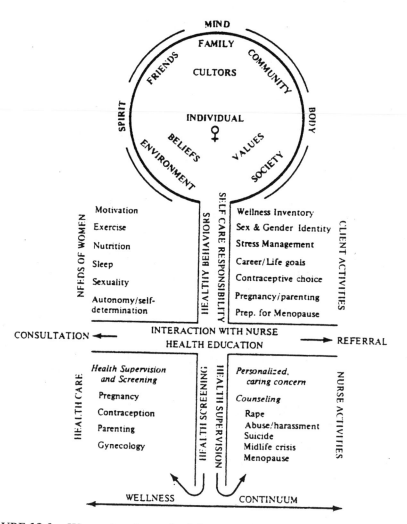

FIGURE 12.1   Women's primary health care model.

an individual woman's definition of her health care needs and her motivation to take health actions. The general health needs of most women of reproductive age center around nutrition, contraception, pregnancy, care of the reproductive organs, sexuality, and work-related conditions. Educational and counseling programs center on anxiety and stress management, sexual assault, abuse or harassment, domestic violence, parenting skills, role identity, accident prevention, drug abuse, and self-care skills. Specific or individualized health care needs will be determined by the woman in interaction with her health care provider (J. E. Thompson, 1990). The older woman will be concerned about menopause, osteoporosis, and maintenance of a healthy body.

PRACTICE OF PRIMARY HEALTH CARE FOR WOMEN

Nurse-midwives incorporate all of the essential components of primary care for women into their practices. This "return" to primary care since the early 1980s for women throughout their lives came at the request of women who had midwifery care during childbirth and who wished to stay with the CNM as a primary care provider for gynecological needs. The majority of a CNM's practice involves women seeking childbearing supervision. For example, an average CNM sees 140 women and attends 10 births a month. About one fifth of outpatient visits to the CNM are for care outside the maternity cycle, including family planning and annual gynecological visits. Since 1996, more than half of all CNMs work in an office/clinic environment, and most list a hospital or physician practice as their place of employment (Paine et al., 1999). A few nurse-midwives own their own birth centers, and some own their own practices and hire an obstetrician for consultation. It is these CNMs who report the highest level of autonomy in practice and the greatest satisfaction with their practices (Higgins, 1996)—one example of the importance of women in control of their lives. Nurse-midwifery care can be found in many settings, including health maintenance organizations, community centers, self-help collectives, and managed care programs (ACNM, 2001b).

The success of CNMs as providers of primary health care services for women can be illustrated by the expansion of practice opportunities for CNMs and the demand for ever-increasing numbers of new CNMs, as demonstrated in the 200% increase in students enrolled in ACNM-accredited programs from 1990 to 1996. Nurse-midwives are best known for their family-centered, partnership model of health care, focusing on wellness and consumer choice. Nurse-midwives receive high marks in satisfaction from women as evidenced by the high rates of return for routine health care as well as keeping prenatal and postpartum appointments (J. E. Thompson, 1997). High-quality care and the "listening to women" approach to interactions also contribute much to the popularity and success of nurse-midwifery care (ACNM, 1994b). If given the chance to think about it, women know what they need, if only we would listen. The midwife's long-honored tradition of being "with women" wherever they are is the hallmark of women's primary health care for the 21st century, as is reflected in the new ACNM logo: "With Women for a Lifetime."

RECOMMENDATIONS FOR THE FUTURE

New plans for financing health-oriented services are needed for full implementation and expansion of the women's primary health care model, or any other health model, for that matter. Nurse-midwives have benefited from years of government support of educational programs. Now it is time for government to support full reimbursement for the quality services provided by all advanced practice nurses working to improve the health of the nation, beginning with its women (ACNM, 1994a, 2001a; Brown, 1992; Ernst, 1996; Paine et al., 1999). If we are to develop and expand primary health services for women that are accessible, acceptable, and affordable, we must work together with women, with lawmakers, and with other health professionals to overcome all barriers to CNM practice (ACNM, 2001a). Given the current constraints in expenditures for health care, the country must carefully choose the most cost- and quality-efficient care providers using a process of caring that results in healthier women and families. Nurse-midwifery care is a premier example of such primary health care for women (ACNM, 2001d).

REFERENCES

American College of Nurse-Midwives. (1989). *Philosophy of the American College of Nurse-Midwives*. Washington, DC: Author.

American College of Nurse-Midwives. (1993a). *Educating nurse-midwives: A strategy for achieving affordable, high-quality maternity care*. Washington, DC: Author.

American College of Nurse-Midwives. (1993b). *Summit II: Visionary planning for health care of women: Listening to the voices of women*. Washington, DC: Author.

American College of Nurse-Midwives. (1994a). *Nurse-midwives: Quality care for women and newborns*. Washington, DC: Author.

American College of Nurse-Midwives. (1994b). *Today's certified nurse-midwife*. Washington, DC: Author.

American College of Nurse-Midwives. (1997a). *Certified nurse-midwives and certified midwives as primary care providers/case managers*. Washington. DC: Author.

American College of Nurse-Midwives. (1997b). *Collaborative management in midwifery practice for medical, gynecological and obstetrical conditions*. Washington, DC: Author.

American College of Nurse-Midwives. (1997c). *Definition of a certified nurse-midwife*. Washington, DC: Author.

American College of Nurse-Midwives. (1997d). *Definition of midwifery practice*. Washington, DC: Author.

American College of Nurse-Midwives. (1997e). *Statement on midwifery education.* Washington, DC: Author.

American College of Nurse-Midwives. (1997f). *Violence against women.* Washington, DC: Author.

American College of Nurse-Midwives. (2001a). *Barriers to nurse-midwifery practice.* Washington, DC: Author.

American College of Nurse-Midwives. (2001b). *Basic facts about certified nurse-midwives.* Washington, DC: Retrieved from www.midwife.org

American College of Nurse-Midwives. (2001c). *Births attended by certified nurse-midwives are on the rise.* Retrieved from www.midwife.org

American College of Nurse-Midwives. (2001d). *Quality and cost-effective care: The midwifery solution.* Washington, DC: Author.

American College of Nurse-Midwives. (2002a). *Core competencies for basic midwifery practice.* Washington, DC: Author.

American College of Nurse-Midwives. (2002b). *Depression in women.* Washington, DC: Author.

American College of Nurse-Midwives. (2002c). *Educational programs accredited by the ACNM Division of Accreditation as of 1/02.* Washington, DC: Author.

American College of Nurse-Midwives. (2003). *Standards of practice of midwifery.* Washington, DC: Author.

American College of Nurse-Midwives & American College of Obstetricians and Gynecologists. (2001). *Joint statement of practice relations between obstetrician/gynecologists and certified nurse-midwives/certified midwives.* Washington, DC: Authors.

American Nurses Association. (1976). *Scope of primary nursing practice for adults and families.* Kansas City: Author.

American Nurses Association. (1991). *Nursing's agenda for health care reform.* Washington, DC: Author.

Belenky, N. M., Clinchy, B., Goldberger, N., & Tarule, J. (1997). *Women's ways of knowing.* New York: Basic Books.

Bermosk, L., & Porter, S. (1979). *Women's health and human wholeness.* New York: Appleton-Century-Crofts.

Blum, H. (1974). *Planning for change: Development and application of social change theory.* New York: Human Sciences Press.

Brown, S. (Ed.). (1992). *Including children and pregnant women in health care reform.* Washington, DC: National Academy Press.

Choi, M. W. (1981). Nurses and co-providers of primary health care. *Nursing Outlook, 29,* 519–521.

Clarke, S., Martin, J., & Taffel, S. (1997). Trends and characteristics of births attended by midwives. *Statistical Bulletin, 78*(1), 9–18.

Craft, N. (1997). Women's health is a global issue. *British Medical Journal, 315,* 1154–1157.

Ernst, E. (1996). Midwifery, birth centers, and health care reform. *Journal of Obstetric, Gynecologic, and Neonatal Nursing, 25,* 433–439.

Fagin, C. (1992). Collaboration between nurses and physicians: No longer a choice. *Nursing and Health Care, 13,* 354–363.

Family Care International. (2000). *Sexual and reproductive health briefing cards.* New York: Author.

Garrett, S. S., & Garrett, B. (1982). Humaneness and health. *Topics in Clinical Nursing, 3,* 7–12.

Higgins, K. (1996). *The entrepreneurial nurse-midwife.* Unpublished doctoral dissertation, University of Pennsylvania.

Johnson, P., Oshia, S., Fisher, M., & Fullerton, J. (2001). The 1999–2000 ACC task analysis of nurse-midwifery/midwifery practice: A consideration of the concept of professional issues. *Journal of Midwifery & Women's Health, 46,* 313–319.

Kennedy, H. P. (2000). A model of exemplary midwifery practice: Results of a Delphi study. *Journal of Midwifery & Women's Health, 45(1),* 4–18.

Klima, C. (2001). Women's health care: A new paradigm for the 21st century. *Journal of Midwifery & Women's Health, 46,* 285–291.

McKeown. T. (1978). Determinants of health. *Human Nature, 4,* 170–172.

NIH/HHS Expert Panel on the Content of Prenatal Care. (1989). *Caring for our future: The content of prenatal care.* Washington, DC: U.S. Public Health Services.

Paine, L., Dower, C., & O'Neil, E. (1999). Midwifery in the 21st Century: Recommendations from the Pew Health Professions Commission/UCSF Center for the Health Professions 1998 Taskforce on Midwifery. *Journal of Nurse-Midwifery, 44,* 341–348.

Potts, M. & Walsh, J. (1999). Making Cairo work. *Lancet, 353,* 315–318.

Roberts, J. (2001). Challenges and opportunities for nurse-midwives. *Nursing Outlook, 49,* 213–226.

Scully, D. (1980). *Men who control women's health: The miseducation of obstetrician gynecologists.* Boston: Houghton Mifflin.

Scupholme, A., DeJoseph, J., Strobino, D. M., & Paine, L. L. (1993). Nurse-midwifery care to vulnerable populations. *Journal of Nurse-Midwifery, 37(5),* 341–347.

Thompson, J. B. (1980). *Nurse-midwives and health promotion during pregnancy.* Unpublished doctoral dissertation, Columbia University.

Thompson, J. B., & Thompson, H. 0. (1981). *Ethics in nursing.* New York: Macmillan.

Thompson, J. E. (1990). Health education during pregnancy. In I. R. Merkatz & J. E. Thompson (Eds.), *New perspectives on prenatal care.* New York: Elsevier.

Thompson, J. E. (1996). Women are dying: Midwives take action. In ICM/WHO/UNICEF, *Strengthening midwifery within safe motherhood.* Geneva: WHO.

Thompson, J. E. (1997). Midwives: Listening to women. *Nursing Spectrum, 6(8),* 8–9.

Thompson, J. E. (2002). Midwives and human rights: dream or reality? *Midwifery, 18,* 188–192.

Thompson, J. E., Fullerton, J., & Brogan, K. (2002). Essential competencies of midwifery practice: Phase I. *Midwifery.*

Thompson, J. E., Oakley, D., Burke, M., Jay, S., & Conklin, M. (1989). Theory building in nurse-midwifery: The care process. *Journal of Nurse-Midwifery, 34,* 120–130.

Thompson, J. E., & Thompson, H. O. (1985). *Bioethical decision making for nurses.* Norwalk: Appleton-Century-Crofts.

Thompson, J. E., & Thompson, H. O. (2001). Ethical aspects of care. In L. V. Walsh (Ed.), *Midwifery: Community-based care during the childbearing year* (pp. 489–500). Philadelphia: Saunders.

Tresolini, C. P., & the Pew-Fetzer Task Force. (1994). *Health professions education and relationship-centered care.* San Francisco: Pew Health Professions Commission.

United Nations. (1996). *Platform for action and the Beijing declaration.* New York: Author.

U.S. Department of Health & Human Services. (1991). *Healthy people 2000: A report on health promotion and disease prevention.* Washington, DC: Author, Pub. No. 91-55071.

U.S. Department of Health & Human Services. (1996). *Healthy people 2000: A progress review.* Washington, DC: Author.

U.S. Department of Health & Human Services. (2000). *Healthy people 2010: Understanding and improving health.* Washington, DC: Government Printing Office.

Welch, H. (1996). Nurse-midwives as primary care providers for women. *Clinical Nurse Specialist, 70*(3), 121–124, 143.

Woods, N. F. (1995). Women's bodies. In C. I. Fogel & N. F. Woods (Eds.), *Women's health care* (pp. 374–389). CA: Sage.

Young, D. (1993). Crisis in primary care: Will midwives meet the challenge? *Birth, 20*(2), 59–60.

Chapter 13

NURSE ANESTHETISTS: EVOLUTION FROM CRITICAL CARE PRACTITIONERS TO ANESTHESIA PROVIDERS

William P. Fehder

Nurses have been providing anesthesia care to patients since the inception of anesthesia, discovered in the United States in the mid-19th century. Surgeons realized that their reputations depended upon not only the success of the surgery but the patients' survival of anesthesia, and they sought out the most dependable provider of anesthesia, who was often the nurses they trusted with their patients' care. The quality of care provided by nurse anesthetists was excellent.

The professional issues that nurse anesthetists faced, and continue to deal with, were similar to those for other advanced practice nurses. Some of those issues are level of education for entry into practice, establishment of national organizations for program accreditation, national certification standards, collegial relationships with other health care providers, and types of employment arrangements. A brief look at the history of nurse anesthetists in the United States illustrates the context of anesthesia practice in this country. This chapter discusses the scope of practice for the certified registered nurse anesthetist, how that practice has evolved, and what the future might hold for nurse anesthesia.

ANESTHESIA AND NURSES: HISTORICAL CONTEXT

The Early Days

It is commonly accepted that anesthesia was discovered in the United States in the 1840s. At that time, traveling showmen and itinerant professors of chemistry demonstrated the euphoria-producing effects of inhaling ether (termed *ether frolics*) and nitrous oxide (termed *benders,* and the probable derivation of the term *on a bender.* The recreational use of these agents became especially popular among students of chemistry on college campuses as well as in the offices of young medical practitioners (Thatcher, 1953).

Although the subject of some controversy, three men are credited with the recognition of the anesthetic properties of ether and nitrous oxide: Crawford W. Long, a Georgia physician and Horace Wells and William T. G. Morton, New England dentists. Long may have observed, and indeed participated in, ether frolics during his medical studies at the University of Pennsylvania in Philadelphia. Through observation, Long came to the realization that the euphoria produced by inhaling ether and nitrous oxide rendered participants insensitive to pain. On returning to Jefferson, Georgia, Long performed surgery on patients while they were under the influence of inhaled ether, although he did not make any attempt to publicize his practice beyond this rural community.

Wells and Morton, originally dental partners in Boston, observed the ability of nitrous oxide to produce insensitivity to pain during "laughing gas" exhibitions and realized that painless tooth extraction could be a financial boon to their practice. However, Wells' attempted demonstration of the analgesic properties of nitrous oxide for dental extractions to surgeons at Massachusetts General Hospital was a failure due to technical problems. Morton went on to team up with Boston professor Charles T. Jackson to develop successful methods for delivering ether as an anesthetic for surgery. Morton's work with ether as an anesthetic culminated in the successful demonstration of anesthesia to surgeons in the surgical amphitheater of the Massachusetts General Hospital, known ever since as the "ether dome." Morton then obtained a patent on the use of ether for producing anesthesia. News of the anesthetizing properties of ether spread throughout the world, leading to the investigation of the anesthetizing properties of other substances such as chloroform, which resulted in an abrogation of Morton's patent. The acceptance of anesthesia for surgery in the United States led to the question of who would provide the anesthesia for patients.

The Search for an Anesthesia Practitioner

Surgeons determined who would provide anesthesia to their patients, and initially the job of anesthetizer was given to whoever was available—from medical students to surgeons-in-training to the janitor. Often the task of anesthetizing patients was given to the referring physician as a means of recompense by the surgeon. Physicians, however, were often more interested in observing and learning surgical technique than in monitoring the physical status of the patients, resulting in high death rates during surgery. Surgeons needed a clinician who would be satisfied with a subordinate role, would be willing to make anesthesia a primary interest, would not be interested in learning surgical technique, and would accept comparatively low pay but have the aptitude and intelligence to develop the skill of providing smooth anesthesia and relaxation. They found just such a person in the Catholic hospital sister .

Although it is not known who the first nurse anesthetist was, the earliest recorded one is Sister Mary Bernard, who was called upon to assume the duties of anesthetist at St. Vincent's Hospital in Erie, Pennsylvania . It could be said that the tradition of Catholic nuns being trained to administer anesthesia throughout the Midwest began professional anesthesia care in the United States.

The Sisters of St. Francis established St. Mary's Hospital in Rochester, Minnesota, for Dr. William Worrell Mayo, a surgeon. Believing that nurses were capable of providing anesthesia, Dr. Mayo instructed two nurses, Edith and Dinah Graham, in anesthesia technique. From this beginning, the Mayo Clinics became a magnet for surgeons to observe skilled surgery and anesthesia. Many were so impressed by the work of Alice Magaw, who succeeded the Graham sisters as anesthetist, that they sent their nurses to observe and learn from her. Magaw published articles describing her practice of anesthesia and was given the title "mother of anesthesia" by Dr. Charles H. Mayo. In her famous paper published in 1906, Magaw stated that nurse anesthetists were noted for patience, and the ability to pay attention to the patient during a long operation while avoiding conversation, concentrating on the surgical technique, and other distractions from caring for the patient . The Mayo Clinics served as a center for the dissemination of information about nurse anesthetist practice throughout the country.

Early Nurse Anesthesia Education Programs

Dr. George W. Crile, a prominent surgeon in Cleveland, was responsible for acquiring nurse anesthetists at Lakeside Hospital and then University Hospitals of Cleveland, which are now part of the teaching hospitals of Case Western Reserve University. In 1908, Crile asked Agatha Hodgins to become his personal nurse anesthetist. Hodgins perfected the administration of nitrous oxide-oxygen anesthesia, and surgeons who came to Lakeside Hospital were so impressed with this technique that they asked her to train nurses from their own clinics. Hodgins helped train physician and nurse anesthetists until the United States entered World War I, when she went to France as part of the Lakeside surgical unit. There she continued educational activities, training British and French physicians and nurses in the administration of anesthesia.

Due to their service during the war, the demand for nurse anesthetists increased greatly, leading to the establishment of many formal nurse anesthesia educational programs in university and major community hospitals throughout the United States. Several legal challenges to the right of nurse anesthetists to administer anesthesia occurred during this period of rapid growth and served to refute the notion that nurse anesthetists were illegally practicing medicine and to establish nurse anesthesia as a professional function of nursing practice (Mannino, 1996). Nurse anesthesia has became more professional through the establishment of formal educational programs. The result is what Davis (1989) termed "the anomaly of American anesthesia," in that two specialties (in almost equal numbers)—one composed of nurses, the other of physicians—deliver anesthetics to patients.

Organizing for Professionalism

Seeking to increase cohesiveness and professionalism within nurse anesthesia, Agatha Hodgins addressed the 1930 biennial convention of the American Nurses Association (ANA), suggesting that the ANA provide a separate section for nurse anesthetists within their organization as they had for the National League of Nursing Education and the National Organization of Public Health Nurses. Her attempts to negotiate such an arrangement with the ANA were rebuffed, resulting in a long-standing schism between nurse anesthetists and the general nursing community. In 1931, Hodgins went on to establish the National Association of Nurse Anesthetists, predecessor of the current American Association of Nurse Anesthetists (AANA). In this way, the oldest specialty nursing association in the United States was founded.

The nurse anesthetist organization originally met during the American Hospital Association conventions for the purpose of placing better qualified nurses in the field, providing continuing education, and giving protection and recognition to nurse anesthesia practitioners. In June 1945, the association administered the first qualifying exam, and the credential of certified registered nurse anesthetist (CRNA) was granted to those nurses who passed. The establishment of this examination and credential made nurse anesthesia the first nursing specialty for which certification was available (Bankert, 1989).

In 1952, the American Association of Nurse Anesthetists established national educational standards through an accreditation program for schools of nurse anesthesia, and the AANA was recognized as the accrediting agency by the United States Department of Health, Education and Welfare in 1955. Early action to meet the need for recognition, that is, creation of the CRNA title, minimum practice qualification standards with a national examination, and curriculum standardization through accreditation, placed nurse anesthesia at the forefront of advanced and specialty nursing practice.

MODERN NURSE ANESTHESIA EDUCATION

Program Accreditation

Begun in 1952 under the auspices of the AANA, accreditation has been governed since 1975 by a fiscally autonomous multidisciplinary body under the corporate structure of the AANA, the Council on Accreditation of Nurse Anesthesia Educational Programs/Schools. The Council on Accreditation establishes standards addressing administrative policies and procedures, institutional support, curriculum and instruction, faculty, evaluation, and ethics. Accreditation provides quality assurance through continuous self-study and review of educational preparation. Programs are accredited periodically by means of a self-study and a visit by a team of reviewers and may receive up to 10 years' accreditation status. Graduation from an approved program is one prerequisite of eligibility for the national certification (AANA, 2001a).

Building on a firm foundation of undergraduate nursing education and critical care nursing experience, all current nurse anesthesia educational programs are between 24 and 36 months in length and must offer a master's degree. The requirement that nurse anesthesia education be at the master's level was implemented by the Council on Accreditation for all students enrolling in programs as of 1998. The 85 accredited nurse anesthesia programs in the United States are affiliated with schools of nursing, allied health, or medicine. The diversity of educational affiliations stems from the schism that occurred in 1930 between nursing and nurse anesthesia as well as the views of some nursing educators who, influenced by physician colleagues, did not view anesthesia as the practice of nursing and denied the programs' placement within schools of nursing.

Recently, with the advent of more advanced practice nursing roles, the ANA and other nursing groups have supported the AANA in preserving its professional rights. Commonality of interests has fostered an increasing reconciliation between the two groups. The AANA is an ANA organizational affiliate and a member of the ANA's National Organization Liaison Forum, which consists of more than 70 national nursing organizations and serves as a platform for addressing important issues that affect nursing and health care in general. Indeed, in recent years prominent nurse anesthetists have been accorded recognition by being elected as Fellows of the American Academy of Nursing (FAAN).

Educational Structure

Candidates for admission to nurse anesthesia educational programs must be registered nurses with an appropriate baccalaureate degree (most often a BSN) and must have at least a year of professional experience in an acute-care setting. As programs have become more popular, minimal requirements for admission have been raised beyond those required for accreditation, such as additional years of acute-care experience in specific types of intensive care units and increased scores on standardized tests such as the Graduate Record Exam. Although the basic curriculum is prescribed by the Council on Accreditation, programs differ from each other for many reasons.

Some long-standing programs have evolved over the years to meet increased educational standards: from hospital-operated diploma programs to baccalaureate programs and, finally, to the master's degree now required. Thus, some programs, especially rural ones, are more loosely affiliated with a degree-granting institution that assumes responsibility for its own didactic instruction and an affiliating college or university providing the additional curricular content to meet the master's degree requirements. Other programs are housed directly within a university or college that provides all required courses with students affiliating at a hospital for clinical experience. Some small programs have established a consortium to pool educational resources and thus provide higher quality instruction in anesthesia-related areas and use clinical affiliations to provide students with the wide diversity of clinical experiences required to be a versatile practitioner.

Another spectrum of difference among anesthesia programs is the timing of clinical experience vis-à-vis didactic instruction. Many programs provide integrated didactic instruction with a gradually increasing clinical experience, believing that one reinforces the other and results in a superior outcome. In this type of educational model, students spend 3 to 4 days a week in the classroom and 1 to 2 days in the clinical area initially, reversing the proportion to 4 days of supervised clinical practice with 1 day of classroom instruction for the last year of instruction.

Another model used by several programs, especially those conducted by the military services, provides a concentrated period of all classroom instruction followed by up to 2 years of supervised clinical practice, often at a distant affiliating clinical site. In this model, students continue to interact with each other and didactic faculty, often through on-line education and seminars.

Curricular Requirements

Most students entering nurse anesthesia education are experienced intensive care nurses and the curriculum builds on that experience as well as on prior nursing education. Most nurse anesthesia programs range from 45 to 75 graduate credits in courses specifically related to anesthesia. The minimum science curriculum provides 30 semester credit hours of instruction in anatomy, physiology, pathophysiology, pharmacology, chemistry, biochemistry, and physics. Courses provided in anesthesia practice include induction, maintenance, and emergence from general anesthesia; airway management techniques; pharmacology of anesthetic agents and adjunctive drugs; and anesthesia for special populations such as pediatrics, geriatrics, and obstetrics. The basic anesthesia curriculum is rounded out by course content based on the type of institution housing the program. If the institution is a school of nursing, then nursing courses such as nursing research, health policy, and health promotion might be included in the curriculum. The clinical component of the nurse anesthesia curriculum is much more extensive than that for other advanced practice nursing specialties. This is in part due to the high degree of manual dexterity required to skillfully insert endotracheal tubes, to insert invasive monitoring lines (intravenous, arterial, central venous, and pulmonary artery), and to perform all types of regional anesthetic blocks, such as spinals and epidurals.

Nurse anesthetists administer all types of anesthesia: general, regional, local, and conscious sedation. They use all available anesthetic agents and adjunctive drugs. Nurse anesthetists maintain patients' homeostasis in the face of existing disease and/or surgical challenges by monitoring and interpreting data from sophisticated monitoring devices, determining the need for and implementing fluid and blood therapy, managing patients' airways and ventilation, and recognizing and correcting any complications that occur during the course of the anesthesia and obtaining consultation as needed. Nurse anesthetists are often called upon to provide airway and ventilatory support and manage resuscitation for cardiopulmonary arrest or serious injury.

CRNAs take care of the patient's needs before, during, and after surgery. Preoperatively, CRNAs perform a physical assessment, participate in preoperative teaching, and plan for the patient's anesthetic needs by preparing for anesthetic management. Intraoperatively, the CRNA induces and maintains anesthesia to keep the patient pain free while monitoring vital signs and maintaining a homeostatic state. Postoperatively, the CRNA oversees recovery from anesthesia and follows the patient's course from recovery room to the patient care unit. Patient teaching in the immediate postoperative period is often ineffective due to the anterograde amnesia produced by commonly used anesthetic drugs such as midazolam; thus patients often are not able to remember what they are told. The CRNA, therefore, will provide vital postoperative teaching to the patient's family, especially if the patient had an untoward or unusual reaction to anesthesia that will need to be communicated to future anesthesia caregivers, such as difficulty with airway management, unusual reactions to muscle relaxants, or malignant hyperthermia. Continuity of patient care is ensured by the extensive report the CRNA gives to the postoperative care nurse. The CRNA who cared for patients who remain in the hospital postoperatively usually visits them the next day and on subsequent days if they experienced problems or complications related to their anesthesia.

To prepare to meet the requirements of this exacting clinical specialty, each student must administer a minimum of 450 anesthetics, representing at least 800 hours of anesthesia time under the direct supervision of a CRNA or a physician anesthesiologist. Actual student experiences far exceed the minimal requirements: The average is 773 cases and 1,595 hours of clinical experience for each student. There is currently no postgraduate residency system in nurse anesthesia, so the beginning CRNA must be prepared to perform all anesthesia services to all ages and types of patients. A process of professional socialization concurrent with classroom and clinical education is necessary to enable the student to assume the role of nurse anesthetist.

Issues In Professional Socialization

Nurse anesthesia programs accept applicants who are well-educated, experienced acute-care nurses and then educate them for the role of nurse anesthetist. As with other nursing specialty programs, there may be an initial identity crisis associated with leaving a senior practice status and assuming a new student role. More important, nurse anesthesia has been identified as a subculture of nursing. In a process of professional socialization to the subculture of nurse anesthesia, students have to give up parts of their personal and professional cultures—a sometimes difficult process. A desire for increased professional autonomy is a primary reason identified for seeking a career in advanced practice nursing and is particularly germane to nurse anesthesia. However, the professional socialization required to accomplish autonomy in practice is very difficult.

Nurse anesthesia practice builds upon the ability of the critical care nurse to assess unstable patients rapidly and implement immediate action if needed. The anesthetic state produced renders patients physiologically defenseless and often unable to breathe for themselves. The CRNA who has artificially produced this defenseless state in the patient is faced with the responsibility and accountability for regulating all of the patient's physiological needs in the face of the stress of surgery. CRNAs must continuously monitor patients through observation, interpreting data produced by electronic devices and analysis of hemodynamic and laboratory data and making constant adjustments to the anesthesia regimen using the critical thinking skills necessary for clinical competence. Actions are often taken rapidly after quick but careful consideration of available data.

The new level of autonomy and accountability for the care of a patient by the student nurse anesthetist can be overwhelming and a profound stressor. The ability of the student to succeed in this highly stressful situation depends, in large part, on the professional socialization process through which the student identifies with and acquires the behaviors and attitudes of the "aspired to" advanced practice group by early exposure to professional role models during clinical education. Professional socialization includes taking on the organizational goals, social mission, and knowledge advancement espoused by the group. Role modeling by both physician and nurse anesthetists is invaluable as a tool for professional socialization and often influences the choice of future practice setting as well as professional behaviors. Through expert modeling, students achieve the ideals of safe and ethical practice, maintenance of current knowledge through continuing education, and pursuit of advanced academic degrees.

Continuing Education and Recertification

As early as 1967, the AANA recognized the need for recognition of continued professional excellence and established a recertification program, encompassing clinical and didactic experiences, through which the CRNA could demonstrate current knowledge in nurse anesthesia practice. The voluntary recertification evolved and became codified in 1978 when the membership of the AANA voted to establish the Council on Recertification of Nurse Anesthetists, which became responsible for accrediting continuing education programs and establishing criteria for practitioner certification. The council established objective criteria to determine if an individual nurse anesthetist is properly licensed, has engaged in the practice required to maintain an adequate level of skill, has obtained sufficient continuing education credit to keep current with advances, and has avoided mental, physical, and other problems that could interfere with the practice of nurse anesthesia. Currently, CRNAs are recertified biennially after satisfying the requirements of the Council on Recertification for 40 hours of accredited continuing education, current licensure that is appropriate to the state in which the CRNA practices, and an attestation to the lack of mental and physical impairment. All U.S. states and federal agencies such as the military services and the Department of Veterans Affairs require current recertification to continue practice as a CRNA.

THE ANESTHESIA PRACTICE ARENA

Today, more than 28,000 actively practicing CRNAs administer approximately 65% of the 26 million anesthetics given each year in the United States (AANA, 2001b; Garde, 1996). Nurse anesthetists are the sole anesthesia providers in more that two thirds of all rural hospitals in the United States providing 70 million rural Americans access to anesthesia care. In inner cities, CRNAs also provide a significant amount of the anesthesia delivered. Nurse anesthetists provide services in conjunction with other health care professionals such as surgeons, dentists, podiatrists, and anesthesiologists in diverse settings ranging from hospital operating rooms to physician's offices under a variety of employment arrangements. Commensurate with the level of responsibility, CRNAs are one of the best-paid nursing specialties with a reported median annual salary of $105,000 in 2000 (AANA, 2001b). Shortages of nurse anesthetists have resulted in recent increases of salary in different areas of the country. Shortages of CRNAs have resulted in curtailment of elective and diagnostic procedures requiring anesthesia and sedation especially in outpatient settings. AANA President, Deborah A. Chambers, expressed concern in November 2001 that nurse anesthesia faculty and students in military reserve status would be called up for active duty resulting in a disruption of nurse anesthesia education programs and an exacerbation of the CRNA shortage (Chambers, 2001).

CRNA Practice Settings

CRNAs practice anesthesia in every state and territory of the United States as well as in all branches of the U.S. military service, the public health service, and the Department of Veterans Affairs. The nature of employment arrangements for CRNAs has been changing due to changes in reimbursement for anesthesia services. In 1975, 69% of nurse anesthetists were employed by hospitals, which built their cost into the hospital overhead structure as they did with other hospital nursing services (Shumway & Del Risco, 2000).

In 1989, CRNAs acquired independent billing rights under the Medicare system, but many hospitals were unable to manage the billing process or coordinate it with anesthesiologists who were already billing Medicare; thus hospitals were not able to capture the cost of CRNA salaries. At the same time the Health Care Financing Administration decided to initiate reductions in anesthesia reimbursement rates for all providers. These market changes resulted in hospitals terminating CRNA employment and instead contracting for nurse and physician anesthesia services to reduce cost. Thus, the number of hospital-employed CRNAs was reduced to 37% of all CRNAs (Shumway & Del Risco, 2000). At the same time, the employment of CRNAs by anesthesiologist groups increased from 20% of all CRNAs in 1975 to almost 38% in 1997 (Shumway & Del Risco, 2000). Nurse anesthetists practicing in CRNA-only groups or contracting independently has increased during those same years from 8% to 15% (Shumway & Del Risco, 2000). At the same time, the proportion of CRNAs who practice in surgicenters and physicians offices has increased only slightly from 2% to 3.7% during those years. Supervision of CRNAs by anesthesiologists is another factor that has produced changes in practice settings for CRNAs.

Supervision and Collaboration

Despite the political battles waged between their professional organizations, the American Society of Anesthesiologists (ASA) and the American Association of Nurse Anesthetists, CRNAs have functioned in a relatively professional manner. Both anesthesiologists and CRNAs function in a dependent role to the surgeons on whom they rely to provide patients and cases. CRNAs are legally responsible for their own practice under each state's nurse practice act and can be supervised by the operating surgeon if required by regulations. However, CRNAs have often functioned as employees of, or have been supervised by, anesthesiologists, who might also be employees of the hospital. With few exceptions, anesthesia departments functioned smoothly and efficiently under such arrangements. Many anesthesiologists have served as clinical and didactic faculty members for nurse anesthesia programs. Significant financial incentives often fueled such arrangements because anesthesiologists could bill for their supervision of several anesthetic procedures performed at the same time by several CRNAs. Medicare permits CRNAs to be reimbursed for their patient care and also permits anesthesiologists to be reimbursed for the medical direction of the anesthesia performed by several CRNAs at the same time.

In 1982, the ASA introduced a mode of practice termed the *anesthesia care team* (ACT) and published a statement in which it defined anesthesia as the practice of medicine, stating that every anesthetic should be given under the direction and supervision of an anesthesiologist (Lester & Thomson, 1989). Furthermore, it set seven tasks that the anesthesiologist must complete for medical direction to occur: write the preoperative assessment, prescribe the anesthetic plan, be present for induction and emergence, make frequent checks throughout the anesthetic, remain physically available during the anesthetic for immediate diagnosis and treatment of emergencies, refrain from personally administering a concurrent anesthetic, and provide postoperative care.

In an attempt to reduce Medicare fraud, Congress set essentially the same requirements for reimbursement of medical direction by anesthesiologists by enacting the Tax Equity and Fiscal Responsibility Act (TEFRA) in 1982. This insurance reimbursement regulation has been misinterpreted as a standard of care in anesthesia practice. The AANA lobbied to obtain a new federal rule that would eliminate the necessity for anesthesiologist supervision for Medicare reimbursement of CRNA services. After much wrangling between the ASA and the AANA, the final draft regulation was published in the *Federal Register* January 18, 2001 (66 FR 4674). However, a Bush administration moratorium on the implementation of all rules promulgated during the last days of the Clinton administration resulted in a delay and reexamination of the supervision rule. Finally, a compromise rule was adopted November 13, 2001, allowing each state's governor to decide to opt out of the supervision regulation, thereby shifting this battle to the individual states (66 FR 56762). As of June 2002, Iowa, Nebraska, Idaho, Minnesota, and New Hampshire have opted out of anesthesiologist supervision of CRNA Medicare practice. As with all groups of advanced practice nurses, CRNAs will continue to struggle with issues of professional autonomy into the foreseeable future in national, state, and local arenas. The close relationship nurse anesthetists have with surgeons and their patients remains a strong force in favor of CRNAs. The acquisition of research skills through advanced education, along with an academic and clinical research agenda, will also serve to foster the professionalism of nurse anesthetists in the mind of the public.

THE NURSE ANESTHESIA RESEARCH ARENA

As with any other advanced nursing practice specialty, there has been an increasing appreciation of the importance of research in the field of nurse anesthesia. A discipline such as nurse anesthesia must strive to provide patients with the most effective and efficient services possible. This can be accomplished by the development of a relevant body of knowledge that improves the practice of the CRNA and serves the secondary goal of enhanced professional stature. The need for dissemination of knowledge was recognized by a founder of the discipline, Alice Magaw, who regularly gave talks about her research in anesthesia practice to the Olmsted County Medical Society that were also published in the Minnesota state medical journals. Through her extensive case reports and methodological papers, Magaw disseminated her research findings to a wide group of physician and nurse anesthetists, promoting safe and effective anesthesia practices. Although nurse anesthesia certainly had a strong evidence-based foundation, research took a back seat to other professional issues such as the right to practice, curricular standardization, and organization for recognition and protection.

More recently, the mandated evolution of nurse anesthesia education programs into the graduate education framework resulted in an increase in program requirements for scientific inquiry, statistical methods, and faculty-guided student research. This addition of a scholarly requirement, along with university faculty requirements, has resulted in an increased demand for higher education in nurse anesthesia faculty. The number of doctorally prepared CRNAs is increasing to meet the increased expectations on faculty, with a net increase in research activities in nurse anesthesia.

Recognizing a need to advance nurse anesthesia as a profession through education and research, the AANA established the AANA Education and Research Foundation in 1981. The AANA Foundation (as it is now called) promotes research by nurse anesthetists by funding research workshops, publication workshops, researcher awards, and research grants. Through a mentorship program, the foundation also supports CRNA doctoral students. Among other priorities, the foundation has set nurse anesthesia outcomes research as among its highest priorities.

THE FUTURE

As with nursing in general, nurse anesthesia faces the problem of an aging of its workforce. The average age of CRNAs is more than 40 years old. This is probably due to two factors: the decreased interest of high school graduates in entering nursing schools, resulting in a decline in the number of nurses available to enter anesthesia school, and a decline in the number of nurse anesthesia programs. The result has been an increase in the number of CRNA position vacancies and a commensurate increase in salary in many areas of the country. As the average age of CRNAs in practice increases, the yearly proportion that will retire will exceed the entry into practice of new graduates. The AANA has recognized this problem and has been able to stabilize the number of nurse anesthesia programs for now. The AANA also has an aggressive campaign to encourage nurses to consider anesthesia as a career choice through presentations at National Student Nurses Association conventions. While the shortage of CRNAs has been a temporary financial boon, if the shortage should become more severe it could result in the increased development of a third type of anesthesia provider, such as the anesthesia assistant.

The increased educational requirements to enter the field and the desire for increased professional recognition have resulted in some interest in making the clinical doctorate the academic credential for entry into the field of nurse anesthesia. At the present time, anesthesia program directors do not feel that there is adequate infrastructure support to permit the clinical doctorate to be mandated. Programs housed in strong academic settings are exploring optional clinical doctorates for nurse anesthesia students. Many program directors who are not currently doctorally prepared are now enrolling in doctoral programs in preparation for an anticipated increase in academic requirements. Thus, there is a steadily increasing interest in moving toward a clinical doctorate as the entry credential for nurse anesthesia practice.

CONCLUSIONS

Nurse anesthetists will continue to face many of the same challenges that are common to other advanced nursing specialties. The increasing cohesiveness between nurse anesthetists, other advanced practice nurses, and the general nursing community is fostered by common goals and interests. Approximately 50% of nurse anesthesia programs are affiliated with nursing schools and offer their students Master's in Nursing degrees (AANA, 2002). This proportion is likely to increase as states continue to enact legislation mandating a master's degree in nursing for advanced nursing practice. It is likely that more programs will offer optional clinical doctorates to students enrolled in nurse anesthesia programs beyond the two that currently have such offerings. Although there is a shortage of all anesthesia providers, the excellent patient outcomes and the availability of CRNAs in all communities will ensure the continuing viability of nurse anesthesia as a career choice for nurses. Building on the firm foundation of critical care nursing, CRNAs will continue in their long and distinguished tradition of caring for the patient through all phases of surgery.

REFERENCES

American Association of Nurse Anesthetists. (2001a). List of recognized educational programs by Council on Accreditation of Nurse Anesthesia Programs. *American Association of Nurse Anesthetists Journal, 69,* 492–500.

American Association of Nurse Anesthetists. (2001b). *2000 American Association of Nurse Anesthetists membership survey.* Park Ridge, IL. American Association of Nurse Anesthetists.

American Association of Nurse Anesthetists. (2002). List of recognized educational programs by the Council on Accreditation of Nurse Anesthesia educational programs. *American Association of Nurse Anesthetists Journal, 70*(6).

Bankert, M. (1989). *Watchful care: A history of America's nurse anesthetists.* New York: Continuum.

Chambers, D. A. (2001). President's message. *American Association of Nurse Anesthetists Newsbulletin, 55*(10), 2.

Davis, A. B. (1989). Anesthetist and anesthesiologist: Technology in the social context of a medical and nursing specialty. *Transactions & Studies of the College of Physicians of Philadelphia, 11,* 123–134.

Garde, J. F. (1996). The nurse anesthesia profession. A past, present, and future perspective. *Nursing Clinics of North America, 31,* 567–580.

Lester, R. A., & Thomson, W. A. (1989). Perceptions of CRNAs: Current and future roles—Part II. *American Association of Nurse Anesthetists Journal, 57,* 417–425.

Magaw, A. (1906). A review of over 1,400 surgical anesthesias. *Surgery, Gynecology and Obstetrics, 3,* 796–799.

Mannino, M. (1996). Legal aspects of nurse anesthesia practice. *Nursing Clinics of North America, 31,* 581–589.

Shumway, S. H., & Del Risco, J. (2000). A comparison of nurse anesthesia practice types. *American Association of Nurse Anesthetists Journal, 68,* 452–462.

Thatcher, V. S. (1953). *History of anesthesia with emphasis on the nurse specialist.* Philadelphia: Lippincott.

Waugaman, W. R., & Lu, J. (1999). From nurse to nurse anesthetist: The relationship of culture, race, and ethnicity to professional socialization and career commitment of advanced practice nurses. *Journal of Transcultural Nursing, 10,* 237–247.

Chapter **14**

ROLES OF NURSE PRACTITIONERS IN THE U.S. DEPARTMENT OF VETERANS AFFAIRS

Karen R. Robinson and Robert Petzel

In these times of integrated delivery systems and escalating health care costs, there is an increased interest in the use of providers who can deliver cost-effective care that results in quality outcomes (Carroll & Fay, 1997; Carter, 1997; Hadley, 1996; Hylka & Beschle, 1995; Mundinger, 1996; Naylor et al., 1999). In many integrated health care systems, nurse practitioners (NPs) are stepping forward as providers who are able to provide quality care at a reasonable cost (Lang, Sullivan-Marx, & Jenkins, 1996; Robinson, 2000). Nurse practitioners are experts at disease prevention and health promotion and are competent in diagnosing and managing illness. It has been estimated that nurse practitioners are prepared to provide 90% of the services primary care physicians provide (Mundinger, 1999). A study of 1,316 primary care patients, randomly assigned to either nurse practitioners or physicians, found patient outcomes comparable in the two groups (Mundinger et al., 2000).

The U.S. Department of Veterans Affairs (VA), like other health care systems, recognizes that nurse practitioners provide compassionate, competent, quality, and cost-effective care. Headed by the Secretary of Veterans Affairs, VA is the second largest of the 14 Cabinet departments and operates nationwide programs of health care, financial assistance, and national cemeteries. From 54 hospitals in 1930, when created by Executive Order 5398, VA's health care system now has 163 hospitals, with at least one in each of the 48 contiguous states as well as Puerto Rico and the District of Columbia. VA operates more than 850 ambulatory care and community-based outpatient clinics, 137 nursing homes, and 73 comprehensive home-care programs. VA health care facilities provide a broad spectrum of medical, surgical, and rehabilitative care. VA has experienced considerable growth in the medical system workload over the past few years. The total number of patients treated increased by over 11% from 2000 to 2001; more than twice the prior year's rate of growth. Of the 25.3 million veterans, more than 3 of every 4 served during a war or an official period of hostility, and 6% are female. Vietnam-era veterans account for the largest segment of the present veteran population. The median age of all veterans is 58 years, and the median age of female veterans is 45 years. More than 4.2 million veterans received care in VA health care facilities in 2001; it is estimated to increase to 4.5 million in 2002. VA's outpatient clinics registered approximately 42.9 million visits in 2001 (http://www/va/gov/opa/fact/docs/vafacts.htm).

Of the veterans receiving care in the VA, 33% are 65 years of age and older, 66% earn below $20,000 annually, 60% have no health insurance, and 80% are unable to work. VA is used annually by approximately 75% of all disabled and low-income veterans (http://www.va.gov/opa/fact/docs/vafacts.htm). Major illnesses of these individuals include pulmonary disease, coronary artery disease, congestive heart failure, cancer, pneumonia, diabetes, substance abuse, and mental illness, to name a few.

VA employs about 36,000 registered nurses (RNs); of that number, 2,250 are nurse practitioners or 6.25% of the RN workforce. Nurse practitioners are employed in settings such as inpatient and outpatient psychiatry/mental health, primary care clinics, home-based primary care, critical care, employee health, community health, geriatrics, women's health, orthopedics, endocrinology, dermatology, surgery, and cardiology. The primary purpose of nurse practitioners in the VA is to provide direct patient care to assigned patients through assessment, planning, clinical decision making, direct and indirect interventions, and evaluating and assessing patient response. Nurse practitioners obtain health histories, perform physical examinations, manage essential and preventive care, and educate patients and their families. They may also be involved in educating staff, research activities, and administrative responsibilities. They manage chronic diseases, such as heart disease, hypertension, and arthritis, and also treat acute, episodic illnesses. Nurse practitioners order and interpret laboratory and diagnostic procedures and prescribe drugs and nonpharmacologic treatments (VA Fact Sheet, 2002). Some nurse practitioners perform procedures such as flexible sigmoidoscopies.

Many of VA's women veterans' health coordinators are nurse practitioners. They provide annual gynecological examinations and follow-up medical procedures. Others deliver employee health care at VA and other work sites or care for special groups of patients with HIV infection, multiple sclerosis, and cancer. Through home care, they help decrease the need for hospitalization, continue the patients' education about their illnesses, and impart self-care skills (VA Fact Sheet, 2002). VA nurse practitioners also provide health care to veterans in substance abuse treatment programs because these patients are at greater risk for infectious diseases such as hepatitis C, chemical-related diseases such as alcoholic cardiomyopathy, and mental illness. Clinicians, including nurse practitioners, who are familiar with addiction medicine, enhance positive outcomes in managing the health problems of this patient population (H. Beazlie, personal communication, January 9, 2002).

The majority of nurse practitioners in the VA have a master's degree, a national certification, and a license as a nurse practitioner. Individuals meeting these criteria may function as licensed independent practitioners. They do not require supervision by a physician, physician countersignature of their orders, or countersignature for their care plans. The VA does continue to employ some nurse practitioners who were educated through other training programs and are not master's prepared. These individuals may have a more limited scope of practice (Under Secretary for Health, 1997, 1999). In VA, 97% of nurse practitioners have prescriptive authority (VA Fact Sheet, 2002).

BACKGROUND

In the United States, the nurse practitioner role developed as a result of the primary care physician shortage in the 1960s and 1970s (Bigbee & Amidi-Nouri, 2000). In 1973, the VA added 43 nurse practitioner positions to admission areas—the first major use of nurse practitioners in the VA. In 1975, VA issued a policy statement outlining appropriate functions for nurse practitioners. There are now 2,250 nurse practitioners working in the VA (VA Fact Sheet, 2002).

Prior to 1995, an ad hoc task force was appointed to address advanced practice nurse (APN) issues in the VA. Their first task was to collect demographic information about the advanced practice nurse workforce. In

September 1995, the APN Advisory Council was established as a subcommittee of the Nursing Board of Directors for the Nursing Strategic Health Care Group, VA Central Office, Washington, D.C. This Advisory Council addressed issues specific to advanced practice nursing (nurse practitioners and clinical nurse specialists) and drafted official documents for the VA (B. Westfield, personal communication, July 3, 2002).

VA established prescribing authority for advanced practice nurses under a federal regulation in 1995, at a time when many states did not grant prescriptive authority for advanced practice nurses (General Guidelines, 1995). This allowed the VA to further maximize the utilization of advanced practice nurses in clinical care. Prescriptions or medication orders written by duly authorized advanced practice nurses within their approved scope of practice no longer required a physician cosignature. However, the individual's scope of practice needed approval by an appropriate facility-based authorizing body such as the Clinical Executive Board or the Medical Executive Committee. This authority remains in effect and has been recently endorsed by Anthony J. Principi, Secretary for VA, and while 49 of 50 states now have prescriptive authority for nurse practitioners, the federal regulation expands that authority in some cases (B. Westfield, personal communication, July 3, 2002).

With the transition of the VA from an inpatient-based system to one that is driven by primary care, there has been a significant increase in the utilization of nurse practitioners. The APN Advisory Council serves as a resource center for VA Central Office and the VA health care facilities in the appropriate utilization of nurse practitioners and clinical models for nurse practitioner practice. The Council currently has representatives on the Multidisciplinary Practice Advisory Council to address common practice issues of advanced practice nurses, physician assistants, and clinical pharmacy specialists.

Today there are diverse options available for nurse practitioners employed in the VA. Nurse practitioners contribute to the science of nursing. VA's advanced practice nurses and nurse researchers advise the National Nurse Executive Council (NNEC) on VA clinical guidelines and performance measures that relate to nursing practice. They have the full support of Cathy Rick, Chief Nursing Officer, Nursing Strategic Health Care Group, VA Central Office, Washington, D.C. Ms. Rick states, "I hope to have them help us with nursing's agenda and continue to move nursing forward. I feel strongly about recognizing nurse practitioners for their contributions, but also want to take advantage of their expertise to move the system and advance the profession—quite frankly, to contribute to the profession at large, not just within the VA" (C. Rick, personal communication, December 20, 2001).

The VA health care system has a long history of supporting nurse practitioner education by providing tuition funds to individuals for academic study. The master's-level advanced practice nursing program was established by the Office of Academic Affiliations in 1981 to attract clinical nurse specialist and nurse practitioner students to the VA. Direct funding support continues to be offered to advanced practice nursing students who do their clinical experience at VA facilities. Students must be enrolled in the academic institutions that are affiliated with VA. A minimum of 120 hours of clinical experience at the VA facility is required for funding support ("Affiliated Associated," July 2001). From October 1, 1999, through September 30, 2002, a total of 854 nurse practitioner students were funded by this program. An additional 287 students have been offered funding for fiscal year 2003 (October 1, 2002 through September 30, 2003) (F. Kennedy, personal communication, September 4, 2002).

In 1997, VA linked with the Department of Defense (DoD) to implement one of the earliest and most successful distance learning nurse practitioner education programs in the nation. Local facilities indicated that tuition reimbursement was insufficient to meet their growing needs for nurse practitioners. In response, VA collaborated with the Uniformed Services University of the Health Sciences (USUHS) in Bethesda, Maryland, to implement the novel Distance Learning Post-Masters Certificate Program for Adult Nurse Practitioner education. Of approximately 685 clinical nurse specialists employed by the VA, 60 have attained certificates as adult nurse practitioners through this program, which capitalizes on VA's state-of-the-art video teleconferencing capability, partnered with a rigorous USUHS nurse practitioner curriculum. Unique to this accredited curriculum is the absence of a residential requirement for the clinical practicum at the teaching campus. Rather, each VA facility provides one class coordinator and several clinical preceptors to supervise student practice. Faculty from USUHS oversee clinical practice, visit each site, and use distance learning modalities to maintain contact with preceptors. At the conclusion of this 18-month program, students are eligible to take the national nurse practitioner certification exam. To date, students have attained a 98% pass rate on the exam and have assumed a number of primary care roles (C. Beason, personal communication, January 2, 2002).

The VA Employee Incentive Scholarship Program (EISP) was established by Title VIII of Public Law 105-368, Department of Veterans Affairs Health Care Personnel Incentive Act of 1998. Under this authority, VA may award scholarships to employees pursuing degrees or training in health care disciplines for which recruitment and retention of qualified personnel is difficult, and also pay their reasonable expenses, such as registration, fees, books, materials, and supplies. This program would assist those employees desiring to become a nurse practitioner. There is a period of obligated service.

EXAMPLES OF VA NURSE PRACTITIONER ROLES

With the support of former and current VA leaders as well as programs such as the VA/DoD Distance Learning Post-Masters' Certificate for Adult Nurse Practitioners and other tuition-support funding assistance, a variety of nurse practitioner roles have evolved in the VA.

Nurse-Managed Primary Care Delivery Clinics

Nurse practitioners have been attracted to primary care in increasing numbers, working as supervised employees of physicians, in collaborative practices, or in solo practices. The collaborative model described by Mundinger (1994) appears to be attractive to many nurse practitioners in primary care settings. In the model, nurse practitioners are mainly responsible for the diagnosis and management of uncomplicated illness and provide the education, counseling, and management of disease prevention and health promotion, using primary care physicians as consultants and referral sources. The physician provides diagnosis and treatment for unstable, complex, or life-threatening diseases. This model gives physicians time to provide the services and judgments that are needed at the highest level of knowledge.

Based on the Under Secretary for Health's information letters, which stress optimal use of nurse practitioners in the delivery of primary care, a review of the literature, and the information gathered from three contacts reported in the literature, VA Health Care Veterans Integrated Service Network (VISN 13) established nurse-managed primary care delivery clinics (Robinson, 2000; Under Secretary for Health, 1997, 1999). At that time, VISN 13 included all VA medical centers and clinics located in the states of Minnesota, North and South Dakota, and one clinic in Wisconsin. The VISN has now expanded to include Iowa, Nebraska, and part of Illinois. These community-based outpatient clinics (CBOCs) use nurse practitioners as independent practitioners with prescriptive authority with a goal of delivering a cost-effective, efficient, high-quality health care system.

To qualify as a nurse-managed CBOC, the following criteria must be met:

- use a master's-prepared nurse practitioner with national certification as a primary care provider

- have a qualified registered nurse as a case manager on site
- ensure that credentialing and privileging are in place, including prescribing authority
- provide for ancillary help and access to medical records, laboratory, pharmacy, and radiology services
- establish outcomes research in the future
- establish academic partnerships

Initial clinic sites included Chippewa Valley, Wisconsin; Fergus Falls and Maplewood, Minnesota; and Grafton, North Dakota. Staffing includes a nurse practitioner, a registered nurse, and a clerk, with total FTE (full-time equivalent) ranging from 4 to 6.5. Some sites also have a licensed practical nurse. Panel sizes for each nurse practitioner range from 750 to 900 patients. These clinics provide primary care to veterans, most of whom are new to the VA system. Patient satisfaction survey results are excellent; patients appreciate the availability of these clinics in their communities and are complimentary of the care they receive.

Testimony to the U.S. Senate Committee on Veterans Affairs in regard to the VISN 13 nurse-managed clinic innovation (U.S. Senate Committee on Veterans Affairs, 2001) led to the U.S. Senate and House of Representatives passing, and President George W. Bush subsequently signing, nurse recruitment and retention legislation, which establishes an evaluation of nurse-managed health care clinics in the VA. Patient satisfaction, provider experiences, cost of care, access to care, and functional status of patients receiving care are to be evaluated in VA nurse-managed clinics located in three different geographic service areas. A final report is to be submitted by July 23, 2003, to the Committees on Veterans'Affairs of the Senate and the House of Representatives (Department of Veterans Affairs Health Care Programs Enhancement Act of 2001, H.R. 3447, Pub. L. No. 107-135, Sec. 123, January 23, 2002).

Acute Care Nurse Practitioner Role

As a result of the downsizing of medical residency programs, reallocation of more residency slots to primary care settings, and the difficulty in filling existing acute-care residency slots, the management of hospitalized patients has changed. Nurse practitioners are assuming this role in increasing numbers (Richmond & Keane, 1996). Roles of acute-care nurse practitioners vary considerably. For example, one model has nurse practitioners delivering care to disease-specific population groups (e.g., cardiology, diabetes, cancer). Another model incorporates a problem-based approach to care, with nurse practitioners providing specialized wound care, managing acute and chronic pain, providing nutritional support, and/or managing urinary incontinence.

In 1994, the VA Medical Center in Salt Lake City, Utah, successfully implemented the nurse practitioner role in the surgical intensive care unit (SICU) (see chapter 18). The individual in this role orders appropriate laboratory and radiographic studies and performs procedures such as intubation as well as placement of central lines, arterial lines, pulmonary artery catheters, and chest tubes. The SICU nurse practitioner's caseload includes up to 10 surgical intensive care patients. In addition, he or she sees patients on the surgical units; provides follow-up care for four to six patients who have transferred out of the intensive care unit; and provides support to neurosurgical, cardiothoracic, urology, ear-nose-throat, and orthopedic services, as well as interim support to vascular and general surgery services. The SICU nurse practitioner is an educator to patients, families, nursing staff, medical students, and residents and participates in clinical research projects and rounds. Administratively, this individual assists the intensivist and SICU nurse manager with the development and writing of unit policies and procedures (Jarvis, 2002). Over the past 8 years, this role has become well established at the Salt Lake City VA Medical Center. In fact, a second nurse practitioner has been added to the SICU, and a total of five inpatient nurse practitioners are employed by the medical center.

Case Management/Nurse Practitioner Role

The cardiology section at the Zablocki VA Medical Center in Milwaukee, Wisconsin, includes case management (general and specialty cardiology), patient and staff education, preoperative cardiology clearance examinations, and management of the 23-hour Chest Pain Evaluation Program in the nurse practitioner's role. As a case manager, the nurse practitioner works with other members of the team to ensure continuity of care for the cardiac arrhythmia patient population. In collaboration with the cardiology fellows and staff physicians, the nurse practitioner evaluates both inpatient and outpatient consults to the service, developing and implementing a plan of care. Evaluations often include follow-up stress testing, echocardiograms, loop recorders, and Holter monitoring. Preprocedure history and physical examinations are performed, and follow-up for patients with pacemakers and implantable cardioverter defibrillators are provided in a weekly nurse-run device clinic (B. Hammer, personal communication, January 2, 2002).

In the educator role, the nurse practitioner educates patients and their families about specific cardiac rhythms and the reasons certain diagnostic tests and interventional procedures are recommended. He or she also conducts preventive and medication education. Staff education is also an integral part of the role.

The overall goal of the 23-hour Chest Pain Evaluation Program is to safely, effectively, and accurately evaluate patients with chest pain. A chest pain decision tree walks the provider through various steps. The nurse practitioner's role is to monitor the overall program, provide monthly in-services to the rotating cardiology team, assist in tracking admissions, and work to eliminate process barriers.

The following outcome measures were established and tracked to demonstrate effectiveness of the 23-hour Chest Pain Evaluation Program:

1. No acute cardiac intervention within 30 days of discharge from the program
2. No unscheduled readmission for chest pain or a cardiac event within 30 days of discharge from the program
3. No deaths due to a cardiac event within 30 days of discharge from the program
4. A decrease of 30% in the total number of patients admitted for chest pain
5. Length of stay for patient with moderate risk for myocardial ischemia is 23 hours or less
6. A decrease of 50% in the direct cost per case for patients at moderate risk

Since implementing the program in July 1999, steady progress has been made each quarter to achieve success. Last quarter's results indicate that each of the aforementioned outcome measures has been met (B. Hammer, personal communication, August 26, 2002).

Compensation and Pension Examination Program

The VA comprises the Veterans Benefits, Veterans Health, and National Cemetery Administrations, which have important linkages in terms of providing veteran services. One such linkage is related to veterans' applications for compensation and pension (C&P) for injuries or medical conditions associated with their military service. A major factor in determining a veteran's C&P status is a clinical examination, which can be conducted at most VA medical centers. Results of this examination are critical indicators of a veteran's health and burial benefits.

Traditionally, physicians have performed these examinations. After a review of the C&P guidelines, the New York Harbor VA Healthcare System (NYHHS) determined that nurse practitioners could perform general medical examinations, as well as some other nonspecialty examinations.

In the spring of 1997, the NYHHS implemented its initiative to have nurse practitioners conduct certain C&P examinations (Miller, 2000). The purpose of this initiative was to enhance the efficiency of the C&P examination process without compromising quality. In an effort to accomplish this goal, NYHHS (1) developed an exportable model that utilizes nurse practitioners to provide general medical C&P examinations and (2) evaluated the impact of this practice on quality, cost, and veteran and staff satisfaction (Miller, 2001). The nurse practitioners perform the examinations and maintain a collaborative agreement with the C&P physicians, who are available for consultation.

At the New York campus, the use of nurse practitioners decreased the turnaround time for examination completion from an average of 40 days to 20 days within 18 months of the program's implementation (Miller, 2001). In addition to providing a competent C&P assessment and improving timely service, utilizing the nurse practitioners in this role also increased patient satisfaction. Of 188 general medical examinations completed from January 1997 to February 2000, 128 were performed by nurse practitioners and 60 by physicians. Patients showed higher satisfaction with nurse practitioners on all nine satisfaction questions asked by the independent research firm hired to conduct the telephone interviews. For example, when rating the overall quality of the service, veterans who were examined by a nurse practitioner rated the examination a 7.7 (on a scale of 1 to 9 where 9 was "Extremely Satisfied"), compared to a 6.9 rating for veterans examined by a physician; the difference was statistically significant. Interestingly, there was no significant difference in patient satisfaction with nurse practitioners and physicians for patients 50 years of age and older. Patients under 50 years of age reported significantly higher satisfaction with nurse practitioners.

Approximately 24 VA medical centers currently have nurse practitioners performing C&P examinations. In addition to the NYHHS, some of the other medical centers are located in Minneapolis, Minnesota; Ann Arbor, Michigan; Oklahoma City, Oklahoma; Lexington, Kentucky; Memphis, Tennessee; Loma Linda, California; Milwaukee, Wisconsin; Syracuse, New York; Richmond, Virginia; Miami, Florida; Providence, Rhode Island; and Columbia, Missouri (E. Miller, personal communication, August 14, 2002).

The patients perceive the nurse practitioners as having exceptional interpersonal skills, and appreciate their holistic perspective. Nurse practitioners are adept at providing preventive care and patient education, are able to detect unrecognized disease, and are willing to facilitate the entry of veterans into care at the VA. While not part of the C&P examination process, these extra services have helped to make the veterans feel that they had a complete examination. In addition, the volume of claim appeals has decreased, and satisfaction with the entire process is enhanced (Beason & Hynes, 1998; Miller, 2000).

Complementary and Alternative Medicine (CAM) Integrative Health Program

In the last decade, Americans have been seeking a new approach to health care that emphasizes not just treatment of disease symptoms but how to stay healthy in body, mind, and spirit—holistic health care. Two national telephone surveys, conducted over 6 years, indicated an increase in the use of CAM therapies from 33.8% to 42.1% within the United States (Eisenberg, Davis, et al., 1993; Eisenberg, Kessler, et al., 1993). In 1998, the VA awarded a contract to assess the current state of CAM therapy use. Findings revealed that veterans, like the general public, believe that CAM products are not harmful and that some veterans are using the therapies (Klemm Analysis Group, Inc., 1998).

In 1997, a nurse practitioner at the VA Medical Center in Salt Lake City, Utah, proposed a program to offer and integrate nonpharmacological holistic therapies and self-help methods with traditional medical care. After developing a business plan and receiving necessary approval, the clinic officially opened in April 2001. CAM modalities offered in the Integrative Health Clinic and Program include acupuncture, hypnosis, guided imagery, education and information on herbal medicine and nutritional supplements, meditation, qigong movement, prayer groups, yoga, nutritional counseling, and weight management. A 6-week series of classes on new strategies and insights into mental/emotional well-being and resiliency in chronic illness is conducted. In addition, the nurse practitioner provides hypnotherapy to assist with chronic pain control, stress management, habit control, smoking cessation, and weight control. A monthly educational series of 1-hour lectures on CAM modalities is offered to all providers, staff, and patients.

The nurse practitioner at the Salt Lake City Medical Center continues to develop the Integrative Health Program and investigate the addition of efficacious modalities to the program. The plan is to evaluate the integration of CAM modalities with traditional medicine in the management of certain medical conditions. Further program development is being considered for preoperative, intraoperative, and postoperative guided imagery stress reduction, massage, and biofeedback (S. Smeeding, personal communication, December 27, 2001).

Currently the program has received over 300 referrals, with the number of new referrals increasing to the present 5–8 per day. The program has been well accepted by patients, providers, and staff. Primarily through the interventions of acupuncture and hypnosis, significant improvement in the quality of life has been reported for chronic pain patients (S. Smeeding, personal communication, August 22, 2002).

Employee Support Program

Advanced practice psychiatric mental health nurses, such as the psychiatric-mental health nurse practitioners, are ideally suited to coordinate VA's employee support programs. This role offers a unique opportunity for a nurse practitioner to capitalize on his or her expertise related to health promotion and disease prevention and to use clinical and research skills. As a program specialist, the nurse practitioner conducts a workplace analysis to identify the needs of employees, management, and the organization. Through these proactive approaches, the individual can create a healthy work environment that promotes staff morale, facilitates a drug-free workplace, and reduces workplace stress.

Nurse practitioners provide state-of-the art services that enable employees and their immediate families to deal with crisis, grief, stress, and mental health issues. Major responsibilities of the nurse practitioner include crisis intervention, grief work/counseling, relapse prevention, organizational consultation, and health education. Ideally, this service is provided within a medical center because it provides easy access to services and the nurse practitioner is familiar with the organizational culture. Confidentiality is the core of a successful employee support program because of the sensitive nature of employees' and managers' problems or stressors. Deborah Antai-Otong, MS, PMHNP, RN, CS, the Program Specialist/Coordinator of the VA Medical Center program in Dallas, Texas, emphasizes that expert interpersonal and group dynamic skills are crucial to the program's success. These skills are vital because the individual works closely with supervisors, management, and various parties to address service issues, mediate problems, and offer strategies that facilitate healthy conflict resolution (D. Antai-Otong, personal communication, January 4, 2002).

Gerontology/Extended Care Centers

Many VA gerontology nurse practitioners are employed in extended care centers that offer patient services such as skilled nursing care, rehabilitation therapies, reconditioning, radiation therapy, complex medical management, wound care, prosthetic training, management of geropsychiatric conditions, respite services, end-of-life care, spinal cord injury care, and comprehensive general geriatric evaluation and management. In these settings, nurse practitioners manage chronic diseases as well as diagnose and treat acute diseases with a focus on the holistic approach to meet the medical, social, and functional needs of older patients. In addition, nurse practitioner activities include admission screening; history and physical examinations; prescribing medications, treatments, and procedures; program development; patient and staff education; local, state, and national leadership in committees related to nursing practice; preceptorship for graduate nurse practitioner students; and research. Prescribing and admitting privileges can be included in their scope of practice (E. Boger, C. DePew, P. Lawrow, & J. Hager, personal communication, January 8, 2002).

In many VA settings, gerontology nurse practitioners lead the interdisciplinary health care team that collaboratively manages the veterans' care. The health care team consists of nurse practitioners, physicians, nurses, chaplains, dietitians, psychiatrists, pharmacists, and recreational, physical, and occupational therapists.

Home-Based Primary Care

In some parts of the country, nurse practitioners are doing home visits to provide necessary primary care to their veteran patients. This is beyond the traditional "visiting nurse" concept. Nurse practitioners perform the same duties as they would if they were in the clinic setting; however, in addition, they are providing increased access to care for those patients who have difficulty traveling for appointments.

The VA Medical Center in Denver, Colorado, has a program that utilizes a multidisciplinary approach to provide primary health care and support services to an aging, chronically ill veteran population (L. Kehm, personal communication, December 31, 2001). By providing this care, the need for hospitalization, nursing home care, emergency department, and outpatient visits are reduced. Those most likely to benefit from this program include patients with complications following stroke, congestive heart failure, chronic obstructive pulmonary disease, dementia, and diabetes. In addition, many individuals who do not have a caregiver or who have behavior problems, are at high risk for falls, have complicated medication regimens, or have poor pain management achieve positive outcomes from this program.

The Denver VA Home Based Primary Care Team consists of three nurse practitioners, a social worker, a dietitian, an occupational therapist, and a pharmacist. A comprehensive initial assessment is completed in the home, which includes physical, psychosocial, nutritional, functional status, and environmental components. An interdisciplinary, individualized treatment plan is established for each patient and reviewed by the team on a regular basis. Patient and caregiver education, advance directive discussion, and appropriate referrals to various community agencies are included in the plan. Coordination of care with outside agencies such as hospice, visiting nurse services, and mental health agencies is ongoing. The nurse practitioners are responsible for maintaining current pharmacy profiles and diagnostic/laboratory testing, as needed. Frequency of the home visits is based on patient needs and may vary from month to month. The program maintains a census of 76–80 patients.

When the Denver group compared hospitalization by 50 patients one year prior and after enrollment in the Home Based Primary Care Program, they found days of hospitalization decreased from 370 to 190 (58% decrease), intensive care unit days decreased from 21 to 17 (20% decrease), days in a nursing home (excluding respite care) significantly decreased from 421 to 58 (86% decrease), and emergency department visits decreased from 116 to 27 (77% decrease). In addition, specialty appointments, including pulmonary, urology, cardiology, and podiatry, decreased from 235 to 123 (48% decrease), and no-show appointments decreased from 117 to 48 (59% decrease). Medication costs increased approximately 4%; however, outcomes were improved and polypharmacy decreased. Changes also were noted in behavior management and in preventive measures such as lipid management and diabetes control. The group estimated a total savings of $120,482 from visit reduction (L. Kehm, personal communication, August 26, 2002).

Mobile Health and Wellness Program

The Mobile Health and Wellness Program, initiated in 1997, is a nurse-administered program providing health screening, education, and risk identification/stratification to veterans residing within the service area of the VA Medical Center in Salem, Virginia (Beason & Hynes, 1998; Therien, 2000). Objectives of this program include increasing awareness of disease prevention and health maintenance, improving access to health care for all eligible veterans, increasing VA market penetration, and enhancing community partnership. Staffing of this nurse-administered program includes a nurse practitioner, a licensed practical nurse, one health technician, and two administrative or clerical staff (Therien, 2000).

During the health screening, interested veterans are enrolled in the Salem VA Medical Center system and informed of its scope of services. Veterans are provided with necessary education to prevent, and provide better coping measures for, high-risk disease. Services include weight, blood pressure, cholesterol, and blood sugar checks. Patient education, especially for heart disease, high blood pressure, cancer, and diabetes, and lifestyle screenings for factors that could contribute to disease or accidental injury are offered. Immunization status is obtained.

Nurse Executive/Nurse Practitioner

During the last 25 years, the nurse executive role has evolved from a front-line operations and supervisory role to a powerful executive-level position in today's complex health care organizations (Sorrells-Jones, 1999). The nurse executive plans with individuals at the corporate level about what the organization should be and creates strategies for his or her areas of responsibility. Long-range thinking and planning drive the daily operations (Barnum & Kerfoot, 1995).

An ability to deal with rapid change, an entrepreneurial spirit, and the skill to deal with many diverse individuals and groups are requirements for today's nurse executive. Nurse executives at the VA Medical Centers in Salt Lake City, Utah, and Albany, New York, certainly possess a spirit of entrepreneurship. Brian Westfield is not only the nurse executive of the Salt Lake City tertiary care medical center and primary consultant to the VA Central Office on advanced practice issues, but also, as a nurse practitioner, provides primary care to his assigned panel of patients two afternoons each week. Susan Burkhart-Jayez, Albany VA Medical Center, as a nurse practitioner, conducts compensation and pension examinations one morning each week. She states this allows her to be connected to the veterans and to determine best practices as well as what improvements are needed. Both individuals are members of the senior management team in developing a strategic plan for their organizations; at the same time, they are able to offer a perspective on whether the plan is practical and effective in the clinical setting (S. Burkhart-Jayez, personal communication, August 1, 2002; B. Westfield, personal communication, January 14, 2002).

Outpatient General Surgery

At the VA Medical Center in Dallas, Texas, the nurse practitioner is a clinician, educator, researcher, consultant, and administrator. As a clinician, the nurse practitioner provides direct patient care in the outpatient surgical setting by performing activities such as history and physical examinations on day surgery patients, initial interviews and assessments of outpatients consulted to surgery from other disciplines, postoperative follow-ups, and minor clinic procedures. In the educator role, the nurse practitioner conducts education for patients, families, and staff. As a researcher for the surgical service, the nurse practitioner is actively involved in the assessment, diagnosis, and follow-up of patients who are candidates for or already enrolled in surgery studies such as laparoscopic versus open repair of inguinal hernia. In the nurse practitioner's administrative role, he or she reviews all abnormal radiology reports for surgery to ensure appropriate follow-up and consultation have been implemented. In addition, the nurse practitioner reviews and completes the majority of general surgery outpatient consults to ensure that patients are scheduled to the appropriate surgery clinic for evaluation and/or follow-up (T. Armitage-Clark, personal communication, January 4, 2002).

SUMMARY

As we move into the 21st Century, the world of health care continues to be in a state of dramatic transformation. Demands for higher quality and patient satisfaction, greater accountability, lower costs, and improvement in patient outcomes are driving the system. VA nurse practitioners employed in roles such as those described in this chapter have come forward to provide safe, highly skilled, cost-effective care that has resulted in high patient satisfaction and positive outcomes for the veteran patients. We believe these providers are valuable contributors to the success of our delivery system.

ACKNOWLEDGMENTS

The authors extend sincere appreciation to Cathy Rick, MSN, RN, Chief Consultant, Nursing Strategic Health Care Group, VA Central Office; Charlotte Beason, EdD, RN, Program Director, Nursing Strategic Health Care Group, VA Central Office; Deborah Antai-Otong, MS, PMHNP, RN, CS, Dallas VAMC; Tara Armitage-Clark, MSN, RN, CS, ANP, Dallas VAMC; Henry Beazlie, MSN, RN, CNP, Louis Stokes Cleveland VAMC, Wade Park Unit; Estella Boger, MSN, RN, NP, Fargo VAMC; Susan Burkhart-Jayez, MS, RN, NP, Albany VAMC; Charlotte DePew, MS, RN, C-ANP, Minneapolis VAMC; Julia Hager, MAN, RN, C-GNP, Minneapolis VAMC; Beth Hammer, MSN, RN, NP, Milwaukee VAMC; Darcy Harr, MSN, RN, NP, Fargo VAMC; Sabrina Jarvis, MS, ACPN, FNP, CCRN, Salt Lake City VAMC; Linda Kehm, MSN, CA, ANCC, Denver VAMC; Fortune Kennedy, EdD, RN, Office of Academic Affiliations, VA Central Office; Patricia Lawrow, MPN, RN, C-NP,

Minneapolis VAMC; Elvira Miller, EdD, RN, VA New York Harbor Healthcare System; Mary Ramar, RN, MA, CNAA, Nursing Education Program Manager, Health Care Staff Development & Retention Office; Sandra Smeeding, APRN, CNS, FNP, Salt Lake City VAMC; Jan Therien, MHSA, RN, Salem VAMC; Brian Westfield, MS, RN, NP, Salt Lake City VAMC; Joyce Nicholas and Diane Nordeng, Library Service, Fargo VAMC. Without this group's valuable assistance and expertise, this chapter would not have been possible.

REFERENCES

Barnum, B. S., & Kerfoot, K. M. (1995). *The nurse as executive* (4th ed.). Gaithersburg, MD: Aspen.

Beason, C. F., & Hynes, D. M. (1998, November 3). Improved outcomes for compensation and pension examinations utilizing nurse practitioners VAMC New York. In C. F. Benson & D. M. Hynes (Eds.), *Enhancing veterans healthcare through innovations: Report of the innovations in nursing initiative review task force*. Washington, DC: Department of Veterans Affairs.

Bigbee, J. L., & Amidi-Nouri, A. (2000). History and evolution of advanced nursing practice. In A. B. Hamric, J. A. Spross, & C. M. Hanson (Eds.), *Advanced nursing practice: An integrative approach* (2nd ed., pp. 3–32). Philadelphia: Saunders.

Carroll, T. L., & Fay, V. P. (1997). Measuring the impact of advanced practice nursing on achieving cost-quality outcomes: Issues and challenges. *Nursing Administration Quarterly, 21*(4), 32–40.

Carter, M. A. (1997). The promise of nurse practitioners. *Nursing Administration Quarterly, 21*(4), 19–24.

Department of Veterans Affairs Health Care Programs Enhancement Act of 2001, H.R. 3447, Pub. L. No. 107-135, Sec. 123, January 23, 2002.

Department of Veterans Affairs. (2002). *Facts about the Department of Veterans Affairs*. Available: http://www/va/gov/opa/fact/docs/vafacts.htm

Eisenberg, D. M., Davis, R. B., Ettner, S. L., Appel, S., Wilkey, S., Van Rompay, M., & Kessler, R. C. (1998). Trends in alternative medicine use in the United States, 1990-1997: Results of a follow-up national survey. *Journal of the American Medical Association, 280,* 1569–1575.

Eisenberg, D. M., Kessler, R. C., Foster, C., Norlock, F. E., Calkins, D. R., & Delbanco, R. L. (1993). Unconventional medicine in the United States: Prevalence, costs, and patterns of use. *New England Journal of Medicine, 328,* 246–252.

General guidelines for establishing medication prescribing authority for clinical nurse specialists, nurse practitioners, clinical pharmacy specialists, and physician assistants. (1995, March 3). VHA Directive 10-95-019.

Hadley, E. H. (1996). Nursing in the political and economic marketplace: Challenges for the 21st century. *Nursing Outlook, 44,* 6–10.

Hylka, S. C., & Beschle, J. C. (1995). Nurse practitioners, cost savings, and improved patient care in the department of surgery. *Nursing Economics, 13,* 349–354.

Jarvis, S. (2002). *SICU nurse practitioner.* Unpublished manuscript.

Klemm Analysis Group, Inc. (1998). *VHA CAM practices and future opportunities.* Retrieved from http://vaww.va.gov/med/patientcare/primary/cam.cfm

Lang, N. M., Sullivan-Marx, E. M., & Jenkins, M. (1996). Advanced practice nurses and success of organized delivery systems. *American Journal of Managed Care, 2,* 129–135.

Miller, E. D. (2000). Improved outcomes of veterans' compensation and pension examinations using nurse practitioners. *Nursing Clinics of North America, 35,* 519–525.

Miller, E. D., & the VA New York Harbor VA Healthcare system. (2001). *A national initiative to improve compensation and pension examinations through the use of nurse practitioners: Final report.* New York: VA New York Harbor VA Healthcare System.

Mundinger, M. O. (1994). Advanced-practice nursing—Good medicine for physicians? *The New England Journal of Medicine, 330,* 211–214.

Mundinger, M. O. (1996). New alliances: Nursing's bright future. *Nursing Administration Quarterly, 20*(3), 50–53.

Mundinger, M. O. (1999). Can advanced practice nurses succeed in the primary care market? *Nursing Economics, 17,* 7–14.

Mundinger, M. O., Kane, R. L., Lenz, E. R., Totten, A. M., Tsai, W., Cleary, P. D., Friedewald, W. T., Siu, A. L., & Shelanski, M. L. (2000). Primary care outcomes in patients treated by nurse practitioners or physicians. *Journal of the American Medical Association, 283,* 59–68.

Naylor, M. D., Brooten, D., Campbell, R., Jacobsen, B. S., Mezey, M. D., Pauly, M. V., & Schwartz, J. S. (1999). Comprehensive discharge planning and home follow-up of hospitalized elders. *Journal of the American Medical Association, 281,* 613–620.

Office of Academic Affiliation, Department of Veterans Affairs. (2001, July). *Affiliated associated health education programs.* Available: http://www.va.gov/oaa/AHE_EdOpportunities.asp#Nursing

Richmond, T. S., & Keane, A. (1996). Acute-care nurse practitioners. In J. V. Hickey, R. M. Ouimette, & S. L. Venegoni (Eds.), *Advanced practice nursing: Changing roles and clinical applications* (pp. 316–333). Philadelphia: Lippincott.

Robinson, K. R. (2000). Nurse-managed primary care delivery clinics. *Nursing Clinics of North America, 35,* 471–479.

Sorrells-Jones, J. (1999). The role of the chief nurse executive in the knowledge-intense organization of the future. *Nursing Administration Quarterly, 23*(3), 17–25.

Therien, J. (2000). Establishing a mobile health and wellness program for rural veterans. *Nursing Clinics of North America, 35,* 499–505.

Under Secretary for Health. (1997, July 7). *Information letter: Utilization of nurse practitioners and clinical nurse specialists.* Washington, DC: Department of Veterans Affairs.

Under Secretary for Health. (1999, February 24). *Information letter: Utilization of nurse practitioners and clinical nurse specialists.* Washington, DC: Department of Veterans Affairs.

U.S. Senate Committee on Veterans Affairs. (2001, June 14). *Looming nurse shortage: Impact on the Department of Veterans Affairs.* 107th Congress (testimony of Dr. Robert Petzel).

VA fact sheet. (2002, April). Retrieved from http://www.va.gov

VOICES FROM THE FIELD

Although the nurse practitioners' role has grown and expanded, the unique voice of the nurse practitioner in interaction with patients, families, and colleagues remains foundational. How to maintain the unique application of nurse practitioner services in a cost-conscious and erratic health care delivery environment raises great challenges and successes. In Part III, we provide you with first-hand accounts of nurse practitioners and physicians who speak about their successes and challenges from their own practices.

New to this section is a chapter by Colagreco and Kirton, who succinctly outline the "nuts and bolts" of the business and regulatory aspects of their practice. Their "how to" perspective on the operations of practice is a fresh and accurate account of licensing, contracting, and payment mechanisms that is very useful for the student and the practicing clinician. The new chapter by Beidler and Torrisi portrays how family nurse practitioners close gaps in community health care across underserved and culturally diverse arenas to change how health care is delivered. In this section also we present updates from four key voices from the field, nurse practitioners and physicians who tell their stories of interaction with patients, families, other practitioners, and health systems.

Jarvis' account of the early development and endurance of a nurse practitioner in a surgical intensive care unit portends the current growth of acute and critical care nurse practitioners models and informs us of the pioneering efforts that nurse practitioners often have taken to change care in health systems. Bill Kavesh, one of the early physician supporters of geriatric nurse practitioner practice, poignantly describes and advises us about the way physicians and nurse practitioners must relate to one another in interdisciplinary practice from his experience in home care and long-term care.

Boland and Leib write about how they have built a mutually trustful and respectful collaboration to share accountability and to jointly make decisions in day-to-day experience with patients and families. In her updated chapter, O'Sullivan adds new research and perspectives on behavioral health, presenting a first-person account of her NP practice with adolescents over many years. Stracuzzi and Rinke, in their chapter on advanced practice nursing in home care, lay out an exciting experiment in providing much-needed primary care to homebound and frail adults. Unique to this role is the focus on patients who are truly homebound and who have had little or no access to primary health care prior to the intervention of this home care model of practice.

Chapter **15**

THE VOICE OF EXPERIENCE: THE NUTS AND BOLTS OF ADVANCED PRACTICE FOR NURSE PRACTITIONERS

Joseph P. Colagreco and Carl A. Kirton

NURSE PRACTITIONER STATUS

Nurse practitioners, clinical nurse specialists, nurse-midwives, and nurse anesthetists are uniformly referred to as advanced practice nurses (APNs). An APN is "a registered nurse, currently licensed in (a) state, who is prepared for advanced nursing practice by virtue of knowledge and skills obtained through a post-basic or advanced educational program of study acceptable to the board of nursing" (Ryser, 1999, p. 351). The scope of practice for all APNs is regulated by state nurse practice acts.

Each state determines whether APNs practice under "certification" or a "second licensure." If the state issues second licenses to nurse practitioners, those licenses are held by the practitioner in addition to their registered nurse licenses. In most states, the board of nursing establishes the criteria that must be met for a nurse to be certified or licensed as a nurse practitioner. In only six states, the board of nurse examiners and the board of medical examiners jointly regulate advanced nursing practice (Pearson, 2002, p. 12).

Nursing has the sole authority to determine nurse practitioners' scopes of practice in 44 states and the District of Columbia. Yet in all but 12 states and the District of Columbia, nurse practitioners have some requirement for physician collaboration or supervision (Pearson, 2002, p. 12). These requirements are the legislative results of organized medicine to limit nursing practice.

NURSE PRACTITIONER CERTIFICATION OR LICENSURE, TITLES AND CREDENTIALS

Certification and Licensure

Nurse practitioner students and employers of APNs are often confused by the lexicon of advanced practice. Consider the following questions from a prospective employer:

1. Are you state certified?
2. Are you nationally certified?
3. Who certifies you?
4. Are you licensed?
5. What do your credentials indicate about your practice?

Given the range of certification and licensure regulations across states, it is no wonder that advanced practice nursing students, prospective employers, and the public at large are confused regarding the answers to the aforementioned questions.

Many students have asked if we can delineate the difference between a license to practice and certification. The National Council of State Boards of Nursing (2001) explains it as follows:

> Licensure is the process by which an agency of state government grants permission to an individual to engage in a given profession upon finding that the applicant has attained the essential degree of competency necessary to perform a unique scope of practice (while) certification is another type of credential that affords title protection and recognition of accomplishment, but that does not include a legal scope of practice.

It is important to recognize that there is no national nurse practitioner licensure examination. States that issue a second license require that the nurse practitioner who is seeking second licensure be certified by a national nursing certification body. So, states that issue second licensure for nurse practitioner practice rely on the national certifying bodies to test the competencies of nurse practitioners in their states. For example, Arkansas provides second licensure only for APNs who are nationally certified. In contrast there are states, such as New York, that do not require national certification as a condition to practice as a nurse practitioner. In New York, the state department of education certifies nurse practitioner programs. Graduates of accredited programs are deemed state certified upon completion of the approved program and after filing required documents specified in the state law.

National certification is attained by examination of qualified APNs by national professional organizations. These organizations seek to ensure national rather than state uniform competency in advanced practice. National professional organizations are authorized by the National Commission for Certifying Agencies (NCCA) to confer recognition of a standard of APN professional practice through certification. Competencies are tested through written examination. Generally speaking, national certifying organizations set their standard above the minimum essential level of practice necessary to ensure public safety (Fox-Grage, n.d.). A qualified applicant must have successfully completed an approved advanced practice program of study. National professional organizations determine the requirements for application for certification from their agency. For example, they might require education at the master's of nursing degree level in order to sit for their certifying examination.

To maintain certification, professionals often must meet certifying organizations' practice and continuing education requirements. For example, the American Academy of Nurse Practitioners requires "a minimum of 1000 hours of clinical practice in the area of specialization and 75 contact hours of continuing education relevant to the area of specialization" to be recertified every 5 years without examination (American Academy of Nurse Practitioners, n.d).

As the marketplace has become increasingly competitive, more employers have begun to require national certification as a condition of employment even when the statute in their state does not require it. This trend reflects the fact that institutions are setting higher standards of practice and the fact that changes in the reimbursement law require APNs to be nationally certified. Medicare requires that nurse practitioners and clinical nurse specialists be nationally certified to obtain a provider number for billing. Certified registered nurse anesthetists (CRNAs) and certified nurse midwives (CNMs) who bill Medicare are not required to have a master's degree in nursing or another field at this time.

Thus, confusion regarding certification revolves first around the differences in the APN state licensure and state certification language codified in state laws, and second in the difference between state and national certification. The credential granted to nurse practitioners for advanced practice under state statute as determined by the board of nursing or the boards of nursing and medicine jointly, and recorded in the nurse practice act of the particular state, can be either a second license or a certification. National certification is separate from state certification and is akin to board certification.

Table 15.1 identifies the names, addresses, and Web sites of national credentialing organizations. The decision to seek certification from a particular organization is often based on educational preparation and the professional recommendations.

Nurse Practitioner Title

Title protection is a condition whereby the law designates that no group or person can legally use a particular title or credential in any manner than that which has been defined. When state statute contains this type of language, it is called title protection. When the statute affords title protection for nurse practitioners, only individuals who meet the requirements for certification or licensure as nurse practitioners can call themselves a nurse practitioner.

In 49 states and the District of Columbia, the title nurse practitioner is protected (Pearson, 2002, p. 12). Tennessee is the only state where the title is not protected. In Tennessee, there is no provision within the nurse practice act for use of the title nurse practitioner. In that state, nurse practitioners function under a broad nurse practice act and are not afforded the nurse practitioner title (Pearson, 2002, p. 12).

Credentials

A topic closely related to title protection is that of the legally protected credential of the nurse practitioner. Confusion exists surrounding the correct professional designator to be used when signing documents. When signing prescriptions and other legal documents such as disability forms and chart entries, nurse practitioners should append their name with the legally protected credential cited in the law of the state in which they are licensed or certified to practice (Miller, 1999, p. 51). Credentials issued by national certifying bodies are not legal designators. Credentials issued by national certifying bodies can be supplemental to the legal designator, but they in no way replace the designation required by the state when signing professional legal documents. The legal designator does not need to be

TABLE 15.1   National Credentialing Organizations

Organization	Address and Telephone Number	Web Site	Credential Conferred
American Nurses Credentialing Center	600 Maryland Avenue, SW Suite 100 West Washington, DC 20024-2571 Phone: 800-284-2378	http://www.nursingworld.org/ancc/	Advanced Practice Registered Nurse, Board Certified (APRN, BC) The advanced practice nurse can use APRN or attach the BC (Board Certified) component to the designation required by the state in which he or she practices.
American Academy of Nurse Practitioners	American Academy of Nurse Practitioners Certification Program Capitol Station P.O. Box 12926 Austin, TX 78711 Phone: 512-442-5202	http://www.aanp.org E-mail: certification@aanp.org	Nurse Practitioner Certified (NP-C)
National Certification Board of Pediatric Nurse Practitioners	416 Hungerford Drive, Suite 222 Rockville, MD 20850-4127 Phone: 301-340-8213	http://www.pnpcert.org/	Certified Pediatric Nurse Practitioner (CPNP)

(continued)

TABLE 15.1   National Credentialing Organizations (continued)

Organization	Address and Telephone Number	Web Site	Credential Conferred
ACNM Certification Council, Inc. (ACC)	ACNM Certification Council, Inc. (ACC) 8201 Corporate Drive, Suite 550 Landover, MD 20785 Phone: 301-459-1321 Fax: 301-731-7825	http://www.accmidwife.org/ E-mail: info@ACCmidwife.org	Certified Nurse-Midwife (CNM)
National Certification Corporation (NCC)	National Certification Corporation (NCC) P.O. Box 11082 Chicago, IL 60611 Phone: 312-951-0207	http://www.nccnet.org/	Women's Health Care Nurse Practitioner (RNC); Neonatal Nurse Practitioner (RNC)
Council on Certification of Nurse Anesthetists	Council on Certification of Nurse Anesthetists 222 S. Prospect Avenue Park Ridge, IL 60068-5790 Phone: 847-692-7050 Certification contact—Linda Vitek Phone: 847-692-7050, ext. 3092 Fax: 847-692-7082	http://www.aana.com/ E-mail: certification@aana.com	CRNA

attached to documents that are not within the legal scope of practice, e.g. such as publications. In the case of publications, a nurse practitioner who is certified by the American Nurses Credentialing Center could append his or her name with the credential APRN, BC (advanced practice registered nurse, board certified; ANCC, n.d.).

Each national certifying organization confers its own credential upon individuals who meet criteria designated by that organization. In addition to the names and addresses of national credentialing organizations, Table 15.1 identifies the corresponding APN credential issued by each credentialing body.

To identify the legal title and credential needed in a particular state, consult the nurse practice act for that state. All nurse practice acts are available on the Internet at http://www.ncsbn.org.

PRESCRIPTIVE PRIVILEGES

Nurse practitioners have statutory or regulatory prescribing authority in all 50 states and the District of Columbia (Pearson, 2002, p. 15). In 13 jurisdictions (Alaska, Arizona, Iowa, Maine, Montana, New Hampshire, New Mexico, Oregon, Utah, Washington, Wisconsin, Wyoming, and the District of Columbia), nurse practitioners have plenary authority to prescribe medications, which means that they have independent authority to prescribe, distribute, and administer medications and medical devices (Pearson, 2002, p. 15). In those states, nurse practitioners are not required to have a formal relationship with a physician in order to prescribe medications. In all of the other states, the law requires nurse practitioners to have some type of formal arrangement with a physician in order to have prescriptive privileges—be it a collaborative or supervisory arrangement (Pearson, 2002, p. 15). In 6 states (Alabama, Florida, Kentucky, Missouri, Mississippi, and Texas) nurse practitioners can only prescribe legend drugs (all drugs other than controlled substances).

Prescribing Controlled Substances

If the state in which the APN will practice includes language in the statute or regulations that allows APNs to prescribe controlled substances, and the APN anticipates writing such prescriptions, she or he must register with the Drug Enforcement Administration (DEA) and obtain a DEA permit and number (DEA number). Forms are available on-line (at http://www.deadiversion.usdoj.gov/drugreg/reg notice.htm) in portable document format

(PDF). APNs can also request applications by calling the DEA in Washington, D.C. APNs must have an advanced practice state certification or license as required by their state to complete the application.

Nurse practitioners can prescribe some or all scheduled drugs in 44 states and the District of Columbia (Pearson, 2002, p. 15). State statutes and regulations vary regarding which schedules of controlled substances (schedules II–V) APNs can prescribe. Information about controlled substance authority by state can be found on the following Web site: http://www.deadiversion.usdoj.gov/drugreg/practitioners/index.html

COLLABORATIVE PRACTICE AGREEMENTS AND PROTOCOLS

Collaborative Practice Agreements

According to Pearson, 2002, 50% of state practice acts require nurse practitioners to enter into some type of collaborative or supervisory arrangement with a physician in order to practice. The nature and scope of this arrangement is outlined in a legal document called a collaborative practice or supervisory agreement. The requirements of the agreement are delineated in the state nurse practice act.

As an example, the New York State Nurse Practice Act requires that nurse practitioners have a collaborative agreement with a physician as a condition of practice. The agreement must include provisions for the following:

- Referral and consultation
- Coverage for emergency absences of the nurse practitioner or the collaborating physician
- Resolution of disagreements between the nurse practitioner and the collaborating physician regarding matters of diagnosis and treatment
- Time frame and process for review of patient records
- Practice protocols

Practice Protocols

In addition to practice agreements, many states require APNs to submit practice protocols to the state regulatory board as a condition of certification or licensure in the state. Practice protocols are "written guidelines used by the nurse practitioner which identify the area of practice to be performed by the nurse practitioner and reflect accepted standards of nursing and medical practice" (New York State Coalition of Nurse Practitioners,

1999, p. 3). State nurse practice acts define the requirements for practice protocols. Individual boards of nurse examiners sometimes reference standard published practice protocols as "approved protocols." In fact, boards of nurse examiners often require such references to be incorporated into written collaborative practice agreements.

When APNs select published standard protocols, they should be careful to select protocols that are flexible rather than prescriptive. Published protocols reflect generally accepted standards for the diagnosis and management of a disease process, but they sometimes lack strong supporting evidence. Published protocols are sometimes inconsistent with the most current evidence-based practice due to the continued explosion of new scientific information. Published protocols can become outdated quickly. Another potential problem with published practice protocols is that some were inadequately researched when formulated. Practice protocols should be flexible and allow for interpretation of the most current literature to afford the best possible delivery of patient care. Nevertheless, published protocols exist and are frequently employed or mandated.

REIMBURSEMENT FOR ADVANCED PRACTICE SERVICES

One of the greatest rewards of professional advanced practice is the accountability and responsibility of promoting and intervening in the health of others. In addition to clinical outcomes for patients, APNs' impact in an institution or to a group practice will also be measured by the revenue generated through their work.

Few Americans pay fully for and directly to their health care provider for services. More than 84% of Americans are covered by one or more health insurance plans, and thus one of the early decisions APNs make after graduation is whether to enroll in any of the payment plans to be reimbursed for their services (The Henry J. Kaiser Family Foundation Online, 2000). The answer to this question depends primarily on the conditions of the APN's employment: whether or not the APN is an independent contractor, an employee, or an employer; and the type of advanced practice in which the APN engages (e.g., nurse practitioner, midwife, or clinical specialist).

APNs must be aware of all payment and reimbursement issues that affect their work. This topic is complex and evolving, and thus this discussion is meant as an initial discourse. Several excellent printed resources and Web sites monitor these developments and should be consulted prior to entering into practice. (See chapter 22).

Medicaid

The Medicaid program, jointly funded by the federal and state governments, assists states in furnishing medical assistance to eligible needy persons. Medicaid is the largest source of funding for medical and health-related services for America's poorest people. In 2001, it provided health and long-term care to 44 million Americans (Center for Medicare and Medicaid Services, n.d.).

In 1989, the federal government established direct Medicaid reimbursement for pediatric nurse practitioners, family nurse practitioners, and certified nurse-midwives. Today 36 state Medicaid programs provide direct reimbursement to all advanced practice nurses. The amount of reimbursement varies from state to state, but in most cases it is 70–100% of physician reimbursement rates.

Under Medicaid legislation, each state (1) establishes its own eligibility standards; (2) determines the type, amount, duration, and scope of services covered; (3) sets the rate of payment for services; and (4) administers its own program. Medicaid policies for eligibility, services, and payment are complex and vary considerably among the states. Nurse practitioners, midwives, and clinical specialists should contact the state agencies responsible for provider enrollment information. State Medicaid program information is available through the following Web site http://statehealth-facts.kff.org (Click on the "Medicaid" link and then follow the Individual state profile tab.)

Medicare

Medicare was enacted in 1965 as one of President Lyndon B. Johnson's Great Society programs. It is a federally funded system of health and hospital insurance for U.S. citizens age 65 or older, for younger people receiving Social Security benefits, and for persons needing dialysis or kidney transplants for the treatment of end-stage renal disease. Medicare is composed of two programs: Part A, which covers inpatient and some other institutional services, skilled nursing facilities, home health care, and hospice; and Part B, which covers professional services.

The Balanced Budget Act of 1997, part of Public Law 105-33, granted direct Medicare reimbursement to advanced practice nurses regardless of geographic setting at 85% of the prevailing physician rate under Part B. Under the previous statute, nurse practitioner reimbursement was restricted to rural areas, long-term care facilities, and services provided incident to services of a physician. Effective January 1, 2001, qualified APNs with master's degrees* and national certifications are eligible for Medicare Part B reimbursement. Fiscal intermediaries, on behalf of the *Center for Medicare and Medicaid Services* (CMS), administer Medicare reimbursement. These intermediaries generally are commercial insurers who contract with CMS to manage the actual reimbursement process. Two types of contractors administer the Medicare program: for Part A, they are called intermediaries; for Part B, they are called carriers. (See chapter 22).

To enroll as a Part B provider in the Medicare program, the APN can visit the CMS site (http://www.hcfa.gov/medicare/enrollment/forms/) to obtain the provider enrollment form (CMS 8551) in PDF format. CMS plans to move to electronic enrollment, but at present the APN must submit the completed application to state or regional carriers to process the application as a new Medicare provider. Once the application has been accepted, the APN will be issued two numbers. A provider identification number (PIN) is used for billing and is issued by each carrier. A second number, a unique provider identification number (UPIN), differs from the carrier-assigned PIN and is reported on claims for referred or ordered services and/or diagnostic tests. The UPIN also enables CMS to collect and combine payment and utilization information for individual providers even when they have multiple practice settings or are members of a group practice. The primary use of this information is to perform statistical analysis and research studies of provider payments and utilization. Thus, it is important that APNs have such numbers to track APN services and contributions in Medicare claims databases.

Requirements for APNs as direct providers of Medicare include adhering to state nurse practice regulations, collaborating with a physician, and having national professional certification. The requirement for physician collaboration applies regardless of whether a state requires APNs to have medical direction, supervision, or collaboration. As direct Medicare providers, APNs are able to bill in all settings for all service codes that pertain to their state-regulated scope of practice, and they receive 85% of the prevailing physician rate for those services.

Prior to enactment of the Balanced Budget Act of 1997, nurse practitioners or certified nurse specialists (CNSs) who were employees of physicians or physician practices could receive reimbursement from Medicare under the Medicare law that covers services and supplies furnished incident to the professional services of a physician. This method of indirect reimbursement was not removed by the Act, and therefore this indirect method

---

* The master's degree in nursing requirement took effect January 1, 2003.

of reimbursement remains an option for APNs. Billing under "incident to" regulations is paid at 100% of the prevailing physician rate but is subject to very specific stipulations of practice.

When billing APN services as incident to a professional service rendered by a physician, APNs cannot bill for services provided to new patients (i.e., patients who are new to the practice or have not been seen by the practice in 3 years) and the physician must be present in the suite of practice at the time that the services are rendered (defined as direct supervision by CMS). Billing incident to physician services is applicable only in community practices and cannot be billed in hospital or hospital outpatient settings. APNs have the option to bill for services under their own provider or bill indirectly incident to physician services on a patient-by-patient basis. They do not have to adhere to one method of reimbursement solely. However, APNs and their employers are subject to strict adherence to the incident to guidelines and are at risk for fraud and abuse review.

A great deal of confusion regarding the language and interpretation of incident to billing exists (Buppert, 2001). The American Nurses Association (ANA) and other professional advanced practice nursing organizations continue to work closely with CMS and legislators regarding these issues. Nursing experts in policy and payment issues suggest that billing for APN services incident to physician services is fraught with risk and should be avoided. (See chapter 22 for more details on this issue.)

Another Medicare option for APNs who are employees of hospitals or hospital clinics is to have their services covered by bundling the cost into the facility charge to Medicare. If they decide on this option, they cannot also bill for their services directly as a Part B provider, but should ensure that their services are being captured by the hospital so that APN services can be valued appropriately.

National Provider Identifier

The Health Insurance Portability and Accountability Act of 1996 (HIPAA) requires the Secretary of Health and Human Services to adopt standards for a unique health identifier for each health care provider. Although not yet implemented, this National Provider Identifier (NPI) will replace PINs and UPINs. Once the change is implemented, all providers currently enrolled in the Medicare program will automatically receive their NPIs from the carrier or intermediary to which they submit claims. Providers who do not participate in Medicare but who participate in state Medicaid plans or other federal programs such as CHAMPUS will also most likely receive

NPIs automatically, but probably on a different schedule. To obtain current information about advances in Medicare legislation, the APN should visit the following Web sites for updates:

http://www.aanp.org/medicare.htm
http://www.nurse.org/acnp/medicare/index.shtml
http://www.nurse.net/medicare/index.shtml

Managed Care

Managed care is a broad term that describes a variety of payment structures and methods of delivering of health care. At the core of managed care plans are the agreements with providers to provide high-quality, cost-effective care. Nurse practitioners' roles and reimbursement in managed care plans vary.

Both the public and private health care sectors have seen an enormous proliferation of managed health care. Therefore, the manner in which these plans are negotiated, particularly in the private sector, has the potential to support or limit the work of advanced practice nurses. Many managed care plans (e.g., Oxford Health, https://www.oxhp.com) list nurse practitioners as providers. Conversely, many still categorically eliminate advanced practice providers as primary care practitioners or consider them "invisible" providers; that is, they are members of group plans or their services are billed under physician providers' numbers.

Consumer protection laws governing managed care organizations are emerging. Nurse practitioners must support these laws—particularly statues that support the consumer's right to freedom of choice of provider. APNs must also advocate for anti-discrimination language in regulatory statues that limit the scope of the nurse practitioner's practice in the health care insurance industry.

If APNs' practice in a setting that contracts with managed care plans, they should contact the local carrier and request information on becoming an approved provider. This is often more difficult than it sounds because some companies still do not recognize APNs. In some cases, it may be the first request the carrier has received, and the plan may be unprepared to handle the request. The APN should be prepared to make many phone calls and provide documentation and supportive information to process the application.

Indemnity Plans

Indemnity plans are also called fee-for service plans or commercial health insurance. Under indemnity plans, reimbursement for nurse practitioners is regulated at the state level.

SELECTING A PRACTICE

Nature of the Practice and Available Resources

Nurse practitioners provide health care services to individuals, families, and communities in a variety of settings. An APN is usually an employee of an organization, but an APN can also be an independent contractor to an organization or can be self-employed in his or her own corporation. Practice settings include tertiary care hospitals, hospital-based clinics, community clinics, industry, offices, private practices, and patients' homes. The patient population, the organization and its culture, and the resources available in the system influence the nature of the work.

Prospective employees should consider their likes and dislikes when selecting a practice setting. They should consider the populations that they will serve and the resources that will be available to them. Consider the following questions:

1. What are the health problems of the individuals and families in the community where I will work?
2. What resources are available in the community to support individuals with their health-related problems?
3. Does the practice employ colleagues who are capable and willing to access those community resources?
4. Will more seasoned professionals mentor the new nurse practitioner?
5. Do the administrators and support staff in the practice understand and support the role of the APN?

Employment Contracts

The APN should consider whether the prospective employer offers an explicit employment contract (either through a professional union contract or an individual employment contract), or if there is only an implicit contractual arrangement regulated by customary human resource and labor relations standards. APNs should remember that all work relationships are contractual; that is, the individual provides specified services for explicit remuneration and benefits. APNs should review their employment agreements. Table 15.2 delineates components of employment agreements.

CLOSING REMARKS

Initiating your first advanced practice position is a challenge and a journey of continued professional and personal development. Seek the advice

TABLE 15.2   Components of Employment Agreements

(a) Work hours–regular work week, on-call requirements, 24-hour responsibility

(b) Salary—Base, increases, incentives/bonus

(c) Benefits—
   • Malpractice insurance
   • Health insurance
   • Retirement plan
   • Disability—Short and long term
   • Paid time off—Vacation, holidays, personal time, emergency time off
   • Allowances for continuing education (time and compensation)
   • Flexible spending account for professional fees, professional publications/journals, pager, cell phone, etc.

(d) Terms and conditions for terminating the contractual agreement

of expert clinicians and partner with them. Join professional organizations and learn through your involvement with others. Network for the future, and seek mentorship. Remember your mission, and outline objectives, actions, and outcomes to measure your perpetual development and success.

Nurses participate in the lives of individuals, families, and communities at times when they are vulnerable or simply developing. APNs' opportunities are vast, and the degree to which they can assist others and themselves in the process of becoming is nearly limitless because they see both through their own eyes and those of the people they assist each day.

REFERENCES

American Academy of Nurse Practitioners. (n.d.). *Certification examination.* Retrieved March 14, 2002, from http://www.aanp.org/

American Nurses Credentialing Center. (n.d.) *Levels of credentialing.* Retrieved March 14, 2002, from http://www.nursingworld.org/ancc/certify/cert/cof-cred.htm

Buppert, C. (2001). Avoiding Medicare fraud, Part 2. *Nurse Practitioner, 26*(2), 34–41.

Center for Medicare and Medicaid Services. (n.d.). *Medicaid.* Retrieved March 14, 2002, From http://hcfa.gov/medicaid/medicaid.htm

Fox-Grage, W. (n.d.) *Nursing regulation: Nursing licensure & certification: APRN: States Study scope of practice & reimbursement.* Retrieved March 14, 2002, from http://www.ncsbn.org/public/regulation/licensure_aprn_statestudy.htm

The Henry J. Kaiser Family Foundation Online. (2000). *Current population surveys: State health facts online.* Retrieved March 14, 2002, from http://statehealth-facts.kff.org

Miller, S. K. (1999). Professional practice. Signatures. *Patient Care for the Nurse Practitioner, 2*(10), 51.

National Commission on Nurse Anesthesia Education. (1990). *The report of the commission on nurse anesthesia education.* Washington, DC: American Association of Nurse Anesthetists.

National Council of State Boards of Nursing, Inc. (2001). Nursing regulation: Licensure & certifications. Retrieved March 14, 2002, from http://www.ncsbn.org/public/regulation/licensure.htm

New York State Coalition of Nurse Practitioners. (1999, August 7) *Letter to members.*

Pearson, L. J. (2002). Fourteenth annual legislative update. *Nurse Practitioner, 27*(1), 10–52.

Ryser, F. G. (1999). Nursing issues. Prescriptive authority: A dilemma facing advanced practice nurses. *Journal of the American Academy of Nurse Practitioners, 11,* 349–353.

MARGINALIZED PATIENTS, FAMILY NURSE PRACTITIONERS, AND NURSE-MANAGED HEALTH CENTERS: CARING FOR RESIDENTS IN PUBLIC-HOUSING-BASED NURSING CENTERS

Susan M. Beidler and Donna Torrisi

Meeting the needs of the uninsured and underinsured is one of the greatest challenges of the U.S. health care delivery system. The challenge reflects the constellation of issues related to insurance eligibility, as well as the lack of consensus regarding whether or not health care is a basic right. The prevailing national perspective is that insurance should be linked either to employment or to eligibility for publicly funded programs. This approach to providing health insurance has been the subject of ongoing, lengthy debate. Meanwhile, an increasing number of individuals and families are without health insurance, and subsequently without accessible and affordable health care. It is well recognized that individuals living in and around public housing developments are among this population.

Residents of public housing developments meet federal poverty guidelines and have several other characteristics that compound their vulnerability. Rogers (1997) identified several factors or determinants of vulnerability. Income has been identified as a major determinant of vulnerability. People who are poor or economically disadvantaged have higher rates of morbidity and mortality (Aday, 1994; Flaskerud, 1998; Flaskerud & Winslow, 1998; Minkler, 1999; Rachlis & Kushner, 1989; Rogers, 1997). Aday (1993) found that low income rates correlate with increased rates of abuse, higher crime rates, increased drug use, and higher rates of teen pregnancy. Decreased functional and mental status, decreased ability to work, and a diminished quality of life have also been associated with low income.

Age has also been identified as a determinant of vulnerability, as is the case with children and the elderly. Children are particularly vulnerable because of their inability to speak for their own needs, and adolescents because of their risk-taking behaviors. The elderly are viewed as vulnerable because of their decrease in physical ability and because they have fewer financial and social supports. Women and children typically constitute the largest percentage of residents in public housing developments. In addition, it is not uncommon to find several generations of individuals and families sharing a residence.

Gender has been found to be a factor, insofar as women tend to be exposed to more stress as a result of their caregiving roles (Aday, 1993; Gitterman, 1991; Rachlis & Kushner, 1989). In most countries, women tend to earn less money than men, which further increases their vulnerability. Childrearing responsibilities and the lack of accessible and affordable day care opportunities frequently preclude female public housing residents from being gainfully employed.

Race and ethnicity are known factors in vulnerability. Blacks and Hispanics, as well as Native Americans, have the highest rates for morbidity and mortality due to diabetes and hypertension (Aday, 1993). In a study by the Commonwealth Foundation, adult minorities were found to be more likely than their White counterparts to be uninsured (Lewin & Altman, 2000). Most of the uninsured were impoverished as well.

PUBLIC-HOUSING RESIDENTS: A PORTRAIT OF THE PEOPLE IN TWO COMMUNITIES

The two communities in Philadelphia referred to in this discussion consist of approximately 4,000 individuals: 60% female, 60% children, 90% African American, and 90% living at or below the poverty level. Thirty percent of the residents are uninsured, while another 60% have medical assistance and the remainder have Medicare or commercial insurance. Though the percentage of elderly is less than 4%, adults age 50 and older resemble the elderly in terms of their health status. It is common for 50-year-old people in these communities to have three or more chronic illnesses. The most common are diabetes (12%), hypertension (18%), hyperlipidemia (10%), and obesity. Nine percent of the population has asthma. Additionally, 20% of adults report having a substance abuse problem, and 21% have a psychiatric disorder such as major depression, bipolar disorder, schizophrenia, or post-traumatic stress disorder. Almost all women over the age of 50 report having been abused by a male partner in their life.

THE MARGINALIZATION OF VULNERABLE POPULATIONS

Closely related to vulnerability is the concept of marginalization. Individuals who are vulnerable have a sense of not belonging. This leads to social isolation and alienation. Furthermore, the low educational level and lack of income that are associated with some vulnerable individuals may lead to ignorance of their rights and result in decreased ability to access resources.

The various factors or determinants of vulnerability are frequently the characteristics that identify those who are not in the mainstream and thus at the margins of society. Marginalization is thus defined as "the process through which persons are peripheralized on the basis of their identities, association, experience, and environments" (Hall, Stevens, & Meleis, 1994, p. 25).

Another property of marginalization is differentiation. There is a potential for stigmatization of those who differ from those in the mainstream. The process of differentiation includes the assigning of negative values to the individuals at the periphery of society. People are frequently differentiated and peripheralized based on visible identifiers such as age, gender, ethnicity, skin color, and in many cases economic and social status.

The appropriateness of public housing developments is open to debate. While it is certainly easier to identify areas of need for public support, residents of these neighborhoods tend to experience further marginalization. Members of mainstream society and even some health care professionals identify residents of these developments not by their street address, but by a derogatory reference—"they're from the 'project.'" While a discussion of the differential health care services that residents of housing developments typically receive is beyond the scope of this chapter, more accessible and culturally competent health care services are necessary to address the disparities that continue to exist.

NURSE-MANAGED CENTERS AND FAMILY NURSE PRACTITIONERS

In July 1992, the Abbottsford Community Health Center (CHC) opened. Initial funding was provided by a federal grant established to improve the health of residents of public housing. For one innovative organization, Resources for Human Development, and a family nurse practitioner, Donna Torrisi, the funding of this initiative allowed a dream to become a reality. While several other public housing-based health centers were established at this time, Abbottsford CHC was the first that was nurse managed and had a nurse practitioner director rather than a medical director.

Abbottsford CHC achieved provider status with several Medicaid managed care organizations (MCOs). However, approximately 2 years into operation, the MCOs were made aware that state health maintenance organization (HMO) regulations required that only physicians be designated as primary care providers (PCPs) in the Commonwealth of Pennsylvania. Donna Torrisi and several other nurse practitioner leaders, legislators, and MCO administrators were able to negotiate with the Pennsylvania Department of Health, Bureau of Healthcare Financing, to have an exception written for this regulation. Each HMO for each nurse-managed health center with which it wanted to contract must request this exception. Eventually, a sister nursing center, Schuylkill Falls Community Health Center, was established at a neighboring public housing development. Both centers eventually established contracts with local Medicaid HMOs through the Community Health Network, a corporation of all of the federally qualified health centers (FQHCs) in Philadelphia. Joint contracting increased the power base from which all of the affiliated health centers could negotiate contracts. Approximately 60% of health center patients are enrolled in Medicaid managed care plans. Both of these public housing-based health centers negotiate a primary care-only rate. Hospital care is contracted with primary care services at local hospitals. Despite this separation of services, HMO utilization reports include total cost per member, which includes specialty care. Repeatedly, the patient panel cost for the nurse-managed centers was lower than the comparison family practice aggregate provider groups. Satisfaction reports from patients to the HMOs were very high, and chart audits by HMO reviewers were excellent.

Nurse practitioners are well positioned to care for marginalized populations. Their theoretical foundation in nursing focuses on individuals and their interactions within society and the environment. The nursing discipline focuses on the maintenance of health and on responses to illness and disease. A strong ethical foundation for the discipline also supports nursing practice with marginalized groups. According to the *Code of Ethics for Nurses* (ANA, 2001), "the nurse, in all professional relationships, practices with compassion and respect for the inherent dignity, worth and uniqueness of every individual unrestricted by consideration of social or economic status, personal attributes or the nature of health problems" (p. 7). Furthermore, the *Scope and Standards of Advanced Practice Nursing* (ANA, 1996) states, "the advanced practice registered nurse employs complex strategies, interventions, and teaching to promote, maintain and improve health and prevent illness and injury" (p. 13).

The Abbottsford Community Health Center (renamed Abbottsford Family Practice & Counseling [AFP&C]) is located within the Abbottsford Homes Public Housing development. Approximately 3,000 individuals resided in the Abbottsford Community in 1992 when the health center opened. The exact number since then is unknown, since it has been determined that a number of "hidden homeless" reside in public housing developments but are not recorded on the lease.

FAMILY NURSE PRACTITIONERS AT ABBOTTSFORD FAMILY PRACTICE AND COUNSELING (AFP&C)

Family nurse practitioners (FNPs) at AFP&C are the primary care providers for approximately 2,000 individuals who reside in or around the health center. For those individuals who have either Medicaid or Medicare, direct third-party payment for services is possible. Individuals who are uninsured are expected to pay for their services according to a sliding fee schedule. However, no one is denied services based on an inability to pay.

The FNPs have a collaborative practice agreement with local physicians. These physicians are available to provide consultation on difficult cases, and they also facilitate the FNPs' prescriptive privileges by serving as their collaborators. Family nurse practitioners practice according to generally accepted practice guidelines that are incorporated into standing protocols.

Family nurse practitioners at these nurse-managed public housing-based health centers need to be culturally sensitive and very flexible. Despite every effort to maintain a schedule for patient visits, no-shows and emergency visits are commonplace. The FNP needs to be skilled in providing a wide range of primary care services. These services include, but are not limited to, prenatal, well-child, and women's health care, including family planning services, pregnancy option counseling, and treatment of sexually transmitted diseases (STDs). Adult medical care, especially management of chronic disease processes such as diabetes and hypertension, is another service provided. Preventive health services are an integral part of the care provided. Both nursing centers integrate behavioral health services into primary care with depression and abuse screening protocols, as well as on-site mental health and drug and alcohol counseling. Mental health services are crucial to the community, and in the past 2 years the size of this department tripled. Two psychiatrists as well as psychologists and social workers and a dedicated outreach worker staff this program that serves adults, adolescents, and children. A variety of support groups are held at the centers: teen support groups, parenting and grandparenting groups, and Peaceful Posse—a group teaching nonviolence for youth. Women, Infants and Children (WIC) health visits and assistance to complete applications for medical assistance and disability are provided. The centers provide free van transportation for health center patients to attend specialist or other health, dental, or social service appointments.

Access to the FNPs is provided through an after-hours on-call system in which all of the nurse practitioners participate on a rotating basis. Due to the proximity of the nursing centers to many of the patients' residences, the FNPs make home visits and coordinate care with other community resources.

Family nurse practitioners average 16 patient visits in an 8-hour session. Most visits last longer than traditional medical office visits because of the time spent listening to patients' complaints and concerns, which frequently involve complex physical, social, and behavioral issues. The FNPs also provide individualized patient teaching, which can be time-consuming as well. When compared to patients of physician groups in the same area, the nursing center patients are seen more frequently and for longer visits.

A HYPOTHETICAL DAY AT THE CENTERS: CHALLENGES AND SUCCESSES

The first patient of a typical day might be a woman described as a grandmother of two school-aged children who came to the center to have the children's immunizations updated. The "grandmother" may very well bear no biologic relationship with the children, but may have assumed custody of them when their mother was incarcerated. The grandmother, also a patient of the center, may have missed several appointments. Although she has hypertension and diabetes and is morbidly overweight, she refuses to schedule another appointment for herself. The FNP attempts to discuss the importance of caring for self as well as caring for children, but the grandmother will have no part of the discussion. The children are examined and immunizations brought up to date. Both children are in need of dental care, but the grandmother states that she is unable to afford the cost of a cab to get the children to the dentist. The van is scheduled to take the grandmother and the two children to their dental appointments; however, there is a two-month wait for the first available appointment.

The next patient might be a young, unwed mother who arrives at the health center without an appointment. She is complaining of a vaginal discharge and itching. Her most recent partner has denied any other sexual partners within the last 4 months, so the patient explains that they have decided not to use condoms. The FNP examines the patient and obtains cultures and specimens to determine the source of the patient's presumed infection. She spends a considerable amount of time with the patient performing contraception and STD counseling and offers confidential HIV testing. The patient refuses and states, "What will be, will be." The FNP reiterates the importance of using condoms and discusses the importance of self-value and self-protection, especially since the patient has three preschool aged children who depend on her in the absence of their fathers.

Another patient walks into the clinic for a blood pressure (BP) check. He is unable to schedule an appointment because he runs his own private taxi service and needs to work whenever someone calls for a ride. At this visit, his BP is extremely elevated, but he refuses to take any medications because he is afraid of the potential side effect of erectile dysfunction, a problem experienced by one of his friends who was treated for high BP. The FNP provides education on the various classes of medications for hypertension and includes an in-depth explanation about side effects. The FNP points out the large number of medications that do not lead to erectile dysfunction. The patient agrees to take a BP medication, but leaves the office without the pharmaceutical samples he was given. The FNP suspects that he had no intent of taking the medication and that he determined that the only way to shorten the visit was to agree to take a medication.

Next is a scheduled patient who returns for a follow-up visit for her polycythemia vera. She needs regular phlebotomies to address this condition. She is overdue for an appointment because she spent the last few months with a relative in Georgia. A brief physical assessment is performed and a complete blood count (CBC) obtained. The patient admits to increasing shortness of breath lately and realizes that she needed to keep this appointment and follows through with her visit to the local hospital.

Factors related to marginality and vulnerability earlier in this chapter are in play for the previous scenarios and represent the types of challenges faced by the FNPs on a daily basis. Many other patient encounters end on a positive note and are reflected in the following actual patient scenarios.

A 26-year-old mother of two was 7 months pregnant, using crack, and had not received any prenatal care yet. An outreach worker, herself in drug recovery, informed the FNP who asked her to "get the patient to me first thing in the morning and we will take care of her together." The mother reported that her two children were born with low birth-weight. She agreed to be examined and to enter into a drug rehabilitation program. The FNP treated the woman for urinary tract and vaginal infections, while the outreach worker spent several hours on the phone locating an appropriate treatment facility. The woman was transported to the program by the health center van, and 2 months later she delivered her first normal birth-weight baby.

In another situation, a 26-year-old mother of three wept as she told her story of struggling with asthma since childhood and of countless nights barely able to breathe and feeling terrified that she would die. She could barely speak through her tears as she spoke of the compassionate care she was receiving from her nursing center nurse practitioner. Her FNP provider had explained to her how to use the inhalers she had been using incorrectly for more than 10 years, and for the first time in her life she felt in charge of her illness.

Another 52-year-old nursing center patient had presented with headaches, backache, and stomachaches approximately 1 year ago. She described how at that time, "my nurse asked me if I was depressed, and I broke down and cried." She added, "I didn't realize how depressed I was since I was feeling that way for so long that I thought it was normal. I just felt violent like I wanted to hurt someone and so hopeless." She then explained how the nurse practitioner took time to talk to her, help her understand her feelings, and see that she was not crazy but suffering from major depression. After treatment, she now feels great, is able to sleep, and has the energy to baby-sit her grandchildren.

Nurse practitioners at the nursing centers routinely screen patients for depression. They have been trained to perform evaluations, differentiate depression from other more complex mood disorders, and treat patients for major depression. Since FNPs began screening routinely more than 2 years ago, over 160 new patients were diagnosed and treated for depression. Seventy percent have had improvement in their symptoms.

Throughout the day, FNPs also take phone calls from patients and family members. For example, in addition to seeing patients like those described in the above scenarios, the nurse practitioner may also need to complete the necessary paperwork to have an elderly patient evaluated by the area office of aging (AOA) for the purpose of being enrolled in a nursing-home waiver program. The program will provide intensive home-based services in an effort to keep the patient out of a skilled nursing facility and in his or her home. In the midst of seeing patients, the FNP may receive a phone call from a family member wanting to discuss the purpose of the waiver program. Because many of the housing center patients do not have regular access to telephones, it may be important to make every effort to speak with patients and family members when they call.

These hypothetical patient scenarios are reflective of actual patient encounters at the nursing centers. The traditional health care delivery system is ill equipped to meet the complex biopsychosocial needs of marginalized patients in the primary care setting. Nurse practitioners and nursing centers are a logical, albeit not complete, solution to the problems elucidated in the case scenarios discussed. Unfortunately, payment mechanisms for the types of comprehensive services provided in these centers are inadequate to meet the overall cost of this type of care.

This model of care has been duplicated, and information management systems are being developed to obtain a larger sampling of the types of interventions provided and outcomes obtained in nursing centers such as these. It is hoped that these efforts will result in more appropriate settings for delivery of primary health care, which will, in turn, reduce the health disparities of marginalized populations in this century.

SAFETY NET PROVIDERS:
THE KEY TO SUSTAINABLE FUNDING

One of the greatest challenges faced by nurse practitioners and nursing centers is maintaining sustainable funding. The federal government continues to identify mechanisms to support these much-needed safety net providers. A well-established mechanism for funding is through designation as a federally qualified health center (FQHC). As was discussed previously, AFP&C received a grant from the Bureau of Primary Health Care (BPHC), Division of Health Resource Service Administration (HRSA) in 1991. This was the inaugural year for this new funding stream, which was specific to residents of public housing. As a grantee of the BPHC, Abbottsford, with Schuylkill Falls following, was designated an FQHC and assumed both the obligations and entitlements associated with this designation.

As FQHCs, the centers are obligated to (1) provide primary care through the entire life cycle, (2) provide care to all patients without regard to ability to pay, (3) provide medications and lab work, and (4) provide behavioral health services, radiology, prenatal care, dental care, and medication either directly or by contact.

The most substantial benefit of the FQHC designation entitles the center to obtain cost-based reimbursement (now called the prospective payment system) for all visits on medical assistance or Medicare patients. For example, if the cost incurred by the center for a patient visit is $100 and the managed care reimbursement is $10 per member per month, the difference is made up in a quarterly reconciliation payment by the State Department of Welfare. The renewable federal grant and the cost-based reimbursement enable the centers to be sustainable. It is therefore incumbent upon nurse-managed health centers that serve the underserved and intend to be "safety net" providers to create a plan from the beginning that will enable them to obtain FQHC status.

Other entitlements for FQHCs allow them to obtain liability/malpractice coverage free of charge for all health center staff under a federal program called the Federal Tort Claim Act. The health centers also may purchase medications from a federal discount warehouse. These medications are used to treat uninsured and underinsured patients.

There are several paths to becoming a FQHC. They include becoming a grantee of the BPHC, applying to become a "look-alike" center, or affiliation with an existing FQHC. It is beyond the scope of this chapter to discuss these routes in detail.

Abbottsford has successfully expanded twice and created two additional FQHC sites. The first was funded by an expansion grant that created the Schuylkill Falls Community Health Center in its public housing community in 1994. The second expansion occurred in 2002 and was born out of a linkage with an academic school of nursing. This site, the largest of the nursing centers in physical space, is The 11th Street Family Health Services of Drexel University. The umbrella name for all three sites is the Family Practice and Counseling Network. The centers are currently in discussion with another academic institution that wishes to relinquish ownership of their nurse-managed center and turn it over to the Family Practice and Counseling Network.

It is an exciting time in the evolution of nurse-managed health centers. These centers, numbering at least 100 nationwide, are primarily operated out of academic institutions and serve low-income and vulnerable people. The National Nursing Centers Consortium (NNCC), of which the Abbottsford director was a founding member, is located in Philadelphia and is a member organization for nurse-managed health centers. The purpose of the NNCC is to support nurse-managed health centers in their capacity to be safety net providers, educate policy makers to remove barriers to independent nurse practitioner practice, and support the centers to become FQHCs. This fledgling organization, under the phenomenal leadership of Executive Director Tine Hansen-Turton, has grown from a local organization supporting nurse-managed health centers in three states to a national organization representing more than 30 nursing centers. Its efforts and accomplishments in supporting nurse-managed health centers is a major factor in the success of centers nationwide as they expand their capacity to care for vulnerable people. The national climate is favorable for nurse-managed centers to proliferate and become FQHCs as a result of President Bush calling for 1,200 new community health center sites over the next 5 years, with a goal of doubling the number of patients served. The NNCC is pushing to have 100 of the new sites designated as nurse-managed centers by the end of this period.

CONCLUSIONS

Nurse-managed health centers and nurse practitioners are well positioned through their philosophical underpinnings and pragmatic functions to provide the type of comprehensive health care services that are needed by marginalized populations in our country. Positive outcomes of care are accumulating. As more of these centers and providers obtain the funding necessary to support their activities, the possibility of decreasing health disparities in our nation exists. To ignore this national resource and move forward with existing, inadequate models of medical care is to accept the status quo.

REFERENCES

Aday, L. A. (1993). *At risk in America: The health and health care needs of vulnerable populations in the United States.* San Francisco: Jossey-Bass.

Aday, L. A. (1994). Health status of vulnerable populations. *Annual Review of Public Health, 15,* 487–509.

American Nurses Association. (1996). *Scope and standards of advanced practice nursing.* Washington, DC: American Nurses Publishing.

American Nurses Association. (2001). *Code of ethics for nurses with interpretive statements.* Washington, DC: American Nurses Publishing.

Flaskerud, J. H. (1998). Vulnerable populations. In J. J. Fitzpatrick (Ed.), *Encyclopedia of nursing research* (pp. 591–592). New York: Springer Publishing.

Flaskerud, J. H., & Winslow, B. J. (1998). Conceptualizing vulnerable populations' health-related research. *Nursing Research, 47*(2), 69–78.

Gitterman, A. (1991). *Handbook of social work practice with vulnerable populations.* New York: Columbia University Press.

Lewin, M. E., & Altman, S. (Eds.). (2000). *America's health care safety net: Intact but endangered.* Washington, DC: National Academy Press.

Minkler, M. (1999, July/August). Poverty kills. *Park Ridge Center Bulletin, 10,* 3–4.

Rachlis, M., & Kushner, C. (1989). *Second opinion: What's wrong with Canada's health care system and how to fix it.* Toronto: HarperCollins.

Rogers, A. C. (1997). Vulnerability, health and health care. *Journal of Advanced Nursing, 26*(1), 65–72.

Chapter **17**

PRIMARY CARE IN THE HOME: THE NURSE PRACTITIONERS' ROLE

JoAnn Hunt Stracuzzi and Lynn T. Rinke

V NA House Calls, a primary care practice for homebound adults, serves over 500 patients in Philadelphia and the surrounding communities. For more than 3 years, this practice has provided care for patients who are no longer able to get to their primary care provider. While most of the patients are elderly, about 20% of the patient population are younger adults with either traumatic injuries or degenerative disorders. Patients are provided with comprehensive primary care by physicians and nurse practitioners using a collaborative practice model. For this underserved population, VNA House Calls has brought health care back to the home.

HOME CARE OVERVIEW

For the last 35 years, the realm of home care has been dominated by the nursing profession. Visiting nurses have been the eyes and ears of the medical community in the home setting, providing valuable insights into patient care. Once patients are discharged from the hospital or sent home after an office visit, physicians have relied on the finely tuned assessment skills of the visiting nurse to help them better understand patients' needs. These nurses understand that patients are affected by their environment—social, cognitive, and physical. Unfortunately, most of these components go unrecognized or ignored in the acute care or office setting. Medicine today barely has the time to examine each patient. There is no time to consider what is going on in the home when each patient is allotted so few minutes. Many questions often go unasked because no one has the time or inclination to go looking for problems. Any nurse with home care experience can attest to the frustration of trying to convey patients' home situations to their physicians. It seems that the components of environment, social needs, and cognition are somehow considered "fluff," and only vital signs and medical findings are of interest to doctors. For millions of patients in the United States, the home care or visiting nurse is the only health care professional who has the opportunity to see the whole patient. So how does the role of the advanced practice nurse work to complement what is already being accomplished in the home care setting by the visiting nurse?

WHAT HAPPENED TO THE HOUSE CALL?

One of home care nursing's major frustrations is the difficulty of getting physicians to participate in the plan of care. The homebound elderly constitute the majority of patients in a visiting nurse's caseload. This population can easily be considered medically underserved because they have little access to primary care. While most of these patients report that they have a doctor, many have not been able to get to the office in months for different reasons. These patients use emergency departments of their local hospital for their medical care. Their emergent or urgent problems get addressed, and then the patient is quickly returned to the home because they refuse any long-term care that may be offered to them.

Often these patients are referred to a visiting nurse who has to scramble to find a doctor who is willing to sign the home care orders. This is true especially when the referral comes from the acute-care setting. Patients are left in a state of limbo because the discharging hospital physician will sign only the initial orders and family doctors do not want the responsibility of signing orders when they have not seen the patient in months, or sometimes years. Many of these patients cannot get to the office because they have physical problems that limit their ability to leave the home or to get into their doctor's office. Ambulance transportation is available but is not a covered expense under Medicare guidelines. Only transportation to the emergency department is covered, and therefore many homebound patients go to emergency departments to get care.

In Philadelphia, an urban area of almost 5 million people, there are only a handful of physicians who will make home visits. Many of those who do make home visits do so only in emergency situations. Finding anyone willing to provide primary care at home is almost impossible. It was not until 1998 that the American Academy of Home Care Physicians saw the success of a 4-year effort to improve reimbursement rules recognized by Medicare. Before that (since 1965), the Medicare home health benefit basically excluded physician home visiting services. Some nurse practitioners in rural settings were able to bill Medicare, but the population guidelines for what constituted rural settings were quite stringent. Still other nurse practitioners made home visits for home health agencies without reimbursement (Sullivan, 1992). The Visiting Nurse Association of Greater Philadelphia had been using psychiatric clinical nurse specialists in this way. But with the new reimbursement rules, it became feasible for physicians and nurse practitioners to once again make home visits (Boling, 1998). The problem, however, is that most physicians had found other ways to practice.

The Balanced Budget Act of 1997 granted direct reimbursement to advanced practice nurses for Medicare Part B services. Prior to 1998, nurse practitioners had only been able to be reimbursed in rural areas. The law now permits nurse practitioners to be reimbursed by Medicare for home visits at 85% of the physician rate. Thus, in Philadelphia the stage was set for a new model of primary care practice to emerge, one that understood there was a need for care of the homebound medically underserved patient. There was a means: reimbursement by Medicare Part B. New current procedures terminology codes for home visits were revised and valued higher by Medicare in 1995 through the work of the American Academy of Home Care Physicians, the American Nurses Association, and the American Academy of Family Practice. Finally, advanced practice nurses were poised to provide the kind of care that the medically frail and fragile needed. Nurse practitioners, in collaboration with physicians, were able to provide the primary care that the homebound patient was not receiving.

VNA OF GREATER PHILADELPHIA: A MODEL FOR PRACTICE

In August 1998, the Visiting Nurse Association (VNA) of Greater Philadelphia established one of the nation's first (and the first in a home health agency) collaborative teams of advanced practice nurses and physicians for the express purpose of visiting patients in their homes to provide primary care.

At VNA of Greater Philadelphia, our primary care model is patient driven, comprehensive, and collaborative. At the center are the patent and the primary care provider. Together, in the safety and comfort of the patient's home, the patient, the primary care provider, and often family members work together to understand, diagnose, and then treat the patient's health problem.

The health care services provided are comprehensive in nature. Each new patient receives a 1- to 2-hour visit by a nurse practitioner, who performs a thorough history and physical. In addition to evaluating the patient's psychosocial and medical history, the nurse practitioner can evaluate the patient's environment. A home environment evaluation has long been a valued tool of the visiting nurse. Knowledge about the patient's environment often makes a difference between a noncompliant patient and a successful treatment plan. The nurse practitioner can combine medical knowledge and skills with on-site knowledge of the patient's living situation. As Barbara Bates, MD, who revolutionized nursing with her text on physical assessment, said to nurses many years ago:

> By expanding your knowledge and skills into medicine, and thereby acquiring some of that control, you can in fact expand into nursing. In so doing, you will be bringing the patient the guidance, care, help, understanding, and comfort that he has needed all along and perhaps not received from the physician. . . . By virtue of your having learned more medicine and enhanced your ability to move into a more medical role, the patient may get less medicine. . . . Less medicine, when mixed with more nursing, is probably better medicine (or to translate, better health care). . . . By expanding into medicine, you will need—more than ever before—to increase your consciousness of what nursing is all about. The values of nursing must not get lost in the dominant medical culture. If [they] do, you justly risk the epithet of junior doctor. Our patients do not need junior doctors. They need the knowledge and skills of both medicine and nursing (Bates, 1974, p. 686).

Combining the knowledge and skills of medicine and nursing with the chance to see patients in their own home exponentially enhances diagnostic capabilities. Any health care provider who frequents patients' homes will acknowledge this unconditionally.

Collaborative Practice

Collaboration is the synergistic ingredient in this model. The collaboration between physician and nurse practitioner is only the beginning: collaboration occurs among the primary care provider, the patient, the family, neighbors, the visiting nurse, and other health and social work professionals and paraprofessionals. A strong relationship develops between the visiting nurse and the nurse practitioner because of the complex needs of each patient. In that relationship, one can see the value that each role brings to providing care to this difficult population.

It is usually the expert level visiting nurse who most appreciates the collaborative relationship in which professionals share knowledge and develop strategies to solve problems. These nurses are quick to pinpoint exactly what dynamics in the home are contributing to the success or failure of the plan of care. They also appreciate that the nurse practitioner is an easily accessible resource. The visiting nurses often identify problems that develop and pass along the information to the nurse practitioner who can determine the next step in diagnosing or treating the problem. Nurses have commented that they love working with the nurse practitioners: "I don't know if the nurse practitioners have more time, but they always seem to take more time than the doctors to listen to me. When I talk to a doctor, I always rehearse my speech before I call so I can pack as much information into the three minutes that I have his ear. It is so different with the nurse practitioner. I feel like I can take my time and get through the concerns that I have about the patients." "The nurse practitioners give me their pager numbers and always call back immediately. This is so helpful because we can usually solve problems while I am sitting in the home." Other nurses report that they realize that the nurse practitioner has assessment skills and a knowledge base that is more comprehensive than theirs, especially when it comes to medications: "I always know that I am going to learn something when I am talking to the nurse practitioners. They share what they know in order to help me learn. They want everyone to come along in the learning process so that everyone benefits. If they do not know something, they are quick to get back to me with the information."

The advanced practice nurse in this relationship has the responsibility of creating an atmosphere in which mutual respect can be fostered so that there is a free exchange of information and ideas. Most advanced practice nurses will admit readily that they can clearly remember when they were in the visiting nurse role trying to get information to and from the physician. Those memories translate into a commitment to a true collaboration.

Day-to-Day Operations

Patient Perspectives

Most referrals come from word of mouth through family, friends, and neighbors. Since the inception of the program, we have had a consistent waiting list. Generally, patients on the waiting list have not been seen by a physician for months or even years, and thus waiting for 1 to 2 weeks for a home visit is not usually an inconvenience. Recently, we have committed to see each new patient within 1 week and we will make room in our schedule to see the patient even sooner if the referral source feels that the patient needs more urgent care.

The initial visit is made by the nurse practitioner. In addition to the usual paperwork (consents, insurance information), a thorough history and physical (H&P) is done. Much time is spent determining what medications have been prescribed in the past and what medications the patient is actually taking. Medicine bottles are examined to see when the scripts were last filled, and if noncompliance is suspected, pill counts are done with permission. In addition, the patient is asked about use of vitamins and herbal supplements. Throughout the H&P, the nurse practitioner assesses, evaluates, and teaches the patient and caregiver. Patients unanimously confirm that the nurse practitioner's visit is the longest any primary care provider has ever spent with the patient. The nurse practitioner also performs a short mental state examination, often conducts an electrocardiogram and a pulse oximetry test, and performs other tests as indicated. In addition, a nutritional assessment and depression screen are completed. Following the H&P, and depending on the patient's chief complaint, the nurse practitioner orders laboratory tests and diagnostic studies and modifies the patient's medication regimen.

Within the following week or two, assuming there is no emergency medical need, the physician visits the patient. The physician visit focuses on the patient's medical needs and includes an evaluation of the treatment plan indicated by the nurse practitioner. Patients are strongly urged to call the office if they are having any symptoms or problems. The clinicians often have to reinforce this point because patients are not used to the idea that they have the right to call the office any time, including nights and weekends. Since the primary care model is patient driven and home based, it is explained to the patients that the earlier they call with a possible problem, the sooner we can initiate treatment to prevent a hospitalization, which is one of our primary goals.

The patient is visited by the nurse practitioner or physician as often as necessary (generally every 7 to 10 days) until the patient's status is stable. Then, as in an office setting, the patient is scheduled for a home visit every 4 to 6 weeks.

About 15% of the patients are referred to a psychiatric clinical specialist, usually for depression. The psychiatric clinical specialist provides psychotherapy, behavior modification, and psychotropic medication management. Often patients also require traditional visiting nurse services, in which case appropriate referrals are made.

The vast majority of patients remain VNA House Calls patients until they die or are placed in a nursing home. Very few are hospitalized (1% of the census on any given day), and, if hospitalized, the stay is very short. Our hospital length of stay is approximately 4 days, compared to 6.5 days for the Medicare population at large.

Clinician Perspective

The clinicians set up their visiting schedules weekly, allowing for three to five emergent visits per clinician per week, on average. The nurse practitioners generally schedule five to six visits a day and admit four to six new patients a week to the practice. The physician schedules the same number of visits a day, including four to five new patients who have been admitted to the practice the previous week by the nurse practitioners.

Each clinician generally starts his or her day in the field. The office manager, medical assistant, and support staff manage the office and take phone calls from patients, families, nurses, physicians, and others. These three office staff members provide critical support to the clinicians while they are in the field. In addition to manning the phones, the office staff manage the clinical records, process bills, prepare laboratory reports to be reviewed by the clinicians, call paramedics, and arrange for laboratory work. Basically, they do everything anyone working in a doctor's office or clinic would do. The medical assistant may also go out to draw blood or collect other specimens; however, his time is generally fully utilized in the office.

The clinicians come back to the office at the end of the day. They have the opportunity to follow up on phone calls that have been forwarded to them during the day and to finalize any studies for the patients that were seen that day. They can discuss anything unusual with the physician and the office manager. Once a week, the clinicians hold a case conference reviewing the status of patients they have visited. Generally, patients are visited by the advanced practice nurse two to three times for every one physician visit; however, all the core clinicians know the status of each patient. Visiting nurses are welcome at the case conference to discuss patients that they are seeing.

The case conference is often interrupted by phone calls through the end of standard office hours (about 5:00 P.M.). When the answering service is put on, clinicians can then focus on treatment plans for the patients and can evaluate how effective they have been. Decisions can be made to order new medications or more laboratory tests, or an extra home visits can be planned. The case conferences are actually focused on two areas: patient care and teaching. Both physicians and nurse practitioners assume teaching and learning roles—this is collaboration. Once a month, the team meets to review patients who are receiving Medicare Part A home health services and, where appropriate, to document and bill for care plan oversight under Medicare Part B. Since at any one time approximately one third of the patients are receiving Medicare Part A home health care, this can be a significant source of revenue.

Consultations

A small but growing part of our practice is the provision of in-home nurse practitioner visits and consultations to patients treated by community physicians. In these cases, the patient has a primary care provider other than the VNA physician but cannot get to the provider's office. We are very sensitive to the physician community and aim to be very "physician friendly." The nurse practitioner consultation is valuable to the primary care provider who desires more information than the visiting nurse can provide. At the same time, the community physician is not threatened with losing the patient to the VNA primary care practice. The nurse practitioner may see this patient only once or continue visits until the patient is well enough to get to the physician's office. Sometimes the patient never recovers the ability to return to the primary care provider's office and we work with the physician to gradually transfer the patient to our in-home service. These consultations are billable services under the Medicare Part B guidelines.

The psychiatric clinical nurse specialists (CNSs) also provide consultation services to community-based primary care providers. The psychiatric CNS with an expertise in geropsychiatric issues and pharmacology often works very effectively with the community primary care provider to manage the patient's psychiatric problem at home, particularly through medication management and behavioral modification. Community-based providers are generally very satisfied with the outcomes achieved when the psychiatric CNS is called in for consultation. Psychiatric CNSs contribute to the comprehensive care of the homebound patient (Rinke, 2000).

ADDITIONAL ROLES FOR NURSE PRACTITIONERS IN HOME CARE

Most health care systems in the Philadelphia area are composed of an acute care hospital, physician practices, and a home care agency. Nurse practitioners are employed by the health care systems to work in the hospital, emergency departments, occupational health centers, or critical care settings. They are also utilized in the primary care offices to provide acute, chronic, and episodic care. Rarely, however, are nurse practitioners found in home care settings regionally or nationally. Especially in a time when seamless health care is important, opportunities do exist for nurse practitioners to provide home visits to help keep patients from "falling through the cracks." This is an expanding area of practice for nurse practitioners in the Philadelphia area.

Once a home care agency determines that a patient needs to be closed to skilled nursing (because of Medicare Part A guidelines) and the patient still does not have a primary care provider, the VNA House Calls nurse practitioner is in a good position to continue to provide primary care services. Prior to the visiting nurse closing the patient to home care services, the patient could receive nurse practitioner referral and a home visit under Medicare Part B. Depending on the patient's needs, a follow-up visit might be weekly, biweekly, or monthly. These patients would have telephone access to the nurse practitioner to report any change in condition, and additional acute visits could be made if needed. Close monitoring by the nurse practitioner would prevent unnecessary, and costly, emergency department visits, and any time a skilled need developed, the patient could be referred back to the home care agency, which could once again provide nursing services under Medicare Part A. In this scenario, the nurse practitioner fills the void that is often left in physician follow-up. Frequently follow-up does not occur, and the patient once again ends up needing costly emergency care. Presently we are not familiar with any health care system using this nurse practitioner model, but we suspect that it would be cost-effective to the system and beneficial to the patient.

CONCLUSIONS

VNA House Calls has been providing home care services using the described model for over 3½ years. We have grown from a practice of about 100 patients to about 500 patients. We continue to grow. Each week we receive approximately 10 referrals for new patients. We estimate that we have cared for close to 1,000 patients since we began. Each day our commitment to provide primary care services to the homebound population of Philadelphia is reconfirmed. We are often encouraged by our patients, their families, and the health care community at large. We try to educate every physician, pharmacist, visiting nurse, social worker, family member, friend, and clergy that we talk to about our practice. We have even advertised our program on the sides of buses to help get the word out.

We have learned that not only is each patient unique, but so is each patient's caregiving situation. We have become better practitioners through knowing what "home" looks like for our patients. Our patients have chosen to remain in their homes until their death, and we understand how important that decision is. Some of the patients we see improve dramatically, and they can be referred back to their former health care provider because they are able to leave their homes. Most of our patients remain homebound because of the physical limitations that cause them to be referred to us initially. They live each day in their homes where they are happy to remain. Many of our patients are eventually referred to hospice care because they have decided that they have had enough hospitalizations and they seek palliative care only. As primary care providers in the home care setting, our role varies as much as our patients vary. We provide care that ranges from helping one patient live well while helping another patient die well. This is the role of the nurse practitioner in home care.

CASE VIGNETTES

Of the hundreds of patients that we see, the common patient diagnoses are those in any outpatient population. Coronary artery disease, congestive heart failure, diabetes mellitus, cerebral vascular accident, degenerative joint disease, peripheral vascular disease, multiple sclerosis, traumatic brain injury, spinal cord injuries, dementia, and Parkinson's disease are the most prevalent. In addition, patients have all of the most common acute episodic problems. We work to educate patients and their families in health promotion strategies. Our goal is to keep all patients well, in particular our homebound population. The following cases present a glimpse into the rewards of caring for people in their homes.

Vignette 1

E. L. is a 66-year-old woman who suffered an intracranial hemorrhage at age 46, leaving her without any motor function or speech. Following this incident, she was cared for at home by her husband and three children until the untimely death of her husband 17 years ago. After her husband's death, she was placed in a nursing home and her children were cared for by family members. At the time of the original nursing home admission, a 10-year-old daughter vowed that as soon as possible she would find a way to bring her mother home to care for her. That day occurred 20 years later. E. L.'s daughter, now a woman of 30, found a way to care for her mother at home.

This patient was referred to our practice 2 years ago by the local agency on aging that was financially overseeing her care through a nursing home waiver program. When I first visited the home, the patient had been home for over 2 weeks with no support services in place. Since her care was long term and she had no skilled needs, she was not referred to a visiting nurse agency. Her daughter was a very willing caregiver, but she had many practical questions and needed direction in managing her mother's daily care.

A complete history revealed that the patient was discharged on antihypertensive medication and aspirin. She had a gastrostomy tube in place and was receiving all medication and nutrition through the tube. In addition, her daughter was concerned about her mother's continuous cough and was having difficulty with the mechanics of the tube feedings, which were set up as a continuous feeding. On examination, E. L.'s blood pressure was found to be elevated.

Time was spent reviewing how to care for a bed-bound patient, including bathing, skin care, and the need for frequent position changes. The hospital bed did not have a preventive overlay mattress, so one was ordered. The daughter was observed using the pump that was delivering the nutritional formula to the patient, and corrections were made. An alternative feeding schedule was proposed that thrilled the daughter because she was checking the patient so frequently through the night that she was not getting needed sleep. In addition, a mucolytic was prescribed, with instructions to the daughter to call after a few days if the cough did not resolve.

Because the patient's blood pressure was elevated on initial examination, visiting nurses were ordered to monitor the pressure while the nurse practitioner adjusted the medications. During their visits, the nurses also helped the daughter to gain confidence in caring for her mother. Within a few short weeks, E. L. was stable. The visiting nurse closed the case, and E. L. was receiving excellent care from her daughter. We continue to make monthly visits, with intermittent visits for acute problems. E. L.'s daughter comments at each visit that without our care she would not have been able to fulfill the promise that she had made to her mother and herself years ago.

Vignette 2

L. S. is a 55-year-old mentally challenged woman who has lived at home with her parents since birth. Her mother is 80 years old. L. S. was referred to our practice because her behavior was more and more withdrawn. At the time of the referral, she spent day and night in her upstairs bedroom. A history revealed that L. S. had not been downstairs since she fell down the stairs about 3 years before, resulting in a wrist fracture.

Her mother now reports that L. S. spends most of her time in bed and is amused by the television all day. The caregiver is also caring for her husband, who is 10 years her senior. He stays on the first floor of the home because he is unable to climb stairs.

After two visits to the home, it was apparent that L. S. would not permit any examination to be completed. We were able to get a blood pressure and pulse, which were normal. L. S.'s mother was very concerned that L. S. had had no medical exam in years. The last time L. S. went to a family doctor, the mother was asked to never bring L. S. back to the office because she caused such a disturbance. After a long discussion, the mother agreed to medicate the patient so that a complete examination could be performed.

Medication was given 1 hour prior to the next scheduled visit later that week. At the visit, a more complete examination was performed. All findings were within normal limits, and the mother's worries were relieved. An antidepressant was offered, and a referral was made to a social worker. The social worker came to the home to help the family connect to a community agency with resources for mentally challenged individuals.

Today a recreational therapist comes to the home and is working to help L. S. overcome her fear of leaving her room. When appropriate, a physical therapist will be ordered to work with L. S. on stair climbing. In addition, plans have been made for L. S.'s care in the event of her mother's illness.

Recently L. S. developed an acute respiratory infection, and medication was prescribed. L. S. responded to the medication and recovered quickly. L. S.'s mother was grateful that an emergency department visit was not necessary because that would have involved sedating the patient so that emergency medical technicians could get her on a stretcher to get her out of the house. Instead L. S.'s care was handled promptly and there were no serious complications caused by the delay in care.

Vignette 3

V. J. an 88-year-old man, returned to his home following a second stroke. He had been hospitalized for 1 week and then was in a transitional care unit for a few days. One year previously, following his initial cerebrovascular accident, he had been through rehabilitation and was able to ambulate in the home with a walker and the assistance of his daughter. The recent stroke, however, left him bed-bound and unable to communicate. The patient's history was obtained from his wife and daughter because of V. J.'s inability to participate in the interview.

At the initial visit, it became clear that the family had unrealistic expectations of the potential for V. J.'s recovery. His wife's initial question was when her husband would walk. I quickly realized that since V. J. had recovered from the initial stroke, his wife assumed that he would recover from this event as well. Before any further discussion, I asked to examine V. J. so that I would be better able to answer her questions.

V. J. was clearly not functional as result of the devastating stroke. His profound limitations precluded admission for rehabilitation. Lack of rehabilitation was one of the wife's chief concerns. She felt that V. J. was cheated of an opportunity to recover. On examination, V. J. was febrile with a normal blood pressure. He was lying flat in the bed under a heat duct that was blowing hot air directly onto his face. His lips were dry and cracked, his tongue was coated, and he was having some difficulty breathing. He had scattered rhonchi with a productive cough of yellow sputum. His heart rate was rapid but not tachycardic. His abdomen was soft, nontender, with positive bowel sounds. He was discharged with a Foley catheter, and his urine output was low and concentrated. He had a patent feeding tube. The family was giving the correct amount of feeding per the discharge instructions, but there was no instruction given about the need for additional water.

Laboratory tests for blood and urine were sent. The family was educated about the patient's need for hydration, and the bed was repositioned in the room to move the patient away from the vent. The wife had a humidifier and agreed to use it. Finally, a discussion ensued about V. J.'s future. We discussed the respiratory infection, and the family agreed to antibiotics. We also discussed V. J.'s poor prognosis, and the family presented me with a living will, which indicated that the patient did not want mechanical resuscitation. The family did not want the patient sent back to the hospital either. We discussed caring for V. J. to keep him comfortable, and I brought up the subject of hospice care. The wife and daughter agreed to consider it. Prior to our discussion, they believed that hospice was only for patients with cancer. Visiting nurses were arranged in the interim. This visit lasted about 2½ hours, and by the time I left I felt confident that the family now knew what to expect in regard to V. J.'s condition. When I returned to the office, I received a call from V. J.'s daughter saying that she and her mother both agreed to hospice care. Within three days, V. J. died in his home with the care of his wife and daughter and the hospice nurses. Later, when I told my colleagues about this family, one commented, "It is a shame that the patient did not get to see the doctor before he died." I replied, "Maybe, but wasn't this family fortunate to have a nurse practitioner?"

REFERENCES

Bates, B. (1974). Twelve paradoxes: A message for nurse practitioners. *Nursing Outlook, 31,* 686–688.

Boling. P. A. (1998). Physicians in home care: Past, present, and future. *Caring, 17,* 10–15.

Rinke, L., & Holt, S. (2000). Primary care in the home: The time is now. *Home Health Care Management and Practice, 12*(3), 1–9.

Sullivan, E. (1992). Nurse practitioners and reimbursement. *Nursing and Health Care, 13,* 236–241.

Chapter **18**

SURGICAL INTENSIVE CARE UNIT NURSE PRACTITIONER

Sabrina D. Jarvis

BACKGROUND

Although I have practiced in a variety of acute-care settings, including medical, surgical, emergency, and intensive and critical care nursing, I wanted to develop a new area of practice. Over the past 8 years, I have worked to develop the role of the surgical intensive care nurse practitioner. This has been a challenging and interesting career development.

In 1990, it was not my original intent to continue working in the acute-care setting once I had completed my graduate education. I graduated from a family nurse practitioner master's program and began working in hospital-based home health. I quickly realized that while I enjoyed home health nursing, I truly missed the acute-care setting.

At the time, there were no inpatient positions for acute-care registered nurse practitioners (NPs) at the medical center where I was working. The only openings were in the clinics and in home health. Fortunately, the master's program I attended had a core program that provided the educational background I needed to also function as a clinical nurse specialist (CNS). Over the next several years, I worked as the surgical/surgical intensive care unit (SICU) clinical nurse specialist. I provided clinical support and resource to the staff and surgical nurses and was involved in clinical research, staff development, and patient and staff education. I often helped with patient care in the SICU.

As an advanced practice registered nurse (APRN), my role changed over time to include NP functions. In the evenings I was often called to see unstable patients when the primary physician was not available. I used my nurse practitioner skills to assess, diagnose, and treat the patient until the physician could arrive. I also used my NP education to develop and implement complex plans of care for surgical patients.

In 1994, as the medical center restructured to maintain quality of care despite budget constraints and staffing cutbacks, the emphasis shifted to caseload management and realignment of health care resources. Our affiliation with the medical school was also affected. For many years, there was a resident available to provide patient coverage in the SICU, but this position was eliminated when the medical school residency program changed. In an attempt to provide medical coverage while the surgical teams were operating or away from the unit, I was asked to pilot the role of the SICU NP.

ROLE TRANSITION

At the time, there were no acute-care nurse practitioner programs available in Utah. My first step was to try to find other NPs working in the acute-care setting. I completed a literature review and networked with several nursing education programs providing acute-care educational tracks. This was unsatisfactory because the available literature was very general in role development and the educational programs did not provide consistency in training.

The acute-care nurse practitioner (ACNP) role was relatively new, and there were only 11 programs in the nation providing this education in 1994 (American Association of Critical-Care Nurses, 1999). The NP students' training often appeared to be based on what the physician preceptor was willing to teach, and there was no consistency in the education provided.

I talked with other NPs who were working in such diverse settings as neonatal intensive care and emergency departments. I was interested in clinical competencies and documentation of training. Several of the NPs were in the process of developing their own roles, and there was diversity in both role description and what clinical skills were required for their particular job. I studied the job description for the SICU resident position and met with the SICU nurses and surgeons to determine what role functions they valued.

Initially I met with resistance from both medical and nursing staff. One fundamental problem was the lack of a well-defined, written job description for the SICU nurse practitioner position. I was very cautious and limited the skills I would be willing to learn. The job description was written in general terms to allow for expansion of the role over time. Some of the physicians had not worked with NPs and identified conflicting areas of responsibility. They were concerned that I was learning and performing procedures such as intubation; placement of central lines, arterial lines, pulmonary artery catheters, and chest tubes; reading X-rays; and prescribing vasoactive and cardiac medications. They saw these activities as crossing into the physician practice domain. As I became more comfortable with my role and defined my responsibilities and skills, the physician resistance gradually disappeared.

My relationship with the SICU nurses was also difficult at times as the new role evolved. Many nursing staff members, including the nurse manager, were very supportive. They were patient and understanding as I worked through the transition period and gained the advanced clinical skills I needed to succeed in the role. It was difficult to develop the NP role in the same unit I had served in as a CNS. There was confusion among the nursing staff as to the difference in the roles.

In the new role, I could no longer spend as much time teaching at the bedside and helping with routine patient care. I felt like a neophyte NP, despite having worked as an acute-care NP for several years. Initially I was insecure, made clinical decisions hesitantly, and often sought to validate my decisions with others. I lacked the advanced training to do the complex procedures that were required in the SICU. Initially, I also had to report every intervention to the residents, which added one more step in the communication chain.

Several nurses voiced concerns that I was performing the role of "supernurse" but was unable to write transfer orders or perform the procedures the SICU resident had always done. Some of the nurses did not inform me when there was a patient problem and called the team physician directly rather than involve me.

These problems resolved over time with frank discussion of mutual expectations as I gained the clinical knowledge, skills, and decision-making ability required for the SICU NP position.

ROLE DELINEATION

Initially, there was confusion as I transitioned from the CNS role to the SICU nurse practitioner role. I had been originally trained as a family nurse practitioner but had taken the core courses for the CNS track. These core courses included preparation for the roles of educator, clinical expert, researcher, consultant, and administrator.

As a nurse practitioner student, I had received training in advanced physiology, pharmacology, clinical assessment, diagnosis, and medical management. I was granted prescriptive privileges as an NP and worked in the role in hospital-based home health care for a year before moving to the SICU.

When I assumed the position as the SICU clinical nurse specialist, I functioned in an already established role. Primarily, I served as a clinical expert and consultant to the staff, and assisted with complex patient care. I provided staff education, helped write policy and procedures, and participated in research. My primary role was defined by tradition and by the written CNS scope of practice of the medical center. Over the next several years, I developed a modified scope of practice that utilized my skills as an NP and, in essence, became a blended CNS and NP role—although I did not realize this at the time.

I usually worked in the evenings. If a patient became medically unstable, and the physician could not be reached immediately, I was often called to see the patient. I would diagnose and then treat the patient until the responsible physician could see the patient. This added responsibility was simply accepted and added to my scope of practice but never really identified as a separate role function.

In 1993, the medical center administration requested a written report from all advanced practice nurses to examine scope of practice and role productivity. Only when the report was presented was it realized that I was performing basically a blended CNS/NP role that had evolved over time based on medical center needs and a willingness, on my part, to assume these additional responsibilities.

When I accepted the position as the SICU nurse practitioner, I found myself struggling with role delineation. I understood the five basic subroles of the clinical nurse specialist: clinical expert, consultant, educator, researcher, and administrator. My identified clients were primarily the nurses and the patient care systems supportive of patient care (Mick & Ackerman, 2000; Redekopp, 1997).

The role of the acute-care nurse practitioner has some of the same components found in the clinical specialist role. The American Association of Critical Care Nurses has helped to better define the role and identifies four separate roles for the ACNP, including clinical expert, educator, researcher, and consultant.

The fundamental difference between the CNS and the NP is that the nurse practitioner role and scope of practice emphasize autonomy in medical diagnosis and treatment with legal authority to order diagnostic tests and treatments, and to prescribe medications (Mick & Ackerman, 2000). The CNS defers these activities to physician colleagues.

As stated earlier, in 1994, there was not much information on specific development of the NP role and scope of practice in the SICU and critical care areas. Once the intensive training was completed with the intensivist and the residents, the role evolved. The primary emphasis was on differential diagnosis and medical treatment of critically ill patients and working in close collaboration with the surgeons to provide continuity of care.

This was not an easy process at the beginning. It was difficult because I sometimes inadvertently shifted between roles, confusing the staff. As the NP position developed, the nursing staff actually encouraged the NP activities and would not request my assistance with bedside nursing unless absolutely necessary. Over time, the nursing staff helped to define the NP role and its place within the SICU structure.

As an NP, I focus on teaching patients and families. I continue to teach educational classes, as time permits, and mentor and preceptor staff as well as nurse practitioner and physician assistant students. I am also involved with medical student and resident training.

My clinical practice is research based, and I actively participate in SICU clinical research projects and clinical rounds. Administratively, I assist the SICU intensivist and nurse manager with the development and writing of unit policy and procedures.

It has been an interesting process to develop the SICU NP position. I had to examine the different subroles and then determine their order of importance and the time allotted to each role. Once I understood the major role requirements, I personalized the SICU NP position based on my professional and life experiences. For example, I enjoy teaching, so I am permitted to emphasize this subrole. I have seen this same process of role development with the other nurse practitioners with whom I work. Each one has developed and personalized his or her acute-care NP position.

CHARACTERISTICS AND COMPONENTS

I currently base my practice in the SICU and formally work 10-hour shifts from 1100 to 2130 hours, Tuesday through Friday; however, I actually work 40 to 50 hours a week. My caseload includes up to 10 SICU patients. I often see patients on the surgical wards and provide follow-up care on 4 to 6 patients who have transferred out of the SICU. This caseload is manageable, but very busy. I do not take calls. I work with seven rotating teams who have admitting privileges in the SICU.

The vascular and general surgery teams are large ones and manage their own patients. I provide input on care and manage their patients when these teams are away from the unit. The neurosurgical, cardiothoracic, urology, ear-nose-throat, and orthopedic services are much smaller and are appreciative of the support I provide. I usually do rounds with these teams and participate as a team member. I write orders on these patients and monitor the care provided. Several times a day, I visit with patients and their families. Often, families are in crisis and small issues, if not discussed, become very stressful. A trusting relationship usually develops, and I provide follow-through for any issues that the physician may need to deal with.

I have a close working relationship with the SICU intensivist and review patients with him at least once a day. The intensivist often leads team rounds, which are used as a learning experience for the residents and me. If a problem develops, I routinely consult with the intensivist as needed.

If a patient's condition deteriorates, I will manage the patient and notify the responsible physician. Interventions may include intubation, ordering of vasoactive medications, placement of arterial and central lines, and ordering appropriate laboratory and radiographic studies.

In the evenings there is an inhouse resident or intern who covers the surgical service. They are often busy seeing consults or may need to assist in emergency surgeries. I continue to provide coverage in SICU and will respond to pages from the surgical wards. At the end of the shift, I report off to the resident or intern.

I have developed my job description and maintain a clinical log of advanced clinical procedures I perform. I have also developed clinical competencies and reviewed these with the intensivist. I have clinical privileges established through the medical center's professional board, and each year I update my clinical skills list as I learn new procedures.

Every year, my performance is evaluated based on the federal proficiency system, which is divided into clinical performance and professionalism/leadership activities. The proficiency also includes a current list of my advanced clinical competencies. After a self-evaluation, my proficiency evaluation is completed by the intensivist, SICU nurse manager, and the associate chief of the surgical care center.

CURRENT CLINICAL PRACTICE

Over the past 8 years, the SICU nurse practitioner role has become well established and accepted. It has included the addition of a second nurse practitioner in the SICU to help provide continuity of care 7 days a week.

We work in close collaboration with the surgical residents and are accepted as colleagues. Part of this process has included developing our place within the structured hierarchy that is predominant in medical centers that are affiliated with medical schools. It has been an educational process to understand and appreciate the residents and their training. As nurse practitioners, we have assumed a role in helping to educate and decrease resident workload. Our mentoring of the residents and medical students over the past several years has resulted in their clearer understanding and appreciation of the nurse practitioner role. It is interesting to hear the residents, as they rotate through, orally report on our NP roles to incoming residents, whereas in previous years, we did the introductions.

As the residents rotate through, it becomes a challenge to maintain continuity of care. This challenge is balanced by the availability of the SICU intensivist and attending surgeons, and the strong, permanent relationships we have with other medical center team members, such as social workers, dietitians, occupational and physical therapists, and chaplain services.

There has been a change concerning prescriptive privileges since 2 years ago, when Utah granted NP prescriptive privileging to include Schedule II through V controlled substances. This has had a positive impact on our practice as intensive care nurse practitioners because we order narcotics for the surgical patients.

Over the past 4 years, the role of the nurse practitioner has been increasingly supported and appreciated at the medical center where I work. Where there was once only two inpatient NPs, there are now five, and there is a close network among the medical center nurse practitioners. Also, nurse practitioners recently have been recognized, as a group, by the hospital administration as part of the medical staff.

SUMMARY

The development and progression of the role of the SICU nurse practitioner has been both challenging and rewarding. Over the past several years, I have been fortunate to meet and mentor other nurse practitioners seeking to work in intensive care or trauma areas. These nurse practitioners are defining their own practices and writing contractual agreements.

Information and articles to assist with this process of role delineation are available from resources such as the American Association of Critical Care Nurses (AACN), Society of Critical Care Medicine (SCCM), and the American Nurses Association (ANA). The development of the *Standards of Clinical Practice and Scope of Practice for the Acute Care Nurse Practitioner* (ANA, 1995) has been instrumental in providing the framework for acute-care roles.

Certification in the practicing specialty area is also important. Both my partner and I maintain CCRN, FNP, and ACNP certification. The last year that a nurse practitioner could challenge the ACNP exam without formal college course work was 2001.

It is an exciting time to be a nurse practitioner. As we continue to expand our practices into nontraditional areas, there is a growing wealth of information and practice opportunities.

REFERENCES

American Association of Critical-Care Nurses.(1999). *Acute care nurse practitioner clinical curriculum and certification review.* A. Gawlinski & D. Hamwi (Eds.). Philadelphia: W. B. Saunders Co.

American Nurses Association. (1995). *Standards of clinical practice and scope of practice for the acute care nurse practitioner.* Washington, DC: American Nurses Publishing.

Mick, D., & Ackerman, M. (2000). Advanced practice nursing role delineation in acute and critical care: Application of the strong model of advanced practice. *Heart & Lung: The Journal of Acute & Critical Care, 29,* 210–221.

Redekopp, M. (1997). Clinical nurse specialist role confusion: The need for identity. *Clinical Nurse Specialist, 11,* 87–91.

Chapter 19

PHYSICIAN–NURSE PRACTITIONER RELATIONSHIPS

William Kavesh

M y collaboration with nurse practitioners has returned substantially to where it began almost 30 years ago—in primary care. My first job out of medical residency was as the internist/medical director of a South Boston neighborhood health center, and one of my new activities was providing clinical guidance to a nurse who was just finishing her training as a nurse practitioner at one of the first nurse practitioner training programs in the country. It was a good learning experience for both of us. After a long foray into long-term care (working closely with nurse practitioners there as well), I am again working primarily in the outpatient setting as the director of a primary care geriatrics clinic. In this chapter, I will discuss some of the issues that arise there as well as review physician and nurse practitioner collaboration in home care and nursing home care.

CONTRASTING THE PRACTICE OF GERIATRICIANS AND GERIATRIC NURSE PRACTITIONERS

In many ways, geriatric medical practice reflects a philosophy of patient care that is much closer to the approach used by nurse practitioners than to that of general internal medicine. In my experience, the differences in approach between a geriatric physician and a geriatric nurse practitioner are, in fact, much less apparent than those between a general internist and an adult nurse practitioner. Geriatrics, a specialty dealing with the care of the elderly, especially the frail elderly, requires a more comprehensive approach than the care of many younger patients. While the traditional history and physical examination focuses on immediate organ-centered problems, comprehensive geriatric evaluation also addresses other areas, especially functional, psychological, and social dimensions. In evaluating a patient who falls, for example, a host of questions may arise. Has the patient's cognitive status deteriorated so that he or she now has less safety awareness? Is the patient's vision or hearing becoming impaired, causing the loss of important cues that help maintain balance? Is something going on at home? Is the patient no longer reliably taking medications due to the loss of a caretaker who used to pour them each week? Or are there new stresses due to the illness of a spouse? Has the patient been getting sleeping pills from a neighbor because the neighbor finds them helpful and the patient can't sleep? Geriatric providers, whether physicians or nurse practitioners, spend more time with patients because they have to sort out these issues, because it takes longer to get a history from a cognitively impaired patient, or because the history needs to be taken from both the patient and the person accompanying the patient.

The practice of geriatric physicians and nurse practitioners reflects the similar philosophy of patient care and the unique issues that geriatric patients present. These similarities are evident in a number of indicators. Take, for example, lengths of outpatient visits. When we asked an observer to count the number of minutes that patients spent with geriatric physicians or nurse practitioners in our clinic, the time was the same—about 30 minutes. That is a lot of time in an age where the push for efficiency sometimes clashes with provider concerns about quality. But it also shows that comprehensive care, whether provided by a nurse practitioner or a physician, takes time. Most of our patients think it is time well spent.

Another area of special expertise that nurse practitioners seem to possess in abundance, and that I have noticed increasingly frequently in the past few years, is organizational talent. Whether this has to do with skills they learn as nurses combined with the additional skills needed to approach clinical problems, nurse practitioners develop, run, and monitor new programs with skill and attention to detail. Our clinic quality assurance program was set up by a nurse practitioner, and she continues to run it and look for new ways to improve what we do. The nurse practitioner has the clinical skills to be able to explain the rationale for quality assurance measures to physicians and other clinicians who participate in the program. She also can appreciate the nuances of the issues involved. Most providers understand the reasons for the concept of quality assurance. But when it comes to monitoring the details of what they do, some providers are not always eager to do the work or accept the results of the monitoring process. Our nurse practitioner runs the program in an unobtrusive way, and I, as the director of the clinic, can reinforce the results to physician providers if necessary.

Another nurse practitioner is developing a group visit model for diabetics, who need both education and clinical care. It is this mix of care and education that particularly exploits the strengths of our nurse practitioners. Studies have shown that a key factor in stabilizing diabetes is frequent intervention with educational tools and positive feedback to patients as they move in the direction of desired goals. Nurse practitioners are very good motivators, and their positive interactions with patients can be important in improving compliance. Finally, the organizational aspects of such a program require a good deal of attention to make sure that patients find the overall experience satisfying. One can have a great educational program, but it requires careful implementation to instill an atmosphere of success that will motivate patients to participate. Our nurse practitioner is well equipped to do this.

AMBULATORY PRACTICE

Constructing the Nurse Practitioner's Caseload

A fundamental issue in ambulatory practice, which continues to fuel debate, relates to what type of outpatients should be seen by nurse practitioners. Many of the studies done to compare performance of nurse practitioners and physicians in outpatient settings have evaluated the outcomes of care provided for specific conditions, such as blood pressure control or treatment of urinary tract infections. By isolating a single problem, it is much easier to measure specific outcomes.

However, many patients often present with multiple problems. This is especially the case in geriatrics where many of our patients may simultaneously present with diabetes, hypertension, congestive heart failure, renal disease, and/or chronic obstructive pulmonary disease. The interpretation of symptoms can become very challenging in such a situation. Throw in a little dementia, and things become particularly difficult. The history is sometimes hard to get, and the interpretation of what the patient says may be equally tricky.

Collaborative agreements often contain descriptive material about the types of problems that the nurse practitioner will see. According to many state regulations, such as those in Pennsylvania, the registration process for a nurse practitioner requires that the collaborative agreement with a physician include a description of the guidelines under which the nurse practitioner will practice. Books of guidelines are available. The problem is that these algorithms can never envision all the possible variations that may arise in the care of a particular patient. This is especially a problem for patients who have multiple simultaneous problems.

Should a nurse practitioner be limited to seeing patients with a limited number of straightforward problems that can be managed with simple algorithms? In my collaboration with nurse practitioners, I have never practiced that way. My experience over 30 years has been that most nurse practitioners know their limits and will consult about situations that they feel are beyond the scope of their practice. From time to time, I have found that the nurse practitioner did not pursue something as aggressively as I might. But working in the Department of Veterans Affairs (VA), I also have had the unique opportunity to look over the shoulders of many community physicians whose patients also come to the VA hospital primarily to get medications. Many veterans are now over 65 and are paying hundreds of dollars a month for medicines. So this VA program has been a great boon for them. However, in order to get medications, the veteran cannot simply present outside prescriptions to a VA pharmacy. The veteran must be seen and fully evaluated by a VA provider—a physician or nurse practitioner—and seen at regular intervals just the way a patient receiving primary care at the VA hospital must do. In order to do all this, the VA provider must often review copies of the outside physician's records to understand the rationale for the diagnosis and treatment plans.

What this experience has shown me is that whether a practitioner knows his or her limits appears to me to be more a function of the personality of the person than the particular professional title. I have now seen plenty of physicians who need to be more aware of their limitations, and I have occasionally seen nonphysician providers who also have this problem. Every person providing health care needs to know when to consult with someone else. In the case of nurse practitioners, in our clinic we do operate under guidelines, but they do not cover everything, and the most important thing is for the nurse practitioner and collaborating physician to learn what the upper limit of complexity is that the nurse practitioner can handle. I have to do the same thing. There are patients whose care I share with a consultant. In really arcane situations, such as an oncology patient getting a complex chemotherapy regimen, the consultant may be calling most of the shots and seeing the patient more often than I am. This is similar to the situation with a nurse practitioner. With some patients, the number and complexity of problems is beyond the nurse practitioner's scope of practice, and he or she usually knows it. In those infrequent situations, the nurse practitioner will transfer the patient to me. (New patients are generally assigned to nurse practitioners and physicians at random, so this may not be apparent at first).

If the patient has developed a close, long-term relationship with the nurse practitioner and gets a lot of psychological support from this, we may try to handle the situation with frequent collaborative discussions. I should also note that I sometimes find things that the nurse practitioner was unaware that she had missed. This is also similar to what happens when a general internist or geriatrician shares a patient with a specialist. In the nature of health care, a specialist will know more about a particular organ system than a generalist. With the advent of computerized medical records, we may be able to develop expert systems that scrutinize a provider's note against a set of state-of-the-art standards for each organ system. Some work has been done with computer programs that review emergency department records, and many pharmacies have built-in quality monitors to identify potential adverse drug reactions. But, for the broad practice of general medicine, these systems do not yet exist. For now, we rely on the self-awareness of the primary provider to know when to consult with someone else.

Scheduling Visits

How much time does a nurse practitioner, compared to a physician, need to see a patient? This is one of the major issues that I am currently reviewing at the VA geriatrics clinic where I work. In almost three decades of satisfying collaboration with nurse practitioners, my experience has been that adult nurse practitioners generally are scheduled for longer patient visit times than physicians. I have seen various explanations for this practice. The most common one is that nurse practitioners take a more comprehensive approach—dealing with psychosocial issues and doing patient education. A recent VA regional committee on primary care concluded that primary care nurse practitioners should be scheduled for longer patient visits but gave a different reason, suggesting that they need to spend the extra time talking to collaborating physicians. My experience has been that most nurse practitioners do not need their hands held by a physician for every visit. A review is certainly appropriate for complex problems where the nurse practitioner may feel the need for additional input or in unusual situations that may fall outside collaborative guidelines.

Nurse Practitioner Acceptance

I am aware, as are most of the nurse practitioners with whom I have worked, that nurse practitioners are not physicians, nor do they want to be physicians. They do not get the lengthy training of physicians and do not do intensive residencies. Unless they have immersed themselves in a narrow area of specialization, they do not know as much technical medicine as physicians. But, in my experience, the vast majority know when they risk venturing beyond their scope of expertise as well as physicians do, and their patients are highly pleased with the care they get.

The attitudinal issues are not going to go away easily. Fifteen years ago, I sat on a committee set up by the Massachusetts Department of Public Health to implement a law that authorized prescriptive privileges for nurse practitioners. There were two groups opposed: the Massachusetts Medical Society and the state pharmacists' organization. The medical society insisted that nurse practitioners should not be allowed to prescribe Coumadin because its management was too complex. In my experience, many community physicians do not do an ideal job of managing Coumadin. Pharmacists and nurse practitioners often manage Coumadin clinics. The restriction on Coumadin prescribing was rejected. Physicians also argued that nurse practitioners should not be allowed to prescribe narcotics. That view was rejected in Massachusetts, and I have not heard that this has opened the floodgates to illicit prescribing by nurse practitioners there or in other states where nurse practitioners have been prescribing narcotics for many years.

The best way to put many of these scope-of-practice concerns to rest, I think, is to get more data. In particular, we need more outcomes data looking at emergency department visits, rates of hospitalization, and the like to see if we can discern anything more precise regarding the outcome of nurse practitioner and physician outpatient care. An encouraging beginning was the recent randomized study by Mundinger (2000). However, the young age (mean age 45.9 years) of the participants and the focus on three conditions (asthma, hypertension, or diabetes) limits the generalizability of the results to an older and sicker population. The authors did look at a sicker subset of their study sample and concluded that the care and hospital service utilization outcomes of the nurse practitioner and physician patients did not differ. However, in our clinic at least, both geriatricians and geriatric nurse practitioners often treat patients with concomitant advanced congestive heart failure, renal insufficiency, diabetes, arthritis, and other coexisting conditions that complicate the management and choice of therapies. In these situations, algorithms become harder to construct, and confounding influences are trickier to sort out. But outcomes can still be measured. Such data have existed for over a decade for nursing home care, and they show improved outcomes (Kane et al., 1991). We need more of these data for outpatient care.

Supporting the Practice of Nurse Practitioners

Physicians who collaborate with nurse practitioners in outpatient settings can provide support for the nurse practitioner in a number of ways. First, it is important to be available for consultations about immediate problems. For a brief look at a patient, I may simply ask the patient whom I am seeing to wait a minute or two. If it seems that it will be longer, then I finish with the current patient first. Most of the reviews that I do with nurse practitioners fall into this category. It is also helpful to do systematic reviews of randomly selected patients and use these for teaching purposes. If there is more than one nurse practitioner, they can share in reviewing each other.

The physician also can be helpful in reminding patients that the nurse practitioner is their primary provider. Once in a while, a patient will insist on seeing a physician rather than a nurse practitioner. Our policy is to explain that we do not generally assign patients based on preference, but if someone is insistent, we will occasionally make the switch. My experience is that it is better to bend once in a while. If we are rigid about not allowing a change and then something should go wrong in the future, the patient will have a lot more anger, and angry patients are more likely to find a lawyer.

With regard to litigation, some interesting issues have arisen from the physician perspective. Malpractice rates for nurse practitioners remain very low compared to those for physicians. In Pennsylvania, which the state medical society says is one of the most litigious states in the country, malpractice insurance for a family practice physician may easily run up to $20,000, whereas a nurse practitioner may pay about $500. For the first time, I am hearing from physicians complaining that they are being laid off and replaced by nurse practitioners because the malpractice insurance for the nurse practitioners costs less. Concern is also growing among collaborating physicians about lawsuits against the nurse practitioner that may draw them in. I recently heard a talk to physicians who work with nurse practitioners in nursing homes. The speaker advocated that physicians be very careful to document their review of and agreement with the nurse practitioner's evaluation and plan (Levine, 2002). I have not heard this kind of talk before. What it portends is unclear, but the litigious environment we live in seems to be having a broader impact than many of us expected.

NURSING HOME CARE

Despite some of the concerns physicians may have about legal issues, nurse practitioner-physician collaboration continues to make very good sense in nursing home settings. At the Philadelphia VA nursing home, the nurse practitioners are the primary providers of diagnostic and therapeutic care for their patients. Their caseloads remain luxurious by private sector standards, about 60 patients per nurse practitioner. But the result is that the patients get excellent attention and the complaint rates among their families are extremely low. In addition to writing routine monthly notes, the nurse practitioners also see the patients for any acute problem. They have set up a staggered 10-hour day so that someone is in the facility from 7 A.M. to 6 P.M. This reduces the need for making off-hours decisions over the phone, and the nurse practitioners know each other's patients much better than an on-call physician who may otherwise spend very little time in the nursing home.

The nursing home nurse practitioner performs a number of critical tasks (see Table 19.1). Most importantly, she is the primary onsite provider for the patients under her care. Physicians doing nursing home care generally are engaged in other patient care activities throughout the day, including hospital rounds, office practice, or academic activities. The nurse practitioner is usually the most visible presence in the nursing home. With proper support from the physician, the nurse practitioner evaluates patients and interfaces with families and nursing home staff. Because the nurse practitioner is on-site, acute problems, especially infections in early stages, can be caught quickly and be treated before they are serious enough to require a hospital admission. For this to work, the physician must be readily available to the nurse practitioner, support the nurse practitioner with family and facility administration, and avoid undercutting the nurse practitioner when problems arise.

HOME CARE

Nurse practitioners continue to have the potential to make significant contributions in home care. What continues to surprise me is how few nurse practitioners there are in home care compared to registered nurses. Perhaps this is due to reimbursement strictures. For the purposes of Medicare (Part A) certified home health agency billing, nurse practitioners are viewed as registered nurses. The home care agency collects no more for the nurse practitioner's visit than it would by employing a less skilled, and less expensive, registered nurse.

TABLE 19.1   Role of the Nurse Practitioner in the Nursing Home

1. Primary on-site provider
   - Performs initial evaluation of new admissions
   - Performs periodic routine reviews
   - Takes first call from nursing home staff during working hours for emergency evaluations
   - Is first contact for family members with concerns or questions
   - Arranges transfers to other facilities and discharges
   - Dictates discharge summaries in facilities that require them

2. Relationship to physician
   - Works in collaboration with primary physician
   - Practices within scope of written guidelines
   - Uses telephone and beeper backup by physician
   - Performs regularly scheduled joint rounds
   - Is evaluated by periodic physician examinations and joint review of patient panel
   - Interfaces with consultant physicians as appropriate

3. Relationship to nursing home staff
   - Serves as primary nursing staff contact for patient care issues
   - Interfaces with other nursing home professionals, including dietitians, social workers, and therapists
   - Coordinates management of emergencies and critically ill patients
   - Coordinates hospice support for selected patients
   - Participates in case conferencing
   - Conducts training sessions for staff

4. Relationship to patient's family
   - Establishes communication with family
   - Maintains contact, especially for major changes in condition, issues related to advance directives, possible hospital transfers

Although registered nurses in Medicare-certified home health agencies can do a good deal of surveillance at the home, they are tethered to physicians when it comes to treatment decisions. Thus, they make phone calls, send the ubiquitous Center for Medicare and Medicaid Services home health agency form for the physician's signature on verbal orders that the physician may only dimly recall giving, and generally consult with the physician at frequent intervals regarding changes in treatment. This often may be appropriate because of the level of training that the nurse has. A nurse practitioner is in a very different position. She will have the skills and authority to do evaluations, order lab tests and X-rays at home, and make therapeutic decisions without requiring the physician's immediate concurrence. She also can help coordinate the input of social workers and therapists. (See Table 19.2).

My experience with home care nurse practitioners is that they are quite sophisticated in sorting out issues regarding common home care problems like congestive heart failure, acute and chronic infections, and functional decline. The weekly conference serves as a forum to confirm or refine the initial decision-making process. If the patient needs hospitalization, the nurse practitioner is usually in a good position to make the call and explain to the patient and family why it is necessary. Some home care agencies have dealt with this restriction by setting up a physician home visit subsidiary. The subsidiary can then hire nurse practitioners to work in collaboration with a physician and then bill directly under Medicare Part B (the same section of the Medicare law that authorizes physician reimbursement), just as nurse practitioners have been able to bill for nursing home visits for over a decade. However, this is a cumbersome alternative. I wonder if nurse practitioners are not allowed reimbursement under Medicare-certified home health agency rules because physicians also not allowed reimbursement. In fact, in the past there has been a problem with home health agencies hiring physicians simply to attract referrals from the physician's practice (Kavesh, 1986). This does not seem to be a likely conflict of interest for very many nurse practitioners.

My level of comfort goes up enormously when I am working with a nurse practitioner in a home care setting. If the reimbursement issues were fixed to extend nurse practitioner reimbursement to Medicare-certified home health agencies, the potential for nurse practitioners in home care would grow significantly. (See also chapter 17).

CONCLUSIONS

Nurse practitioners and geriatricians share a common approach to patients, which emphasizes comprehensive evaluation of social, psychological, and functional issues in addition to the traditional history and physical. This approach requires a good deal of time and relies on the input of family members and others who may provide care and support for a disabled or cognitively impaired patient. Because of this commonality in overall approach, I think geriatricians are in a particularly good position to appreciate the more comprehensive approach that has always characterized nurse practitioner education and practice.

TABLE 19.2   Role of the Nurse Practitioner in Home Care

1. Primary on-site provider at the home
   - Performs initial home care evaluation of medical, functional, and social problems
   - Evaluates home environment, safety, and nutritional issues
   - Makes follow-up visits at regular intervals
   - Makes emergency visits as necessary

2. Relationship to physician
   - Participates in weekly patient care conference
   - Provides phone consultation as necessary
   - Performs annual review of patient status
   - Plans for transitions around hospital admission and discharge

3. Relationship to family
   - Educates patient and family
   - Explains advance directives
   - Resolves conflicts
   - Plans for transitions around hospital admission and discharge

Comprehensive evaluation is particularly important in areas such as nursing home care and home care. Nurse practitioners are particularly suited by training to provide this comprehensive care. Patients in nursing homes benefit from the presence of a provider who can communicate easily with the nurses, serve as a nursing role model, and make clinical decisions. The timely presence of a nurse practitioner prevents many hospitalizations because problems are picked up quickly and treatment begun.

Patients and their families in home care benefit from the care of a nurse practitioner who has the time to deal with the many nursing care-related and functional problems in addition to the traditional clinical issues. Home care patients are often disabled or demented. The nurse practitioner is well equipped to evaluate these problems and to communicate with the family about dealing with them. It is a great boon to a geriatric physician to work with a nurse practitioner who has the flexibility to make home visits when the physician's office and hospital practice may be more structured. It is also a great boon to the patients.

REFERENCES

Kane, R. L., Garrard, J., Buchanan, J. L., Rosenfeld, A., Skay, J. C., & McDermott, A. (1991). Improving primary care in nursing homes. *Journal of the American Geriatrics Society, 36,* 359–367.

Kavesh, W. N. (1986). Home care: Process, outcome, cost. In M. P. Lawton (Ed.), *Annual review of geriatrics and gerontology* (pp. 68–73). New York: Springer Publishing.

Levine, J. M. (2002, March). *Medical-legal aspects of nursing home care.* Paper presented at the 25th Annual Symposium of the American Medical Directors Association, San Diego, CA.

Mundinger, M. O., Kane, R. L., Lenz, E. R., Totten, A. M., Tsai, W-Y., Cleary, P. D., Friedewald, W. T., Siu, A. L., & Shelanski, M. L . (2000). Primary care outcomes in patients treated by nurse practitioners or physicians: A randomized trial. *JAMA, 283,* 59–68.

chapter 20

PEDIATRIC NURSE PRACTITIONER AND PEDIATRICIAN: COLLABORATIVE PRACTICE

Carol Boland and Susan Leib

ollaboration is a relationship of interdependence that requires recognition and respect for complementary roles. Eleven years of successful collaboration have convinced us that four components are integral to successful collaboration.

1. Mutual respect. What we mean by mutual respect is that the physician and nurse practitioner (NP) have respect for each other's individual skills and for the unique contribution that each makes to the practice.

2. Trust. Trust is important in terms of the nurse practitioner because he or she needs to be able to trust that the physician will give thoughtful input during consultation, listen to what the problem is, and treat it as if it were his or her own. The physician needs to trust that the nurse practitioner knows his or her own limits primarily in relationship to consulting or referring to the physician as necessary.

3. Shared accountability. Because this is a joint practice, we are both responsible for all the patients in the practice and are equally accountable for them.

4. Joint decision making. The key word here is *joint,* in that if collaboration or consultation is needed, important decisions must be made together.

We write from the vantage point of a nurse practitioner and pediatrician who have worked together for 11 years in private practice in a community of 20,000 in Connecticut. The practice consists of three pediatricians and two pediatric nurse practitioners (PNPs); a second PNP joined the practice in 1997 and was subsequently replaced in 1999. Ten nurses and 15 administrative and secretarial staff support the practice. Patients in our practice are primarily White and middle class. Almost all patients have health insurance, approximately 10% from private pay and 90% through some form of managed care. While pediatric practice is primarily ambulatory, we see newborns and hospitalized children at a 350-bed community hospital.

Our practice originally consisted of two solo physician practitioners. Carol joined the practice as the nurse practitioner prior to Susan coming into the practice. So Carol's role was well established in the practice before we started to practice together. From the beginning, the PNP was introduced to the patients and families as a member of the practice, as someone who could see patients independently. The PNP was seen as an asset to the practice rather than a secondary provider. We have found that it is very important that the nurse practitioner be introduced into the practice in this light.

Another important factor that sets this same tone is that the fee schedule is the same for both nurse practitioners and physicians. When patients comment about the fact that they are paying the same price to see a nurse practitioner as a physician, they are told that the NP is providing essentially the same services as a doctor, and the fee schedule is therefore the same. In addition, overhead is the same in the practice for the nurse practitioner and the physician. The NP has a nurse who works with her. She has lab technicians and secretaries who provide the same services to her that they do for the physicians, and, therefore, the fee should be the same for both the nurse practitioner and the physicians.

Presently in our practice, Carol, the NP, takes after-hour calls once a week, as do the physicians. Due to her own personal choice, Carol does not take calls on weekends. There is physician back-up provided for the NP, but this is also true for one of the older physicians who does not want to admit patients to the hospital.

Since 1991, Carol has seen newborns in the hospital. Carol was one of the first NPs to be given privileges at the hospital where we admit patients. We explain to parents that they may be seeing her on newborn visits in the hospital. We feel it is very helpful to present our model of the NP as on an equal footing with the physician during the early encounters the patient has with the practice.

We have discussed including the NP in administrative and partner issues. When Susan came into the practice, she assumed that she would be a partner at some point; Carol, on the other hand, did not have similar expectations. If an NP is looking at a practice with the idea of becoming a partner, we feel that issue needs to be discussed prior to accepting a position in a private practice. We would offer the same advice to a physician looking into a new practice as well.

We have found several barriers to the idea of Carol becoming a partner. One is psychological in that, as physicians, we find it hard to conceive of a partner who is not a physician. A second barrier is that, on Carol's part, she is not willing to accept the extra responsibility of becoming a partner in a practice in terms of sharing calls more equally and assuming a more active role in the administrative details of the practice. The other barrier is legal. It is unclear under existing Connecticut laws whether the legal structure of a professional corporation allows physicians and NPs to enter into legal partnerships. NPs considering becoming partners in a practice should investigate the legal issues their state.

We would recommend a written practice agreement be negotiated prior to an NP or a physician accepting a position in a collaborative practice. The following points should be included:

1. Specific responsibilities and scope of practice
2. Compensation (salary, benefits, bonuses) and ownership/partnership
3. Resolution of disagreements regarding patient treatment issues
4. Quality assurance responsibilities

INDIVIDUAL PERSPECTIVES ON COLLABORATIVE PRACTICE

Carol

The first position I had after finishing my NP program was as an NP in an outpatient, adult medical clinic where there were five physicians and five NPs on staff. The NPs were basically treated in the same fashion as residents. The physicians were available for consultations and for teaching but were not interested in collaborating. Their role in relationship to the NPs was strictly advisory. My second position was at a Planned Parenthood clinic where I was the sole provider at any given time. There was a physician available by phone for consultation. He also scheduled appointments one afternoon a month to see patients that I felt needed further evaluation.

He was always available in terms of being willing to answer questions, but would take over the cases rather than the two of us collaborating and making joint decisions.

The third practice I joined was a private family practice with an NP already established in the practice, and involved seeing patients by appointment as well as walk-in patients. When I joined the practice I was not introduced as a colleague; my main role was doing some patient counseling and educational programs for the staff as well as seeing walk-in patients. This practice advertised for walk-in patients. However, when people walked in without an appointment, they were discouraged from seeing a physician and were told that the NP was the person who was available to see them. It became somewhat of a penalty to see the NP and it became very difficult to develop a caseload of patients.

Then I interviewed for a position with this current practice. I explained to the physician who wanted to hire me why I felt my role was not as successful as it could have been in the other practice. I felt that if I were going to be an independent provider and contribute to the economic viability of the practice, I needed to be introduced to the staff and patients as a colleague. We accomplished this by developing a pamphlet for the practice that described who I was and what I did. We had a staff meeting with the nurses and receptionists, and I explained my role to them. Most importantly, the physician who hired me spent a lot of time introducing me personally to the patients in the practice. He would introduce me as a colleague, bringing me into the exam room to meet the patient and telling patients I would be doing the same things he did and that they should feel comfortable seeing me for their health care. Also, he began to consult with me for patient issues such as breast-feeding, rashes, and asthma, thereby helping patients to see that I had specific new skills to offer the practice.

Consultation between the physician and me is really an important issue. Basically, I choose to consult for two reasons. One is to confirm my suspicions about a diagnosis or a treatment plan. The second reason is the case of a complicated situation that requires physician input. Whom I choose to consult with depends on many different factors. I may decide to consult with the physician who is generally most familiar with that patient or family. I may consult with a physician depending on his level of expertise in a specific area; some physicians are better at specific problems. Third, and probably the most important reason, is that I tend to consult with the physician who shares my point of view. All providers practice differently. Some physicians tend to do more testing than I like to do or they want to prescribe medication when I am more willing to monitor a child's condition. I will choose to consult with the physician who shares my approach to patient care.

Consultation with specialists has not been a problem. Most have been willing to discuss cases over the phone and see my patients when indicated. Because I have been accepted on only two health maintenance organization provider panels, referrals are made under a physician's name. Most often, the correspondence from the specialist will be addressed to that physician, interfering with my follow-up of the patient. This frustrating communication gap has yet to be remedied. The Connecticut Nurse Practitioner Group, Inc., and the Connecticut State Nurses Association are actively pursuing political and legislative measures to address the exclusion of NPs from provider panels.

The most important aspect of consultation in a truly collaborative relationship is knowing how to consult with a physician without losing your own credibility or having the physician usurp your authority. There is an art to this. Basically, when I need to consult, I ask the patient, "Do you mind if I consult with one of my colleagues on this problem?" I will ask the physician to come in and take a look at the patient. After the physician examines the patient, he or she will always stop outside the patient's room before rendering an opinion. When we have come to a joint decision, I go back to the patient and implement the plan of care. In the past, I have been in situations where, if I ask to consult, the physician says, "Why don't you go on and see your next patient and I will take care of this." This type of situation will destroy your credibility with the patient. They will think the physician has more authority in the relationship.

Conflict in terms of consultation rarely happens in this practice. Because I am a seasoned practitioner, I do not consult often. If I do seek consultation, it usually means I do not know how to proceed with the problem and I am usually going to follow the physician's advice. If I really disagree with that advice, I may seek a second opinion with someone else in the practice. We discuss the patient and come to a mutual decision.

The physicians in the practice often seek consultation from the NPs. We have areas of expertise that are well respected and utilized.

An NP who was a new graduate joined the practice two years ago. Because the practice is truly collaborative and mentoring (we precept NP, physician assistant, and medical students), and because the NP is bright and well trained, she has been able to evolve into a skilled clinician.

Susan

I want to address physician and patient acceptance of pediatric NPs. Physicians' acceptance of NPs depends, to a great extent, on what past experience the physician has had with nurse practitioners. In general, in both my residency training and medical school, I had limited exposure to nurse practitioners. As a resident I had a limited supervisory role of nurse practitioner students both in the emergency department and in the clinic setting and some experience with nurse clinicians and nurse practitioners on the wards in their capacity of dealing with patients. Older physicians have even more limited exposure to nurse practitioners. Lack of exposure definitely affects a physician's acceptance of a nurse practitioner, in the sense of not knowing what they do and what they are capable of.

It probably has been easier for me, as compared to other physicians, to accept an NP because I practice very similarly to a NP in that I have an interest in teaching about developmental and behavioral issues and in empowering parents through patient education. These are areas that nurse practitioners have traditionally focused on. Physicians have usually been more treatment oriented. Carol and I tend to practice very similar care. An older physician or a physician without this kind of focus might have more difficulty integrating an NP into a practice. Initially in our practice, Carol's role included more patient education. However, as she has become busier and as the practice has become busier we really cannot afford for her to do only that. We need her to provide direct patient care and to incorporate the education into her everyday practice.

In terms of acceptance of NPs, patients' opinions are set by how the physician and staff approach the NP. If a secretary says to a patient on the phone, "the doctors are all busy but you can see the NP," that is a very different message than saying, "the NP has a spot available." The tone is set first of all with the secretaries and how they approach it. Our secretaries are very supportive of the NPs, and they do a very good job of directing patients and making them see the positive aspects of seeing an NP. The nurse practitioners' ability to see newborns in the hospital is helpful. The NPs also participate in the practice's prospective parent conferences. So parents meet the NPs at their initiation into the office. Therefore, they know it is expected that NPs will be participating in their care just as will the physicians. We make an effort when we see new patients to describe the NPs' role, explaining what they do in the office, their training, and that they function the way the physicians do.

We have had a couple of complaints in the past. Some patients have insisted that they will see the NP but that a physician must also see them. In these situations, we have explained that NPs discuss with the physicians any issues that they feel they cannot handle, but that otherwise they are perfectly capable of handling patient care. A few patients have called and asked that the physician review NP prescriptions. We have agreed to do this, but we reemphasize quite strongly that the NP has written out the prescription appropriately. The biggest issue generally raised is fees. Occasionally, patients will ask, "why would I see an NP instead of a doctor?" In those cases, I explain that often they do not need a doctor. While my training is more extensive than a PNP's, I do not need such advanced training to manage sore throats and ear infections. If the NPs come across a problem they are not able to handle, the physicians are there to back them up. In most cases, the NPs' training is more than adequate to deal with the general pediatric illnesses and well-child care that we see. More often, rather than globally refusing to see a NP, patients seem to select whether they see the physician versus the NP based on how serious the parents perceive their child's problem to be.

I think what is important is that we continue to assure our patients that the physicians have the utmost confidence in the NPs' capabilities and decision making. We trust that they know their limits, just as we as physicians know our limits in handling more complicated cases. We trust that the NPs will recognize when they need to consult with a physician to provide appropriate care for the patient.

THOUGHTS ON CURRENT AND FUTURE PRACTICE

As mentioned previously, Carol is one of few NPs at our hospital right now to hold privileges in the pediatrics department. Her application for these hospital privileges actually stimulated the department to look at its policies for credentialing nonphysician providers. It then sparked a whole reevaluation of the department's use of providers other than physicians. Carol has also recently been working with the insurance companies and health maintenance organizations, and we have been working with the individual practice associations that have sprung up, in an attempt to get her admitted to the panel of providers so that she can see patients and bill for them under her name rather than under the physician's name. Unfortunately, as providers, we have not gotten very far, although the state nursing associations are working on these issues and Carol continues to work closely with these associations.

We have dealt with the insurance companies by being up-front with them. The NPs are seeing patients. They practice under a physician's supervision, consistent with state law requirements, but are seeing patients independently. Some insurance companies have advised the NPs to bill under a physician's name; others have advised them to bill under their own names. In the future it is possible that insurance companies will allow NPs to bill under their own licenses but for reduced fees. As stated before, this goes against our present office policy of charging the same fees for physician and NP services.

Billing the pediatric NP visits under the physician's name has some implications in terms of managed care because labs and referrals that the NP makes are recorded under the physician's name. This makes it hard to sort out individual utilization patterns, and to determine which practitioner sent the patient for lab work or to a specialist, and creates some issues regarding patient follow-up, but in general it has worked fairly well. Sometimes we have had patients question why a lab bill came back to them in the physician's name when they saw an NP. We have had to explain that these are the insurance requirements.

We have some strong feelings about billing and insurance. The problem has to do with credibility of the individual provider. If a provider is seeing patients and is supposed to be capable of taking care of them, it is very difficult to put someone else's name on the insurance bill. While this may seem like a technicality, little things like this are important to patients because it makes them question whether they really should be seeing an NP versus a physician. At any rate, we do not have a lot of control over the insurance issues right now. In terms of administration within the practice, the NPs are usually included in all decision making regarding how the office is run, and particularly in any decisions that affect practice patterns. We feel it is important to involve the NPs in business decisions as well as in the day-to-day administration of the office.

Nursing staff issues have not been a problem in our practice. Again, this is because of the way that the PNP was introduced right from the start. It was made clear to the nurses as well as receptionists who nurse practitioners were, what they could do, and what kind of expectations the patients and staff should have concerning the NPs' practice. In other practices, however, we have seen NPs run into a wall with nursing staff in terms of staff not wanting to assist the NP in various procedures, such as giving immunizations. Again, we feel that practices can head this off by talking with people, allaying their fears, and letting them know what their expectations should be.

CONCLUSIONS

In summary, a NP and physician who are going to begin a collaborative practice need to discuss and agree upon these specific practice issues ahead of time. They need to do a lot of planning in order to make the collaboration successful, and they need to be sure the nurse practitioner is introduced to the patients and staff as a professional colleague. The nurse practitioner and physician need to understand each other's role. It is important that the physician understands the nurse practitioner's capabilities and limitations. It is especially important that the nurse practitioner work out a method for consulting with the physician on day-to-day patient issues. How such consultations are carried out is, in many ways, symbolic of the face that the practitioners seek to portray to patients.

Chapter **21**

ADOLESCENT FAMILY PRACTICE

Ann L. O'Sullivan

BACKGROUND

My professional career has been spent almost exclusively in positions that combine opportunities for practice, teaching, and research in pediatric primary care nursing. I hope to give you a sense of how my practice has evolved over the years and the degree to which my current practice and teaching have been shaped by the research that has evolved from my practice, by the evolving body of research in the field, and by changes in the regulations on the care of adolescents who become pregnant.

This chapter addresses how my research findings have changed the types of questions that I ask on my first visit with an adolescent mother and her infant, as I seek to achieve a delay in a second pregnancy. Likewise, I will address how research has shifted my focus to concern about overfeeding and obesity as a long-term issue with infants of teenage mothers, as compared to my earlier concerns about injuries from falls, burns, and ingestions. I will share also with you my newest advocacy project (Youth Aid Panel) and encourage you to look for new ways in your community to improve the health outcomes for adolescent parents and their children. This includes examining the impact of new policies at the state, local, or institutional level that have the effect of disrupting established interventions known to improve health, for example, barriers to getting well-child appointments, and issues that we appeared to have solved many years ago.

In the beginning of my career, I worked as a staff nurse at a large metropolitan children's hospital while I completed a master's program as a pediatric clinical nurse specialist. On completion of this program, I accepted a position that combined responsibility as a nurse clinician with that of instructor in the graduate division of a family nurse clinician program. At the same time, I continued a 4-hour-per-week collaborative practice with a pediatrician in order to maintain skills as a nurse practitioner. In 1978, I was accepted as a Robert Wood Johnson Foundation nurse faculty fellow, and spent the subsequent year in the Primary Care Department at the University of Maryland, School of Nursing.

It has been gratifying to continue to maintain clinical and faculty activities since completion of the fellowship program. In 1983, I was able to add research with adolescent mothers and their infants to my faculty role. My practice experiences have included those of a pediatric nurse practitioner and director of the Teen-Tot Program, while faculty activities have centered around participation in a primary care family nurse practitioner program, a pediatric nurse practitioner program, and most recently, a health leadership program. My dissertation capitalized on my clinical interests and consisted of case studies using qualitative methods of interviewing to describe how six adolescent mothers decided to return to school after the birth of their first infant. A number of individuals, including the adolescent mother, the baby's grandparents, and the mother's friends, school nurse, counselor, and gym teacher were interviewed several times until I was able to describe how the adolescent mother made decisions regarding herself and her infant.

Even after 17 years, adolescent mothers' behavior regarding returning to school, delaying second pregnancies, and providing appropriately timed immunizations for their infant continues to provide me with incredible challenges as teacher, clinician, researcher, and community advocate.

PRACTICE WITH ADOLESCENT FAMILIES

Characteristics and Components

The practice with which I am currently involved services the special needs of adolescent families. Located within the ambulatory clinic of a large teaching hospital at their satellite office just five blocks from the main hospital, the practice addresses comprehensive health needs of both the babies and mothers. Presently, most young mothers choose to use the hospital's adolescent clinic or the family planning clinic, also located at the satellite building, for their own care. Formerly funded by the Robert Wood Johnson

Foundation, May D. Rockefeller, The PEW Memorial Trust, and the National Institute of Nursing Research, the project consists of mothers and infants who attend the special care program (the Teen Mother Program) and are followed for 2 years after the birth of their infants. Infants over 2 years of age from former programs are followed on a separate day at the same setting. The level of immunization and the development of the infant, and whether the mother is immunized, has used condoms and hormonal contraception, and has delayed a subsequent pregnancy were the outcome measures at the end of each previous study. Now only the levels of immunizations for infants 2 years of age or less and for children between 3 and 6 years of age are assessed each year.

Our current caseload includes 300 mothers, 15 to 19 years of age, and their babies. The practice consists of myself, a registrar, a social worker, and a pediatrician working together in a collaborative practice arrangement for infant care. Another team made up of a pediatrician, an ob-gyn nurse practitioner, and a social worker give care to the mothers.

Patients see either the pediatrician or the nurse practitioner on their first visit to the clinic, which takes place 2 weeks after discharge of the baby from the hospital. This visit is scheduled in order to make an early assessment of the mother and baby and to provide an orientation to the health setting. The scope of the clinic services and the practice model are described, including an explanation of the home visit, if needed, to the teen mother and baby's grandmother or the women in the adolescent mother's life who help her make decisions. A 30-minute time slot is customarily set aside to allow for adequate interaction and questions. This introductory visit eases the family into the system and helps to prevent use of the emergency department for common problems such as low-grade fever, spitting up, and other primary care problems of the newborn period. An additional 30-minute visit is scheduled for the mother if she would like to be seen on the same night as her infant for her family planning visit.

Who the patient sees after that depends on which of us is free. The nurse aide, after weighing and measuring the infant, places the charts in a rack in the order of arrival at the clinic. Those families with problems with their medical assistance card coverage are seen by the social worker prior to the visit by a clinician. Occasionally, if clients ask to see one or the other of us, we accommodate that request. Then we explain our scheduling procedures to them and explain that if they want to participate in the program, it is to their advantage as well as ours that they see both nurse and physician providers. But there are just some days when somebody wants to see one or the other of us for some personal reason, and the practice group feels it necessary to meet that need.

The nature of the practice is such that probably 95% of the problems could be managed by the skill and knowledge of a nurse practitioner. Nevertheless, while the practice is wellness oriented, what we are trying to accomplish with adolescent mothers is more than providing wellness care. Within this context, and given the aura that still exists around physicians, there is a real need to have a pediatrician integrally involved in the practice. In terms of actual care, however, there is very little that differentiates the pediatrician's practice from my own, either in areas of management or referrals. This degree of overlap between the role of nurse practitioner and physician is not restricted to our practice but seems to be true with pediatric care in general. Pediatricians tend to be easier to work with than other medical providers, perhaps because of the nature of the patients served, the ambulatory work environment, and even the personal preferences of persons choosing pediatric specialization.

Consultation and Referrals Among Providers

Because of the interaction of the client with several health providers, the mechanisms for introducing new management strategies and for referrals must be explicit and adhered to by all of the practice professionals.

In the practice, both the nurse and the physician treat illnesses as they arise, and therefore there is no differentiation in who does the initial screening. Based on our practice model, the pediatrician and the nurse are expected, whenever possible, to deal with the problems at hand. One level of consultation involves the confirmation of findings that must take place during the patient encounter. For example, if I think that a burn ought to be treated with antibiotics, I seek consultation with the physician at the moment. In such a situation, the burn is a medical problem beyond my skill and knowledge and I want to make sure it is managed appropriately. Other kinds of problems for which I might seek immediate consultation include orthopedic problems of the hip or feet and suspected pneumonia in infants under 3 months of age.

A second level of consultation is that of referral to another provider during a return or subsequent visit. If a problem is not urgent and needs more than a 2-minute consultation, the client is asked to make a return visit. This situation typically arises concerning problems of toilet training, spanking, and other disciplinary issues for which the physician might schedule the next or an interim visit with the nurse practitioner. Another example in which we use purposeful alternating visits is in determining the possibility of child abuse. In such a situation, the pediatrician will finish the visit and say something like, "now the next time, I think you ought to come in and see Ann. The routine visit is scheduled for 2 months from now, but we are going to have you come back in 2 weeks because we have some concerns about the things we talked about today."

There are two major reasons for the way that referral patterns have evolved in the practice. In the first place, the pediatrician and I know and feel comfortable with each other and we recognize and capitalize on each other's strengths. Unfortunately, every time a team member changes, this trust, which forms the basis for collaborative practice, must be reestablished. Because of physician mobility and the development of a family planning practice for mothers, the practice has seen changes in pediatricians over the years. Our present pediatrician is a young woman who has two children of her own and has been with us for 3 years. Previously, two of our pediatricians were female (each staying only 6 months during their residency) and one 55-year-old male, who stayed for 3 years. Role negotiation and establishing trust in this practice is therefore a process that absorbs a large amount of both individual and group consultation time.

The second reason underlying our current referral pattern relates to the environment in which we practice. Specialty clinics are accessed only through the primary care referral, based on federally funded managed care. Because these specialty clinics are located at the main hospital, both the pediatrician and I refer problems that in other settings the pediatrician might be more prone to handle on his or her own. This has helped to establish a practice model in which the practice boundaries for the pediatrician and the nurse are virtually identical. I am not seen as less of a provider than the pediatrician because of an inability, for instance, to ligate extra digits with a suture. We both take full advantage of the available specialty support staff.

The Teaching Program

Much of what we do in management of adolescent families involves teaching, both informal (concerning issues such as feeding problems) and formal. While we have always recognized the need for strategy for formal teaching, our initial notion of how to present content has changed markedly since the inception of the program. Originally, we attempted to conduct a class at each clinic visit. We literally shut down the clinic and had the providers and the clients come into the teaching setting. Some patients came at 12:30 P.M., were seen by the social worker and pediatrician, and then attended class, which lasted from 2:00 P.M. to 3:00 P.M. Other patients came at 2:00 P.M. and had appointments scheduled following the class. Constant disruptions further added to the chaotic atmosphere. The providers were rattled, the infants exhausted, and the mothers worried about keeping their appointments. No one could pay attention to what was going on, and it just did not work.

We then tried a series of eight classes. The content was primarily a mother-infant stimulation program in which mothers were encouraged to be the primary teachers for their newborns. This series of classes covered the growth and development phase of the infant, beginning at 5 weeks to 3 months of age and continuing until the child was 14 to 16 months old.

The content was based on a series of 20 classes developed by Dr. E. Badger at the University of Cincinnati. The series has been used successfully for about 20 years in Cincinnati and has been replicated around the country. We incorporated components of those 20 classes into our series, along with additional content intended to build the adolescent mother's self-esteem and to provide additional information about contraception. The series provided for repetition of content. Infant stimulation, strategies for handling and managing a baby, and the importance of the mother as teacher were incorporated into each of the 8 sessions.

Older parents "goo" and "coo," stick out their tongues, play peek-a-boo, and generally carry on a show-and-tell scene with their children. Adolescents are too inhibited to behave this way with their newborns. It takes a lot of work to teach adolescent fathers and mothers the importance of these behaviors to their babies' development. Reinforcement of the class content, therefore, was done during each clinic visit. Regretfully, class attendance was so poor, regardless of the season or time of day, that we have returned to our earliest model of informal teaching. This teaching is done by the nurse practitioner in the clinic room based on the age of the infant present, or by a special discussion after a short video on such topics as safety, birth control, or sexually transmitted diseases. In addition, federal work-study students model appropriate play to develop fine motor and language skills for the infants and toddlers. In addition, our site has become part of the Read-Aloud program, so at each visit, from 2 weeks to 5 years, a book is given to the infant or child, with a prescription for several minutes of reading aloud each day based on the age of the child. Understanding comes in small doses and requires ongoing attention on the part of all the practice participants.

Collaborative Practice Issues

It is the nature of practice with adolescent families that they need a sense of regularity, continuity, and similar expressions of concern irrespective of who is providing their care. These attributes, therefore, become the basis for the group practice.

One of the things that people bring up frequently about interdisciplinary provider groups is that it is difficult for the client to integrate into the group and adjust to the different approaches of group members. Our clientele could, potentially, have such a difficulty but for the fact that we as a team are particularly aware of the problems inherent in interdisciplinary practice. My practice and that of the pediatrician are similar. We ask the same questions and stress the same issues. Therefore, the client has a very similar experience on each visit, and the practitioner's approach does not overwhelm the visit. It is our experience that adolescents can get used to more than one provider as long as the approach remains relatively constant.

The practice is therefore a concentrated effort on the part of four individual providers with special interest in adolescent families. If one of the providers in not interested in adolescents, the practice does not hold together. This becomes especially apparent when an alternate provider substitutes for one of us when we attend meetings or are on vacation.

The importance of uniformity of philosophy and communication style and the ability to come to some general consensus on the management of adolescents are especially visible during the postsession conferences. At the end of each clinic session, the physician and nurse practitioner sit down and go over all of the charts of the families who have been seen that evening to identify problems that have come up since the past visit and to identify special resources that might be needed. We also meet to share information obtained by the social worker, the registrar, and other providers, since by sharing we are able to pull together information not necessarily available to each individual provider.

The decision-making process in the postsession conferences is very fluid. The primary care providers take turns presenting what they have found on history and physical examination of the infant and the psychosocial information they have gotten from the mother. The social worker and registrar add to that profile. Subsequent discussion is aimed at resolving differences in management styles. Sometimes the nurse practitioner or physician is more alarmed by a lack of weight gain or an actual loss of weight than another provider. Sometimes I may want to bring someone back in 2 weeks and the pediatrician would not bring the patient back for 4 weeks. Provider differences in dealing with clinical problems usually are resolved in some compromise agreement. Sometimes it is the nurse who is pushing toward acceptance of his of her position on an issue, and sometimes it is the pediatrician, depending on the issue. The important determinants of the process rest on the ego strengths of the participants. Disagreement is healthy. When my decisions are questioned, it does not mean that the other person is challenging my overall ability or me as a person. Rather, the challenge is to my knowledge or skill in handling a specific incident, and if I am unable to substantiate my position, then the challenge is warranted. The same is obviously true when the nurse practitioner questions the pediatrician's actions. But you cannot challenge people nor can you yourself be challenged unless the participants feel competent in their practice and comfortable with themselves.

The issue of competency and comfort within true, interdisciplinary practice is one that must be addressed from the provider's initial contact with the practice. Practice positions must be filled by people who hold similar practice philosophies. During the hiring process, it is important to identify what the practice group should look like, including the expectations for nurse practitioner, pediatrician, social worker, and registrar. Professional competency, personal self-confidence, trust, and communication are equally important attributes for successful interdisciplinary practice.

Research Findings From 17 Years of Practice

Since 1983, our team has promoted positive parenting by adolescents, particularly adolescent mothers. In the most recent study, we defined this for adolescent mothers as having up-to-date immunization for their infant, and themselves. In addition, we worked with the adolescent mothers to delay repeat pregnancies for the next 18 months in order to enable them to return to school or work, have their uterus return to a prepregnant state, and avoid caring for two infants at the same time.

After four randomly assigned control group studies, we can say that with intensive outreach and follow-up on missed primary care visits, all infants can be up-to-date on their immunizations. And our last project confirmed that we can achieve the same results with up-to-date immunizations for the adolescent mother, when a team provides family planning care for the mother at the same site, but not the same team of providers as the primary care provider for the infant.

But we also found, in our second research project from 1987–1989, that without a case manager/outreach worker on the team, the immunizations will not be current for the infants. And again in 1999–2001, we found that without the services of a case manager/outreach workers, immunization rates of completion dropped by 33%.

New findings from our recent project confirm that five variables differentiate a teen mother at increased risk for a second pregnancy in the next 18 months. These variables include teen mothers who (1) repeated two or more grades in school, (2) never used birth control before their current attempt, (3) never had an abortion, (4) never were injured in a fight (not the teens who run the streets and are subjected to violence), and (5) quit smoking with their pregnancy (a teen mother who took on the parent role early in the pregnancy and wants to be the best mother possible).

Now that we know these five variables, I can use them in my initial assessment of a first-time adolescent mother and her infant in order to alert her to the number of risk factors she has of becoming pregnant in the next 18 months.

Data gathered on injuries to the infants of our adolescent mothers from 1983 to 1996 document that falls, burns, and ingestions were the most frequently noted physical injuries in our teen mother and infant projects. The risk of injury to the infants of urban adolescent mothers was found to be no greater than the risk of infant injury in their community in general (O'Sullivan & Schwarz, 2000).

Perception of Primary Care Practice

Although I am enjoying pediatric practice, I do not think that one can do primary care nursing 9 to 5, 5 days a week. There is a tendency to get bored with full-time practice. When you have seen 98 mothers or young children, and number 99 comes through the door on Friday afternoon at 3 o'clock, it is extremely difficult to listen attentively to the problems at hand. I do not mean to imply that primary care is less energizing for nurses than for other providers. Rather, any full-time practice can become routine or unsatisfying unless, of course, you view it as just a day's work and do not aspire to do anything more. When you do the same job day in and day out, there is a tendency to become stagnant, and your inquisitive tendencies are blunted.

If physicians are more likely than nurses to find satisfaction in full-time practice, their motivation often stems from financial incentives, incentives not operative for most nurses in primary care practice. Furthermore, physicians are more socialized than nurses to engage in entrepreneurial activities. They recognize that in order to develop an ongoing practice, it is necessary to establish a rapport with patients. While some physicians establish rapport because they genuinely care for people, others become somewhat artificial and theatrical in their approach, feeling that this is necessary in order to keep patients.

Lacking the financial incentives, nurses need to seek other ways of making practice exciting and varied. Special projects often serve this purpose. A project, whether administrative, clinical, or teaching, such as precepting students, helps to maintain enthusiasm about practice. Similarly, it is important to develop a special clinical interest, for example, new mothers, single parents, divorced couples, or children of divorced couples. In my own situation, my interest in adolescent families enriches my practice and involves me in new areas of knowledge and with new groups of practice. As a consultant to a national study examining nursing in hospitals, I had the opportunity to speak with staff nurses throughout the country. I was impressed with the differences in the attitudes of those nurses who only did their job and those who took on additional activities, such as committee work. When you give more, you feel better, and you learn more.

For the past 2 years, I have participated in a youth aid panel, a juvenile diversion program that gives first-time juvenile criminal offenders (10–17 years of age) the option of appearing before a panel of community volunteers rather than entering the juvenile court system. A juvenile who completes the contractual obligations imposed by the panel will avoid the stigma and possible adverse effects of a criminal record. Juveniles who fail to complete their obligations are referred to court for criminal prosecution. Unlike the traditional methods of intervention in which the courts assume the decision-making process, the youth aid panel involves the juvenile's family and community in the contracting process. This approach is critical to the prevention and rehabilitation goals that underlie the program. This kind of intervention provides a swift and meaningful community response to delinquent behavior. The key element of this diversion program is to make juveniles understand the seriousness of their actions and the effect that the crime has on their families, their community, and themselves. Juveniles are given a one-time opportunity to participate in the program. The juveniles and their families are very similar to the ones I see in a clinical setting and are often in need of additional education and health services. The program allowed me to learn a great deal more about the community, and I was able to bring a list of resources from the clinical practice setting to the community panel.

While stagnation and job burnout may occur regardless of setting, the problem is more evident in primary care because of the character of most nurse practitioners' practice. In contrast to hospitals, where the routine is less predictable and the patient problems more varied, nurse practitioners in ambulatory settings draw strength and rewards from patients whom they come to know over time. For example, primary care providers for patient populations with chronic illness see their patients frequently, and the patients make the providers feel needed. On the other hand, nurse practitioners who work primarily with well populations—for example, well children and young adults who have episodic and infrequent contacts with a health provider—may not feel as much satisfaction with their practice. For these reasons, it is especially important for nurses in primary care to seek out alternative activities that provide a sense of reward, satisfaction, and recognition.

FUTURE OF PRIMARY CARE PRACTICE

The future of primary care practice for nurses is greatly dependent on the positive resolution of reimbursement issues and prescription issues. Without reimbursement and prescriptive authority, it will become increasingly difficult to sustain nurse practitioners in traditional ambulatory practices. There are already limited job opportunities in some states and in health maintenance organizations, clinics, and the few remaining private physicians' offices. While jobs are still available in rural areas, these too will become scarcer as physicians redistribute from urban to rural settings in search of new practice opportunities.

Nevertheless, there are several trends that may increase future employment opportunities for nurse practitioners.

In the first place, the possibilities for transferring the knowledge and skill gained in primary care into settings that have not traditionally provided health care have increased over the last few years. In truth, the potential practice options are as yet unknown for those nurses sufficiently creative to exploit corporate, industry, community, and church interest in providing health promotion, disease prevention screening, and education for their constituencies.

Secondly, while some nurse practitioners continue to seek work as generalists, there is increasing interest in specialization within primary care. As people familiarize themselves with one area of knowledge, their interests tend to narrow. Typically, nurses have more than one practice interest during the course of their professional careers. In essence, they become specialists in several areas of practice. With each shift in emphasis, they draw on old knowledge, the increasing self-confidence that comes with experience, and the ability to engage in life-long learning gained in their generalist preparation. For example, within my area of practice, I have specialized in the care of the infants and children of adolescent mothers. Truancy and obesity, by necessity, have become areas of special interest to me. Yet, even within this focus, there is ample opportunity for further specialization, not only because of increasing genetic-physical-biological knowledge, but also because of the need to consider changes in psychological and cultural responses in managing adolescent families.

Regardless of practice setting, the notion of flexibility is crucial to nursing practice. One of the positive results of shifting interests among nurses is the recognition that we can never have, nor do we need, all of the answers. I take the position that when I am in a new practice setting, professionals and clients alike have a responsibility to help me learn those things that will help meet their needs. I have become increasingly confident in admitting the things I do not know and seeking answers from others. A spirit of trust, cooperation, and candidness between client and provider is crucial if nurses are to maintain the level of good will that currently surrounds the delivery of primary care.

Another area of collaboration is the use of nurses with primary care skills in tertiary care settings. Nurses can work within institutions on designated units and assume the same authority and responsibility for caseloads of clients that they have had in ambulatory settings, including management of ambulation, nutrition, sleep, and bowel and bladder function—care problems of interest to and best managed by nurses. One current practice in tertiary settings is for nurses with various specialty interests to join together in providing comprehensive care to clients in a manner similar to multispecialty physician group practices. We look to nursing to provide for the whole patient and family. On the other hand, it is unrealistic to expect each individual nurse to be uniformly competent in all areas of practice. Nurses whose skills and interests complement each other should team together.

For example, a primary and tertiary care nurse could assume joint responsibility for a caseload of patients. They would make rounds together and divide the work based on their specialty interests. The tertiary care nurse would assume the major responsibility during the critical care phase of the hospitalization, while the primary care nurse would be more involved during the recovery phase. The services rendered would be documented, and billing would reflect both nurses' contributions and time expenditures.

The most exciting trend I see in practicing as a primary care provider is the use of the theories of behavioral change and the process of change coupled with improved communication skills in an effort to bring about a behavioral change for our clients.

CONCLUSIONS

There are many practice arenas that would potentially benefit from the introduction of nurses possessing primary care skills. Success in exploiting these opportunities will depend on the receptivity of nurses, agencies, and funding bodies.

REFERENCES AND BIBLIOGRAPHY

Dilulio, J., & Palubinsky, B. Z. (1997, Summer). How Philadelphia salvages teen criminals. *City Journal,* 27–40.

Final report on "A Family Model for Teenage Pregnancy Prevention." (1998). National Institute of Nursing Research. (R01NR03565-01). Bethesda, MD: National Institutes of Health.

Final report on "A Trial of Health Promotion with Teenage Mothers." (1993). Philadelphia: Pew Foundation.

Johnson, M., & O'Sullivan, A. L. (2002). The advocate: Children and the courts—Advocacy roles for pediatric nurses. *Journal of the Society of Pediatric Nursing, 7,* 171–174.

O'Sullivan, A. L., & Schwarz, D. (2000). Preventing injuries to infants of adolescent mothers. *Nurse Practitioners Forum, 11*(2), 124–131.

ASSOCIATED WEB SITES

http://www.advocatesforyouth.org
http://www.iwannaknow.org
http://www.hometown.aol.com/mnn1121
http://www.teenshealth.org
http://www.teenpregnancy.org
http://aspe.hhs.gov/hsp/teen/intro.htm
http://www.noah-health.org/english/pregnancy/teenpreg.html
http://www.ama-assn.org/ama/pub/article/3216-6207.html
http://www.noapp.org

PART IV

PAYMENT, POLICY, AND POLITICS

In the midsection of this book, clinicians referred to how their practices are influenced by federal and state regulatory policies. Payment, scope of practice, prescriptive privileges, autonomy, and workforce environments all contribute to a burden of complexity that threatens to limit rather than facilitate innovative health care practice. This is most true for advanced practice nurses, who are uniquely successful in pushing the boundaries of the nursing profession. In this final section, we present four chapters that inform readers about issues that will enable advanced practice nurses to control their practice, move forward, and not allow regulation to impede or determine the boundaries of practice.

Sullivan-Marx and Keepnews, two leading authorities on payment for advanced practice nursing, bring clarity to the vast subject of payment and reimbursement that has leapt forward since the last edition. Achieving Medicare provider status in 1997 opened many new doors for advanced practice nurses in all settings, geographic areas, and age groups and challenged the nature of business and collaborative employment relationships. Advanced practice nurses will find this chapter to be an up-to-date and comprehensive discussion of payment and practice issues.

Similarly, Porcher presents the political landscape of state, national, and professional regulation for nurse practitioners. This chapter provides a roadmap for a beginning or seasoned nurse practitioner to navigate the ever-changing licensing and certification issues. Both historical and current context is described to give readers a fresh perspective on the dynamics of regulation.

In the third chapter, Linda Aiken, a preeminent researcher and leader of nursing and health policy presents her views on workforce and policy influences for advanced practice nursing. Her writings hearken back to the essays in the beginning of this book as she presents three myths that misinform health policy regarding advanced practice nursing. By deconstructing myths regarding shortages, oversupply, and demand for advanced practice nurses, Aiken provides a synthesis of politics, policy, and economics that will reassure and excite the reader.

The final chapter, on academic nursing practice has been significantly revised from the previous edition. In this powerful new version, Evans, Jenkins, and Buhler-Wilkerson reenvision the tripartite mission of schools of nursing as a more complete integration and institutionalization of academic nursing practice reflecting the intentional convergence of research, education, and clinical care. The authors posit that this is a moment of unprecedented opportunity and challenge because there are funds for research and clinical practice and societal recognition of the contribution of nursing. However, the history of and support for academic nursing is far from the benchmarks set by academic medicine.

Together these chapters comprise a comprehensive resource that will motivate readers to overcome challenges for advanced nursing practice and provide the details necessary to do so.

SYSTEMS OF PAYMENT FOR ADVANCED PRACTICE NURSES

Eileen M. Sullivan-Marx and David Keepnews

I n an era of rapid fluctuation in the business and financing of health care, all health care professionals must have skills enabling them to take advantage of practice opportunities and also to overcome threats to their practices. As autonomous providers of health care and members of interdisciplinary teams, nurse practitioners (NPs) and other advanced practice nurses (APNs) make significant contributions in all sectors of health care delivery. With the passage of the Balanced Budget Act of 1997, all advanced practice nurses achieved Medicare professional provider status. With this status came responsibilities for APNs to develop new skills to meet growing demands in practice administration, accurate billing and documentation, and contract negotiation. The purpose of this chapter is to provide the context in which payment policies were developed and an overview of current health care payment structures for APNs.

BACKGROUND

By gaining direct Medicare reimbursement status in 1998, APNs became part of mainstream health care payment. Achieving this status helped to further establish APNs as legitimate independent providers of primary and specialty care. Subsequently, new advanced nursing practices in in-home

391

primary care, acute care, mental health care, and gerontological care have emerged (see chapters 6 and 17). However, despite abundant research demonstrating quality and efficacy of advanced practice nurses, barriers remain that impede utilization of advanced practice nurses in mainstream health care delivery and stifle development of innovative care models (Medicare Payment Advisory Commission [MedPAC], 2002; Sekschenski, Sansom, Bazell, Salmon, & Mullan, 1994).

Baer (1993) noted that advanced practice nurses have the knowledge, and thus the authority and autonomy, to practice. Society, however, has struggled with the recognition of the advanced practice nurse's authority in the health care environment. Payment is one major method used by society to overtly recognize a professional group's authority to practice. Barriers to payment for advanced practice nurses, therefore, often reflect a struggle over professional issues such as scope of practice, prescriptive authority, educational preparation, professional certification, and economic competition. Consequently, legislative and policy initiatives for reimbursement of nurse practitioners developed in a piecemeal fashion and vary from state to state (Abood & Keepnews, 2000; Pearson, 2002). Advanced practice nurses need to be aware that practice and payment are intertwined, requiring ongoing vigilance by nurses and nursing organizations to maintain and expand nursing's contribution to health care delivery.

Regardless of existing barriers to payment, many changes in health care present opportunities for nurse practitioners and advanced practice nurses, including primary care, specialty care, home care, and long-term care (Burl, Bonner, Rao, & Khan, 1998; Hooker & McCaig, 2001; Kane, Flood, Keckhaver, Bershadsky, & Lum, 2002; Mundinger et al., 2000). Attention to the economic forces at work in health care and development of business skills are crucial if advanced practice nurses are to take full advantage of opportunities.

PAYMENT MECHANISMS FOR ADVANCE PRACTICE NURSES

Although advanced practice nurses continue to slowly develop independent nurse-managed businesses, they are most commonly employees in a health care professional group or health system and receive salaries and benefits from their employer. Salaries are based on revenues generated by APNs as well as on the value that they bring to a practice setting in quality, cost, and access to services. Reimbursement or payment for services provided by APNs occurs through several mechanisms. In managed care plans, APNs may receive payment as an identified provider for a panel of patients. APNs who are not identified as the primary provider of care but are employed by a professional practice group receive payment through their employer's managed care arrangement. For example, if an APN is an employee in an independent practice association (IPA) that has a contract with a managed care plan for capitated payment for a group of patients or has an established fee schedule with a managed care plan, the APN's services are covered as part of the professional group's contract.

In the Medicare Part B payment structure, APNs can receive payment for their services in all sites and geographic areas in two ways. First, APNs can bill directly for their services and receive direct reimbursement at 85% of the prevailing physician rate (65% for certified nurse-midwives). Secondly, services provided by APNs may be billed "incident to" physician services at 100% of the physician rate. Incident to billing has specific requirements and is only applicable to nonhospital settings when the physician is available on site. APN services may also be included in Medicare Part A payment to hospitals, skilled nursing facilities, and home care and hospice agencies. Further, each state determines billing regulations for APNs for the Medicaid program and private payer systems (MedPAC, 2002). In the following sections, each of these reimbursement systems and mechanisms is discussed in greater detail.

Managed Care

Consumers and Managed Care

In the late 1990s, there were reports of patients who were most sick switching from managed care arrangements to fee-for-service plans under Medicare (Morgan, Virnig, DeVito, & Persily, 1997). Policy observers suggested that the pendulum had swung from the extreme of excessive care in the fee-for-service era toward far too little care in a managed care era and that the pendulum will soon return to a midpoint of appropriate care (Ginzberg & Ostow, 1997). Over 70% of Americans' health care plans are now covered by some form of managed care (Randel, Pearson, Sabin, Hyams, & Emanuel, 2001).

Consumers continue to express concern through legislative, legal, and ethical venues about the access to and quality of care received from managed care organizations. Resource limits are an integral part of managed care's approach to provide care that is appropriate and cost-effective. American consumers commonly view any limits as a loss of their right to health care. Such views are confounded by escalating media attention on the conflicting scientific research regarding risks and benefits of preventive screening and treatment of diseases. In addition, less attention by the public has been given to the source of managed care policies, those paying for health care, namely, federal and state government and employers (Randel et al., 2001).

Aided by physicians who believed their provider role of advocating for patients was being limited, consumers have urged state legislators to regulate managed care organizations through patients' bill of rights legislation. More directly, patients have also filed lawsuits that ultimately may force managed care to become more forthright in contracts regarding coverage for consumers and increase consumer satisfaction and quality of care (Havighurst, 2001). Patient bill of rights legislation generally (1) includes provisions for a process for consumers to appeal the decisions of managed care organizations, (2) prescribes the availability of care, and (3) requires managed care organizations to pay for certain emergency services (Annas, 1997). In addition, projects to approach managed care problems such as ethical dilemmas, that is, a "conflict in values as the country changes from a patient-centered to a population-centered approach to health care" (Randel et al., 2001, p. 44) have increased understanding, facilitated organizational adjustments, empowered consumers and professionals, and identified best practices in confidential data keeping and coordination of end-of-life care (Randel et al., 2001).

Advanced practice nurses must understand the dynamics in financial, clinical, and administrative agendas in managed care to present themselves as cost-effective and quality-of-care providers. They must recognize, moreover, that managed care is driven by enrollment contracts with employers and consumers. In an environment in which consumers and managed care organizations are less aware of the contributions of APNs or view the APN as an uncommon entity who happens to work with a physician, APNs will have difficulty presenting themselves as a marketable alternative to physicians and may be more successful arguing for their role in value-added services that ultimately benefit employers, consumers, and managed care. In environments in which the APN role is well known by consumers and there is a physician shortage or limitation in access to care, APNs can be successful in marketing themselves as a legitimate provider of primary or specialty health services.

Role of APNs in Managed Care

Changes in health care financing and the restructuring of delivery systems over the last decade have curtailed "solo" practice arrangements and emphasized employment and contractual arrangements for most professional providers. Managed care includes many models that integrate elements of health care delivery and payment (see chapter 7). Managed care models are structured so that financial risk and responsibility for patient outcomes range across a continuum. Preferred provider organizations (PPOs) incur the lowest financial risk to providers, while group health maintenance organization (HMO) models incur the highest financial risk and greatest responsibility for outcomes. Clinician providers who remain independent practitioners, such as in IPAs, and who contract with managed care payers assume a moderate financial risk (Abood & Keepnews, 2000; Buppert, 1999).

In the 1990s, IPAs and PPOs emerged as the predominant physician practice arrangement in managed care, while advanced practice nurses began to develop entrepreneurial independent nursing practices and nurse-managed centers (Lang, Sullivan-Marx, & Jenkins, 1996). (See chapter 25.) Despite efforts to establish independent nursing practices, however, most NPs and APNs are employed by health systems or professional practice groups. As employees, NPs and APNs are one step removed from decisions made by business managers and partners in professional groups or large health systems and often are forced to rely on their physician partners to speak for their issues. It is a daunting but critical task that NPs make certain that health system executives understand APN billing and capture all possible revenues that are appropriate. In addition, APNs must know how to present the value-added contributions of APNs and contribute to the organization's mission through participation on committees relevant to practice and payment.

Advanced practice nurses have been utilized in managed care organizations for preventive services, primary care, coordination of care, and managing the comprehensive care of high-risk and high-need groups. APNs have contributed to cost-effectiveness in managed care by preventing readmissions to hospitals and emergency department visits, reducing patient complications, and providing alternatives to nursing home admissions (Burl et al., 1998; Kane et al., 2002; Lang et al., 1996; Mundinger et al., 2000). APNs who have been successful in negotiating contracts with managed care organizations have done so with careful preparation. APNs have been successful in negotiating with managed care organizations when they identify a need that they can fill with a specific group of patients/enrollees. Strategies for success include meeting with managed care administrators, partnering with other health professionals and health systems, using political support and legal advice, and persisting in the face of denial (Buppert, 2000; "Nurse Practitioner Entrepreneurs," 2002).

Financial Arrangements for APNs

Advanced practice nurses have had a variety of financial arrangements with managed care organizations, ranging from full risk-bearing to receiving a fee for the service provided. Compensation of APNs by managed care organization varies from salary arrangements to reimbursement on a per-member, per-month basis. In the current environment of health care financial restructuring and managed care market penetration, there is considerable variation in the interpretation of state legislation regarding payment for APN services. Decisions to include APNs as providers for a panel of patients are made at the business corporate level and are not necessarily regulated by federal or state law. Efforts to include all groups of health professionals, including APNs, as qualified providers in legislation directed at managed care organizations and patients' bill of rights have been introduced in the U.S. Congress and several states. Such provisions in state insurance laws prohibit managed care organizations from excluding any provider licensed to provide services under state law based solely on type of licensure.

Advanced practice nurses are finding it necessary to work toward passing legislation on a state-by-state basis to ensure inclusion of their services in managed care plans. Twenty-four states and the District of Columbia have enacted legislation enabling some level of inclusion of advanced practice nurses in managed care contracting or payment. Seven other states have legislation allowing APNs to participate in Medicaid managed care plans. Specifically, in Texas and Delaware, HMOs are prohibited from discriminating against APN services; New York has legislation stating that nurse practitioners are qualified as primary care gatekeepers; and Arkansas has included advanced practice nurses as providers in the 1995 Patient Protection Act (Pearson, 2002).

Issues that APNs must address in negotiation with managed care organizations, health systems, or professional practice groups include the following:

- Contract between the APN and employer and payer
- Risk sharing
- Clinical privileges
- Malpractice insurance
- Percentage of payment to collaborating physician
- Participation in bonus payment plans

Medicare

Background

Medicare provides basic health insurance to Americans over the age of 65, and those persons who are disabled or have end-stage renal disease (approximately 38 million Americans). Medicare spending in 2001 represented 13% of the federal budget in the amount of $238 billion and accounted for 19% of the national spending on personal health services. Medicare payments are highly skewed: a small percentage of beneficiaries each year receive the greatest portion of expenditures to cover services. In 1997, 15% of Medicare beneficiaries accounted for 75% of spending (MedPAC, 2001).

Medicare consists of two parts. Part A covers payment made to hospitals, skilled nursing facilities, home care agencies, and hospice. Medicare Part B covers payment to professional providers. Part A is provided to Medicare beneficiaries as an entitlement program through a federal payroll tax; Part B is provided by a voluntary supplementary medical insurance financed by Medicare beneficiary premiums and general tax revenues. Nursing services provided in a hospital system, skilled nursing facility, home health agency, and hospice are covered under Medicare Part A. Medicare Part B covers services of professional providers, including physicians, podiatrists, nurse practitioners, clinical nurse specialists, certified nurse-midwives, certified registered nurse anesthetists, physician assistants, chiropractors, clinical psychologists, social workers, physical and occupational therapists, nutritionists, and speech-language pathologists and audiologists. Medicare Part B also covers laboratory services, outpatient hospital care, and some home health care and supplies (MedPAC, 2001).

In 1983, federal efforts to address growth in Medicare Part A (hospital) expenditures led to the development of a prospective payment system (PPS) based on diagnosis-related groups (DRGs). Following prospective payment enactment, hospital lengths of stay shortened, and care provided on a short-stay or outpatient basis increased. Some have argued that efforts such as PPS only shift the cost of care rather than address core causes of cost inflation (Morgan et al., 1997). Significant shifts in population growth, cost of labor and supplies, and expansion of technology and specialty services further contributed to health care cost inflation.

Federal payment reforms to control rapidly escalating costs of physician services in Medicare Part B began with policy review under the Physician Payment Review Commission (PPRC) in the 1980s. Recommendations from the PPRC, in 1989, led to Public Law 101-239, the Omnibus Budget Reconciliation Act of 1989 (OBRA-89) that established the Medicare Fee Schedule, which sets fees based on resources used. The resource-based relative value scale (RBRVS) is a methodology developed by health economists and adopted for use in the Medicare Fee Schedule by P.L. 101-239 (Hsiao, Braun, Yntema, & Becker, 1988). Prior to this law, physician payment was based on "usual and customary" fees established by regional carriers for Medicare.

Medicare Fee Schedule

In the Medicare Fee Schedule, fee-for-service payment for services provided by health professionals is based on the resource costs used to provide the service. Each service is classified according to the Current Procedural Terminology (CPT) coding system developed by the American Medical Association (AMA) in 1966 (AMA, 2002b). There are over 7,000 CPT codes, of which the most common are the Evaluation and Management Services such as office or outpatient visits for a new patient (99201–99205), ranging from low (1) to high (5) in both complexity and time (AMA, 2002b). To establish the allowable payments for a service, the Center for Medicare & Medicaid Services (CMS) develops a fee schedule for each CPT code using RBRVS methodology and based on recommendations from the AMA Relative Value Update Committee (RUC), professional organizations, carriers, and the public. The fee is established by accounting for the relative work value of the service, the practice cost, and professional liability insurance, each adjusted for geographic location, and using a dollar conversion factor (see Figure 22.1).

Although Medicare has increasingly expanded participation for beneficiaries in capitated payment and managed care plans, fee-for-service plans (in which the provider of the service is directly reimbursed) continue to be a common payment mechanism in Medicare, particularly in rural areas and for the sickest beneficiaries (MedPAC, 2001). In addition, the resource based relative values scale is used by managed care systems to set fee schedules, measure clinician productivity, and analyze value of services provided.

Current Procedural Terminology and Other Billing Coding Systems.   The AMA established the Current Procedural Terminology (CPT) coding system in 1966 to classify physician procedures following the inception of Medicare. CPT codes are established and updated annually by the AMA CPT Editorial Panel. Requests for additions to the CPT coding system are made to the AMA and referred to the Editorial Panel for approval. Since 1993, the American Nurses Association has been a member of the Health Care Professional Advisory Committee to the CPT Editorial Panel. Currently, the CPT Editorial Panel is composed of representatives of the AMA, medical specialty societies, and health professionals (AMA, 2002b).

One of the criticisms of the CPT codes is their limitation to describe only physician services and not the full range of health services provided by, and reimbursed to, all health professionals (Henry, Holzemer, Randell, Hsieh, & Miller, 1997; U.S. Department of Health and Human Services, 1992). There are CPT codes that describe preventive services and counseling; however, they do not specifically describe nursing practice and are

2002 MEDICARE FEE SCHEDULE

Relative Work Value =	0.67
Geographic adjustment =	x 1.023 = 0.68541
Relative Practice Expense Value (nonfacility) =	0.62
Geographic adjustment =	x 1.023 = 0.63426
Relative Value Professional Liability Insurance =	0.03
Geographic adjustment =	x 1.023 = 0.03069
Total Adjusted Relative Value	1.35036
Conversion Factor	x $35.12
Medicare Allowable Charge	$47.43
Nurse Practitioner Fee (85%)	$40.32

FIGURE 22.1   CPT Code 99213, office visit, established patient, level 3, Philadelphia, Pennsylvania.

not generally reimbursed by payers. In response to these criticisms, in 1993 the AMA included other health professionals in the process of developing new CPT codes. Since 1993, the American Nurses Association has had a representative on the Health Care Professional Advisory Committee (CPT HCPAC) to the CPT Editorial Panel and been directly involved in the process of CPT code development and revision.

In addition to CPT codes, services are also billable to Medicare and other payers by using the Health Care Common Procedural Coding System (HCPCS), which includes CPT codes, some codes from the International Classification of Diseases (ICD) system, and other health care codes developed to describe technology and supportive care services. HCPCS codes are generally supportive services and supplies but may have relative work values associated when applicable, such as physician (or practitioner) review of an electrocardiogram with interpretation (G007) (Abood & Keepnews, 2000). ICD codes are largely diagnostic codes but may include some procedures; they do not have assigned relative work values for Medicare purposes. These classification systems were developed for reimbursement of physician services but have been used for all providers (e.g., psychologists, physical therapists) who may provide billable services.

RBRVS Process.   A process to establish relative work values using resource based relative value scale methodology was mandated by Congress in 1988. With the Health Care Financing Administration, the American Medical Association and other medical societies established a process to develop relative work values for each CPT code in 1990. AMA established the Relative Value Update Committee (RUC), composed of AMA members and medical specialty societies to establish a method for professional societies to survey clinicians regarding the value of the work, review the results of surveys, and make recommendations to HCFA/CMS. In 1993, organizations that represent other health care professionals who bill Medicare were added to the RUC process, including the American Nurses Association.

Requests for new or adjusted relative work values for CPT codes are initially addressed through the AMA's relative value update process. Professional specialty societies or groups, the CPT Editorial Panel, or CMS may identify the need for relative work values changes. Evidence to establish or alter relative work values are developed by surveys of practicing clinicians who rate the value of work for a specific CPT code in comparison to a related CPT code using magnitude estimation methodology. Relative work values are scaled estimates of the work involved for a specific code that take into account (1) time, (2) technical skill and physical effort, (3) mental effort and judgment, and (4) psychological stress associated with patient risk (AMA, 2002a). Specialty societies or professional organizations present findings from surveys and their recommendations to either the AMA's Relative Value Update Committee (RUC) or the Health Care Professional Advisory Committee (HCPAC). The HCPAC generally reviews relative work values for services provided by health professionals other than physicians, such as physical therapy services. Recommendations from the RUC and HCPAC are forwarded to CMS. Relative values for the work, practice expense, and professional liability components of a CPT coded service are totaled and multiplied by a conversion factor to determine the allowable Medicare charge for each CPT coded service. Final recommendations for the Medicare Fee Schedule are published by CMS in the *Federal Register* following a public comment period.

The American Nurses Association (ANA) has a representative on both the AMA CPT Editorial Panel and Relative Value Update Committee Process. ANA has a voting seat on the Health Care Professional Advisory Committee that makes relative work value recommendations for health professional services to CMS. ANA also has a voting seat on the Practice Expense Subcommittee of the RUC that in 2000 was charged with making recommendations for relative values for the practice expense component of the Medicare Fee Schedule. This committee establishes relative practice expense values for CPT coded services. The greatest component of practice expense is salaries for nursing and medical assistant personnel.

Since 1995, advanced practice nurses have been directly involved in the development of relative work values for primary care services, psychiatric-mental health services, and specialty codes in critical care, surgical procedures, and continence management. Through the American Nurses Association and other nursing organizations, nurse practitioners and advanced practice nurses have completed surveys to develop relative work values for evaluation and management services and were coalition participants with primary care and mental health professionals to develop new and accurate relative work values for evaluation and management codes, including home visits (Sullivan-Marx & Maislin, 2000).

Direct Reimbursement for APNs under Medicare Part B

Amendments to the Social Security Act passed by Congress and signed by President Clinton as part of the Balanced Budget Act (BBA) of 1997 (Public Law 105-33) gave direct Medicare reimbursement (at 85% physician rate) to nurse practitioners, clinical nurse specialists, and physician assistants regardless of geographic setting. This long-sought legislation was an important opportunity for nurse practitioners and clinical nurse specialists to bill directly for their services in all geographic areas and clinical settings. It is important to note that prior to the BBA of 1997, incremental legislative and policy changes over 15 years were in place allowing nurse practitioners to bill for Medicare services in rural areas and nursing facilities and allowing clinical nurse specialists to bill in rural areas at 85% of the prevailing physician rate. The BBA of 1997 broadened the opportunities for billing by removing geographic area limits and removing limits on direct billing by setting. Billing for NPs and clinical nurse specialists at the lower rate of 85% of the prevailing physician rate was in place prior to the BBA of 1997 and was not changed by this legislation.

When directly billing Medicare Part B, nurse practitioners and clinical nurse specialists are required to collaborate "with a physician which the nurse practitioner or clinical nurse specialist is legally authorized to perform by the State in which the services are performed" (Social Security Act, secs. 2158, 2160).

Medicare law defines *collaboration* as "a process in which a nurse practitioner [read also clinical nurse specialist] works with a physician to deliver health care services within the scope of the practitioner's professional expertise, with medical direction and appropriate supervision as provided for in jointly developed guidelines or other mechanisms as defined by the law of the State in which the services are performed." A clinical nurse specialist, according to Section 1861 (aa) (5) (B) of the Social Security Act, is "a registered nurse and is licensed to practice nursing in the State in which the clinical nurse specialist services are performed and holds a master's degrees in a defined clinical area of nursing from an accredited educational institution. Collaboration with a physician is required for services reimbursed by Medicare even if this is not required by the state in which the service was rendered."

Reimbursement to nurse practitioners and clinical nurse specialists will be covered "only if no facility or other provider charges or is paid any amounts with respect to the furnishing of such services" (Social Security Act, sec. 1861). The intent of this provision is to ensure that Medicare will pay only once for a particular service provided by an NP or a CNS. In order to ensure correct billing procedure, nurse practitioners and clinical nurse specialists will need to be absolutely clear about the source of their salary so that their services are not considered covered under Medicare Part A and also billed under Medicare Part B. In addition to these provisions, APNs must "accept assignment" from Medicare, meaning that APNs must not bill Medicare beneficiaries for amounts greater than Medicare allowable charges for the service provided.

"Incident to" Billing Under Medicare Part B. Prior to the BBA of 1997, nurse practitioners could bill Medicare as physician employees under guidelines for services that were furnished incident to physician services. The BBA of 1997 did not remove the ability of NPs to bill Medicare using incident to mechanisms. Billing incident to in a physician's office setting reimburses the physician practice at 100% of the prevailing physician rate but requires adherence to strict guidelines and is not applicable in the hospital setting. The Medicare Part B guidelines for incident to billing are as follows:

> Incident to services must be provided by employees of a physician under the physician's direct supervision. In addition, the physician must be in the office suite while the service is being provided and be immediately available to provide assistance and direction. The physician also must have provided direct, personal professional services to initiate the course of treatment and must furnish subsequent services at a frequency consistent with active management of the course of treatment. Incident to billing is not allowed for the first visit for a new patient or for subsequent visits that present a new problem. In these cases, physicians must personally examine patients to bill for services at the physician rate; otherwise, services are billed at the nonphysician practitioner rate. (MedPAC, 2002, p. 7)

Certified Nurse-Midwives and Certified Registered Nurse Anesthetists. Certified registered nurse anesthetists (CRNAs) and certified nurse-midwives (CNMs) were not included in the BBA of 1997 legislation because separate legislation was in effect prior to this bill granting them direct Medicare reimbursement. Medicare payment to certified nurse-midwives was established by Public Law 100-203. Payment for services is at 65% of the prevailing physician rate and is made directly to the CNM. No supervision is necessary unless required by state authority. The Medicare Payment Advisory Commission has recommended that "The Congress should increase Medicare payment rates for certified nurse-midwives to 85% of the physician fee schedule. The conversion factor for physician services should be adjusted to make this change budget neutral" (MedPAC, 2002, p. 13).

Certified registered nurse anesthetists provide 65% of all anesthesia services in the United States, and 85% of anesthesia services in rural areas (National Commission on Nurse Anesthesia Education, 1990). Direct Medicare reimbursement to CRNAs was established by Public Law 99-509 in 1986. Congress authorized different payment rates in 1990 (effective in 1996) depending on whether services were medically directed. If medically directed, CRNAs receive 50% of the physician rate and the supervising anesthesiologist receives the other 50%. As of 1996, payment for nonmedically directed anesthesia services provided by a CRNA are paid at 100% of the physician rate for the same service (MedPAC, 2002).

Medicare+Choice Organizations

Medicare also contracts with 180 health plans to provide non-fee-for-service payment for care to beneficiaries under Medicare+Choice. Payment rates are set by county and modified for demographic and health status of enrollees. Medicare+Choice (M+C) plans must report annually to CMS on premiums, quality, and marketing plans. Federal regulations at 42 CFR 422.204 on provider credentialing and rights prohibit M+C from discriminating against any health care professional acting within the scope of license or certification under state law. M+C organizations, however, are not precluded from refusing to grant any health professional participation in the plan as necessary to meet the needs of the plan's enrollees. CMS allows M+C plans to provide services through a network of provider types and does not require M+C plans to include all types of providers, such as advance practice nurses (Kane et al., 2002).

Program for All-Inclusive Care for the Elderly (PACE)

The philosophy of the Program for All-Inclusive Care for the Elderly (PACE) model is to maintain older adults in the community with minimal disruption of their lives. The PACE model is based on the successful On Lok program in San Francisco, which provides a comprehensive, multidisciplinary, community-based program for older adults in their homes with capitated Medicare and Medicaid funding. Initially, a Medicare waiver program, PACE models are now a standard Medicare program (U.S. Department of Health & Human Services [U.S. DHHS], 1999). Services provided include primary and specialty care, adult day care, home care, nursing, social work, rehabilitative services, prescription drugs, and coordination of hospital and nursing home care by PACE staff. Advanced practice nurses can provide specialty as well as primary care medical services. The University of Pennsylvania School of Nursing received approval as a PACE site for its Living Independently for Elders (LIFE) Program in 1997 and provides services to frail, older adults in West Philadelphia using a nurse-managed and interdisciplinary model (see chapter 25).

Medicaid

Medicaid is a federally mandated program that guarantees health care services to low-income families with dependent children and to low-income aged and disabled individuals. Medicaid funds are provided by the federal government and administered by the states. Prior to 1989, reimbursement of advanced practice nurses varied according to individual state policy and legislation. To ensure access to primary care services for low-income families and children, the U.S. Congress passed the Omnibus Budget Reconciliation Act of 1989, establishing direct payment for pediatric and family nurse practitioners in the Medicaid program without the need for supervision or association with physicians or other health care providers. Since 1989, some states have opted to reimburse more broadly than required by federal law and to allow Medicaid payment for all nurse practitioners. Payment for services provided by CNMs has been required by federal law since 1986 (Pearson, 2002).

All states have complied with federal legislation mandating Medicaid coverage of pediatric and family nurse practitioner services in Medicaid programs. A number of states include all nurse practitioners and advanced practice nurses in coverage for their Medicaid programs. The range of payment varies from 70% to 100% of the prevailing physician rate. Twenty-one states reimburse advanced practice nurses at 100% of the physician rate (Pearson, 2002).

In efforts to control cost, many states have received Medicaid waivers under Sections 1115 and 1915 (b) of the Social Security Act to enroll all patients under managed care organizations. States may require Medicaid beneficiaries to access care through a designated primary care provider or enroll in a contracted health maintenance organization. The scope and nature of "waiver" changes vary with each state, requiring political vigilance on the part of nursing in each state to ensure inclusion of payment for services provided by advanced practice nurses (Abood & Keepnews, 2000; Buppert, 2000).

Introduction of Medicaid 1115 waivers to allow states greater control of federal Medicaid funds can potentially exclude APNs from participation as primary or identified providers in Medicaid programs. In the District of Columbia and West Virginia, Medicaid waiver programs exclude nurse practitioners as primary providers or "gatekeepers." Advanced practice nurses have needed to take political action in many states to ensure their continued inclusion in state Medicaid programs. At least eight states have legislation including nurse practitioners in Medicaid managed care plans (Pearson, 2002). Such efforts will need to continue as the federal government seeks ways to reduce costs in the Medicaid program.

Other Federal Programs

Federally Qualified Health Centers

In 1992, federally qualified health centers (FQHC) were established to provide health promotion and preventive services and access to primary care services for Medicare beneficiaries (U.S. DHHS, 1992). Federally Qualified Health Centers originated from community health centers and migrant health centers established under the Public Health Service and include any facility receiving funding from the Public Health Service Act or meeting requirements to receive a grant from this act. Clinics or facilities that meet these requirements but do not receive a public health service grant are called FQHC look-alikes. Services covered in these health centers include health promotion activities usually not covered in the Medicare program, such as annual physical examinations, health screening and diagnostic tests, immunizations, and preventive health education (U. S. DHHS, 1992). Services of "individual practitioners who may be employed in FQHCs, including . . . nurse practitioners, nurse midwives . . . may be covered under Medicare Part B" (U.S. DHHS, 1992, p. 24965). Nurse practitioners working in FQHCs, therefore, cannot also submit billing for Medicare Part B services directly (U. S. DHHS, 1992).

Military Health Insurance

Tricare, a health insurance program operated by the Department of Defense, provides coverage to active duty military personnel, their families, and retired military personnel. Tricare includes three options—Tricare

Prime (an HMO option), Tricare Extra (a PPO option), and Tricare Standard (a fee-for-service option). Tricare Standard is the old Civilian Health and Medical Program of the Uniformed Services (CHAMPUS) program.

All three options include some coverage of nurse practitioner services. Under Tricare Prime, NPs may serve as primary care managers (PCMs). NPs may also serve as preferred providers under Tricare Extra. As a fee-for-service program, Tricare Standard offers the widest choice of providers. Like CHAMPUS, its predecessor, Tricare Standard provides for payment of services by NPs (as well as psychiatric clinical nurse specialists). It does not require referral or supervision by a physician.

Federal Employee Health Benefit Plan

Federal employees can voluntarily receive health insurance by participating in the Federal Employees Health Benefit Plan (FEHBP). Two laws have mandated FEHBP coverage of services for nurses. First, in 1985, Congress mandated reimbursement to all nonphysician providers, including registered nurses, for services provided under this plan.

In 1990, Public Law 101-509 mandated direct payment to nurse practitioners, psychiatric clinical nurse specialists, and certified nurse-midwives for services provided to federal employees participating in this plan. Collaboration or supervision by any other health care provider is not required.

Traditional Indemnity Plan Reimbursement

Payment for advanced practice nurses through private indemnity plan insurance on a fee-for-service basis is regulated at the state level. In the last 20 years, nurse practitioners and other advanced practice nurses have been successful in establishing state legislation supporting reimbursement for their services. Thirty-nine states and the District of Columbia have legislation that either requires coverage or prohibits discrimination against reimbursement to nurse practitioners, certified nurse-midwives, certified registered nurse anesthetists, or psychiatric nurses for services. In three states without legislation, APNs have been able to directly negotiate reimbursement from insurance companies (Pearson, 2002).

State insurance laws address components of health care coverage that include insurers affected (nonprofit and commercial or for-profit), providers affected, or reimbursable services. State laws will vary by type of insurer and whether the benefit to be covered for advanced practice nurse services is mandatory or a mandatory option. In a mandatory option, consumers of health care must request to have APN services included in their coverage. In legislation for mandatory coverage, APN services must be included in coverage. In states where no law exists that covers APN services, APNs have negotiated individually with insurance companies for coverage of their services. Rates of reimbursement vary and may be a percentage of the prevailing physician rate (Pearson, 2002).

ISSUES WITH APNs AND PAYMENT

Medicare

One of the first attempts to ascertain the extent of use of CPT billing codes by otherwise invisible nurse specialists found that use of codes ranged from family nurse practitioners who provided 233 CPT codes to school nurses who performed 58 codes (Griffith & Robinson, 1993). In 1996, Medicare payment to nurse practitioners in the Medicare Fee Schedule was composed of those CPT codes that were directly or indirectly paid to the nurse practitioner at the time, that is, nurse practitioners who billed in rural areas or in skilled nursing facilities. Thus, the most frequently billed codes by nurse practitioners prior to the Balanced Budget Act of 1997 were nursing facility visits. Home visits (Medicare Part B for medical services provided in the home) were least frequently represented because NPs could not bill Medicare for these services except in rural areas.

Payment to advanced practice nurses through "incident to" billing appears in Medicare Claims Data as physician billed, rendering APN services invisible in the federal databases. With direct Medicare billing, APNs can now track services that are billed in federal databases and also track revenue that they have generated in a practice. Tables 22.1 and 22.2 show the ranking of the codes most frequently billed to Medicare Part B by nurse practitioners in 1998 and 1999. In 1999, the first full year that nurse practitioners were able to bill Medicare Part B, nursing facility visits were still the most frequently billed CPT code, and an office visit for a level 3 subsequent visit was the second most commonly billed code. Frequency of billing also increased almost twofold between 1998 and 1999 (U.S. DHHS, HCFA, 1998, 1999). In 2000, 57% of all codes billed by nurse practitioners were evaluation and management (E&M) codes, while 32% of clinical nurse specialist (largely psychiatric services) billable codes were E & M codes (MedPAC, 2002). Between 2000 and 2001, Medicare billing by nurse practitioners increased from $171 million to $254 million, a 49% increase. During this same period, Medicare billing by certified registered nurse anesthetists increased by only 9% from $436 million to $476 million (U.S. DHHS, HCFA, 2001). Thus, as nurse practitioners continue to set up systems for billing under their own provider identifier, rather than under a physician identifier their contribution to Medicare services is becoming clear.

TABLE 22.1   Medicare Part B Payment Data
for Nurse Practitioners, 1998

CPT code	CPT descriptor	Frequency billed
99312	Nursing Facility, level 2, established patient	216,189
99311	Nursing Facility, level 1, established patient	193,250
99213	Office Visit, level 3, established patient	166,767
99212	Office Visit, level 2, established patient	104,448
99203	Office Visit, level 3, new patient	6,336

Professional nursing organizations have established information services and hotlines for questions about correct billing procedures. Gaps in
published material on advanced practice nurse billing have been closed as
new texts have been written and general billing texts now include material
on billing for APN services. Information regarding organizations for advanced
practice nurses can be accessed on the Internet (http://www.nurse.org/
orgs.shtml). The American College of Nurse Practitioners (http://www.nurse.
org/ACNP/medicare/index.shtml\) and the American Nurses Association
(http://www.ana.org/governmentalaffairs) provide updates on payment for
APNs through list serves and Web pages. The Center for Medicare and
Medicaid Services has an extensive web site for professional providers regarding updates on fee schedules and regulations (http://www.cms.gov/physi-
cians). Also, the Medicare Professional Advisory Committee has issued reports
on Medicare billing for advanced practice nurses (http://medpac/publica-
tions/generic_report_display.cfm?report_type_id=1). APNs need to have a
working knowledge of CPT and other coding systems and understand how
to determine payment schedules for individual practices. The AMA and
other resources listed in this chapter are a good beginning to increase awareness of billing and associated fee schedules. Questions that APNs should
be able to answer in their practices include the following:

1. What specific CPT code is used for the specific services provided?
2. What documentation in the patient's record is required for the ser-
    vice that is billed?
3. When is the service provided a billable service? Or is the service
    already included in payment by another source, such as Medicare
    Part A?
4. What resources do I need so that my services are accurately and
    legally billed?

TABLE 22.2   Medicare Part B Payment Schedule
for Nurse Practitioners, 1999

CPT code	CPT descriptor	Frequency billed
99312	Nursing Facility, level 2, established patient	405,293
99213	Office Visit, level 3, established patient	403,461
99311	Nursing Facility, level 1, established patient	321,043
99212	Office Visit, level 2, established patient	218,677
99313	Nursing Facility, level 3, established patient	75,421

Fraud and Abuse

Fraud and abuse by health care providers has been the subject of increasing activity by both federal and state governments over the past several years. Government agencies have devoted increasing resources to investigation and enforcement, and recent federal legislation has increased both the breadth of practices that may be considered illegal and the penalties for violations.

The great majority of NPs are ethical, honest practitioners who would never knowingly commit fraud or abuse. Unfortunately, this is not sufficient protection. NPs need to have a working familiarity with reimbursement laws and with what they are expected to do to avoid legal or regulatory violations.

Some of the more common examples of activities that may be considered fraud or abuse include billing for services that were not actually furnished to the patient, misrepresenting the patient's diagnosis in order to justify or increase payment, misrepresenting services as being medically necessary, billing for services in excess of those needed by the patient, billing for services that were not furnished as billed (e.g., by "upcoding" to a more expensive service), and billing for services that are not covered.

Among its provisions, the federal Health Insurance Portability and Accountability Act (HIPAA) of 1996 (P.L. 104-191) introduced broad penalties for defrauding, or attempting to defraud, virtually any health plan, whether federal, state, or private. HIPAA also prohibits making knowing and willful false statements in connection with the delivery or payment of health care services. It provides for criminal penalties, including fines and prison sentences, for violation of these provisions.

HIPAA also broadened the standards under which civil penalties against providers may be imposed. A provider may be liable for submitting a claim that he or she knows *or should know* is false. If a claim is submitted in a provider's name (e.g., by a billing service), the NP's claim (even honestly) that he or she did not know that the bill reflected services that were not delivered, or that it included services billed at a higher level than actually delivered, is generally not an adequate response to allegations of fraudulent billing. This is one reason why NPs and other clinicians should be aware of what is billed under their names and provider numbers.

Although HIPAA expanded federal laws on fraud and abuse, other significant antifraud laws remain in effect. The Medicare and Medicaid Patient Protection Act of 1987 (42 U.S.C. § 1320a-7b(a)) identifies six types of conduct that are considered felonies and may result in fines of up to $25,000 and/or up to 5 years' imprisonment. Among the prohibited activities is a broadly described one: knowingly and willfully making or causing to be made any false statement or representation of a material fact in any application for any benefit under the Medicare or Medicaid program. This not only prohibits billing for services that were not provided, but also prohibits other false statements with regard to billing, and conduct related to such false statements.

The federal anti-kickback statute (42 U.S.C. § 1320a-7b(b)) prohibits knowingly and willfully offering, paying, soliciting, or receiving anything of value in order to induce furnishing of services under Medicare, Medicaid, or other state health care programs. Violating this law is a felony that is punishable by fines of up to $25,000, imprisonment of up to 5 years, and exclusion from Medicare, Medicaid, and other federal health care programs. The anti-kickback law applies to referrals (e.g., an NP paying another provider for each patient referred to the NP). But it may also apply to other arrangements, such as discounts, rebates, or other reductions in fees. The Office of Inspector General (OIG) of the U.S. Department of Health and Human Services maintains a list of "safe harbors," arrangements that will not be considered a violation of the anti-kickback law. This list is updated periodically through the federal rule-making process, and is contained in the Code of Federal Regulations at 42 CFR § 1001.952.

The federal False Claims Act (31 USC § 3729) is a major source of federal fraud and abuse activity. It imposes civil liability on anyone who submits a false or fraudulent claim paid by the government. Its reach is not limited to health care services; in fact, it was first enacted during the Civil War to address fraud by military contractors. The 1986 amendments strengthened the law and made it clear that it applied to false claims submitted to the Medicare and Medicaid programs. An important feature of the False Claims Act is the fact that it allows a private individual—known as a "qui tam relator" (or, more informally, a whistleblower)—to bring suit in federal court on behalf of the government. If the allegations are proven in court, or result in an out-of-court settlement, the qui tam relator can collect a share of the recovered damages (ranging between 15% and 30%).

Self-referral is another important area of federal enforcement activity. Federal laws (known as Stark I & II) establish limits on a physician's ability to refer patients to clinical laboratories and several other health services in which the physician (or an immediate family member) has a financial interest. The intent of these laws is to avoid referrals made for economic self-interest rather than actual patient need. As written, the laws are specific to physicians; they do not address referrals by NPs. But NPs should be aware of these laws. First, the laws express a clear policy against referring patients based on the provider's self-interest. Second, it is not outside the realm of possibility that the laws may be amended at some point in the future to address self-referral by providers other than physicians. Third, and most immediately relevant, referrals made by an NP (or a physician assistant) may invoke the Stark laws if the physician "controls or influences" the referral. The question of whether an NP is acting independently or under a physician's "control or influence" is answered by examining the specific facts and circumstances surrounding the referral.

SUMMARY

Thirty years ago advanced practice nurses were considered pioneers in health care delivery models, forging a place for themselves in primary care and specialty care. Today, inclusion of APNs in health care systems is increasingly standard practice. Consistent growth in numbers and utilization of nurse practitioners has led to the inclusion of APNs in mainstream health care payment structures. Both business and governmental models of practice have recognized the advantages of including advanced practice nurses in systems of care for cost-savings and quality outcomes. Advanced practice nurses, however, have had a steep learning curve to acquire the requisite business skills and knowledge of reimbursement relevant to their practice. Current emphasis in linking financial responsibility with provision of care and the need to address care of underserved and specialized groups in society have made it inevitable that APNs take an active part in policy and business in order to continue as essential and viable providers of care.

REFERENCES

Abood, S., & Keepnews, D. (2000). *Understanding payment for advanced practice nursing services. Volume One: Medicare reimbursement.* Washington, DC: American Nurses Publishing.

American Medical Association. (2002a). *Medicare RBRVS: The physician's guide.* Chicago: Author.

American Medical Association. (2002b). *Physician's current procedural terminology.* Chicago: Author.

Annas, G. J. (1997). Patients' rights in managed care: Exit, voice, and choice. *New England Journal of Medicine, 337,* 210–215.

Baer, E. D. (1993). Philosophical and historical bases of primary care nursing. In M. D. Mezey and D. O. McGivern (Eds.), *Nurses, nurse practitioners: Evolution to advanced practice* (pp. 102–116). New York: Springer Publishing Co.

Buppert, C. (1999). *Nurse practitioner's business practice and legal guide.* Gaithersburg, MD: Aspen.

Buppert, C. (2000). *The primary care provider's guide to compensation and quality: How to get paid and not get sued.* Gaithersburg, MD: Aspen.

Burl, J. B., Bonner, A., Rao, M., & Khan, A. M. (1998). Geriatric nurse practitioners in long-term care: Demonstration of effectiveness in managed care. *Journal of the American Geriatrics Society, 46,* 506–510.

Ginzberg, E., & Ostow, M. (1997). Managed care: A look back and a look ahead. *New England Journal of Medicine, 336,* 1018–1020.

Griffith, H. M., & Robinson, K. R. (1993). Current Procedural Terminology (CPT) coded services provided by nurse specialists. *Image: Journal of Nursing Scholarship, 25,* 178–186.

Havighurst, C. C. (2001). Consumers versus managed care: The new class actions. *Health Affairs, 20,* 8–27.

Henry, S. B., Holzemer, W. L., Randell, C., Hsieh, S-F., & Miller, T. J. (1997). Comparison of nursing interventions classification and current procedural terminology codes for categorizing nursing activities. *Image: Journal of Nursing Scholarship, 29,* 133–138.

Hooker, R. S., & McCaig, L. F. (2001). Use of physician assistants and nurse practitioners in primary care, 1995–1999. *Health Affairs, 20,* 231–238.

Hsiao, W. C., Braun, P., Yntema, D., & Becker, E. R. (1988). Estimating physicians' work for a resource-based relative value scale. *New England Journal of Medicine, 319,* 835–841.

Kane, R. L., Flood, S., Keckhaver, G., Bershadsky, B., & Lum, Y-S. (2002). Nursing home residents covered by Medicare risk contracts: Early findings from the EverCare evaluation project. *Journal of the American Geriatrics Society, 50,* 719–727.

Lang, N. M., Sullivan-Marx, E. M., & Jenkins, M. (1996). Advanced practice nurses and success of organized delivery systems. *American Journal of Managed Care, 2,* 129–135.

Medicare Payment Advisory Commission. (2001, December). *Report to the Congress: Reducing Medicare complexity and regulatory burden* (pp. 1–48). Washington, DC: U.S. Government Printing Office.

Medicare Payment Advisory Commission. (2002, June). *Report to the Congress: Medicare payment to advanced practice nurses and physician assistants* (pp. 1–27). Washington, DC: U.S. Government Printing Office.

Morgan, R. O., Virnig, B. A., DeVito, C. A., & Persily, N. A. (1997). The Medicare-HMO revolving door: The healthy go in and the sick go out. *New England Journal of Medicine, 337,* 169–175.

Mundinger, M. O., Kane, R. L., Lenz, E. R., Totten, A. M., Tsai, W-Y., Cleary, P. D., Friedewald, W. T., Siu, A. L., & Shelanski, M. L. (2000). Primary care outcomes in patients treated by nurse practitioners or physicians. *Journal of the American Medical Association, 283,* 59–68.

Nurse practitioner entrepreneurs bring care to coastal Georgia. (2002, May). *Nurse Practitioner World News, 7*(5), 1–3, 10–11.

Pearson, L. J. (2002). The fourteenth annual legislative update: How each state stands on legislative issues affecting advanced nursing practice. *Nurse Practitioner, 27*(1), 10–52.

Randel, L., Pearson, S. D., Sabin, J. E., Hyams, T., & Emanuel, E. J. (2001). How managed care can be ethical. *Health Affairs, 20,* 43–56.

Sekschenski, E. S., Sansom, S., Bazell, C., Salmon, M. E., & Mullan, F. (1994). State practice environments and the supply of physician assistants, nurse practitioners, and certified nurse-midwives. *New England Journal of Medicine, 331,* 1266–1271.

Social Security Act, sec. 1861 (aa)(4); *Medicare carrier manual,* secs., 2158, 2160.

Sullivan-Marx, E. M., & Maislin, G. (2000). Comparison of nurse practitioner and family physician relative work values. *Journal of Nursing Scholarship, 32,* 71–76.

U.S. Department of Health and Human Services. (1992). Medicare program: Payment for federally qualified health center services. *Federal Register, 57*(11C), 24961–24985. Washington, DC: U.S. Government Printing Office.

U. S. Department of Health and Human Services. (1999). Medicare and Medicaid programs; Programs of All-Inclusive Care for the Elderly (PACE). *Federal Register, 64,* 66234.

U.S. Department of Health and Human Services, Health Care Financing Administration (1998). *Part B Medicare annual data.* Washington, DC: U.S. Government Printing Office.

U.S. Department of Health and Human Services, Health Care Financing Administration (1999). *Part B Medicare annual data.* Washington, DC: U.S. Government Printing Office.

U.S. Department of Health and Human Services, Health Care Financing Administration (2001). *Part B Medicare annual data.* Washington, DC: U.S. Government Printing Office.

RELATED WEB SITES

http://www.medpac.gov/publications/congressional_reports/jun02_NonPhysPay.pdf (Report on Medicare payment for APNs)

http://nursingworld.org/gova/federal/gfederal.htm#agencies (Reports and information on Medicare and Medicaid payment for APNs) http://www.cms.gov/physicians (All billing and fee schedule Medicare and Medicaid information for health care professionals)

http://www.nurse.org (Central Web site for regulatory and organizational contacts for APNs)

http://www.nurse.org/acnp (Specific Medicare payment issues for NPs)

Chapter 23

LICENSURE, CERTIFICATION, AND CREDENTIALING

Frances K. Porcher

P ublic demand for comprehensive, quality health care flourished during the 1990s. Health care reform ensued, resulting in many changes in our health care system including several regulatory aspects of the advanced practice nurse (APN) role. Significant modifications and revisions were made in individual state nurse practice acts that impacted licensure, certification, and credentialing of APNs. Several states amended their nurse practice acts to expand their legal authority, APN reimbursement status, and prescriptive authority. The concept of second licensure for APNs developed during this time. New options for national certification as an APN were developed, and in many states national certification became a requirement for APN licensure. There continues to be a growing emphasis on credentialing of APNs, especially relative to obtaining hospital privileges or seeking admission to managed care provider panels.

It is the definition of nursing, however, that frames scope of practice. The definition of nursing is especially important for APNs whose practice combines both medical and nursing components. This chapter examines regulatory aspects of the APN role, including methods of regulation, licensure, certification, and credentialing.

METHODS OF REGULATION

The purpose of legal regulation of nursing practice is the protection of public health, safety, and welfare. Regulatory criteria should reflect minimum requirements for safe and competent nursing practice. Legal regulation of nursing practice is the joint responsibility of state legislators and boards of nursing. All state boards of nursing are responsible for enforcement of the state's nurse practice act, licensure and discipline of nurses, and approval of the state's nursing education programs.

The first and least restrictive level of regulation is designation/recognition (National Council of State Boards of Nursing [NCSBN], 1992). Advanced practice nurses with state-recognized credentials are granted permission from the state board of nursing to represent themselves with those specific credentials: NP (nurse practitioner), CNS (clinical nurse specialist), or CNM (certified nurse-midwife). This approach does not involve any inquiry into competence and, accordingly, offers the least protection in terms of public health, safety, and welfare. The right of any APN to practice is not limited.

The second level of regulation, registration, requires APNs to list their names on an official roster maintained by the state board of nursing (NCSBN, 1992). Again, there is no inquiry into competence, and usually scope of practice is not defined.

The third level of regulation, certification (NCSBN, 1992), should not be confused with the meaning adopted by nongovernmental agencies or professional associations to recognize professional competence. In the regulatory sense, certification indicates that individuals have met specified requirements and are therefore "certified." These requirements may vary among states. Boards of nursing often use the professional association certification as a substitute for regulatory certification.

The fourth and most restrictive level of regulation is licensure (NCSBN, 1992). Persons having met predetermined qualifications to engage in a particular profession to the exclusion of others may be granted a license by a regulatory agency or body, such as the state board of nursing. Rules and regulations define the qualifications, scope of practice, and use of the title. Unique to this level of regulation is a high level of accountability and intent to protect public health, safety, and welfare. Licensure defines the requirements for safe nursing practice and validates that the applicant has met those requirements.

In 1986, the NCSBN adopted a position paper on advanced clinical nursing practice, concluding that designation/recognition (level 1) was the preferable method of regulating APNs (NCSBN, 1992). Additionally, educational preparation of APNs was to be at least a master's degree in nursing.

Significant changes in health care, nursing, and society since the mid-1980s prompted the NCSBN to review this position, resulting in a position paper that recommended licensure (level 4) as the preferred method of regulation for advanced nursing practice (NCSBN, 1992). According to the position paper, care activities of APNs are complex and require specialized knowledge and skill, great proficiency, and independent decision making. The potential harm to the public is great unless there is a high level of accountability such as is expected with licensure. Advanced practice nursing is defined as "practice based on the knowledge and skills acquired in a basic nursing education, through licensure as a registered nurse, and in graduate education and experience, including advanced nursing theory, physical and psycho-social assessment, and treatment of illness" (NCSBN, 1992, p. 6).

State boards of nursing are responsible for ensuring that their licensees meet minimum competency levels not only at the time of initial licensure but throughout their careers (NCSBN, 1996). Competence is "the application of knowledge and the interpersonal, decision-making and psychomotor skills expected for the practice role, within the context of public health, safety and welfare (NCSBN, 1996, p. 4). Successful achievement of professional competence for all nurses requires a collaborative approach involving the state boards of nursing, individual nurses, employers, and educators. The issue of ensuring competency in nursing as a regulatory responsibility is echoed in the PEW Health Professions Commission publication "Recreating Health Professional Practice for a New Century" (O'Neil & PEW Health Professions Commission, 1998).

LICENSURE

Nurse practice acts have evolved through four distinct phases: registration acts (1903–1938), definition and scope of nursing practice (1938–1971), recognition of advanced practice nursing (1971–1992), and second licensure for APNs (1992–present). The developmental phases are reflective of the changing roles and responsibilities of nurses as impacted by the health care needs of the time.

In the early 1900s, the first nursing statutes were actually nurse registration acts. A designated board examined the applicant's competency to hold a "certificate of registration," thereby allowing the nurse to use the title RN (registered nurse). The practice of nursing was not defined. North Carolina was the first state to pass a nurse registration act in 1903, followed shortly by New York, New Jersey, and Virginia. By 1923, all states had passed nurse registration acts.

The passage of the mandatory practice act in New York in 1938 marked the start of the second licensure phase. The New York practice act legally defined nursing by defining scope of practice, specifying the education or training necessary for licensure, and prohibiting the practice of nursing without a license (Bullough, 1976). Nursing was narrowly defined to acknowledge dependent care activities pursuant to physician supervision.

This dependent nursing role predominated in nursing practice acts until the American Nurses Association (ANA) proposed the following model definition of nursing in 1955:

> The practice of professional nursing means the performance for compensation of any act in the observation, care, and counsel of the ill, injured, or infirm, or in the maintenance of health or prevention of illness of others . . . the foregoing shall not be deemed to include acts of diagnosis or prescription of therapeutic or corrective measures. (Kelly, 1974, p. 1314)

Although this definition modified requirements for physician supervision for all nursing functions, nurses were specifically prohibited from diagnosing and prescribing.

A decade of change followed in the 1960s, marked by the birth of Medicaid and Medicare, a growing shortage of primary care physicians, the start of the first formal nurse practitioner and physician assistant programs, the Vietnam War, and the emerging women's movement. All of these events contributed to the growing recognition that nursing practice was significantly restricted by state laws.

In 1971, Idaho became the first state to amend the nurse practice act to provide recognition for advanced practice nursing (phase 3). Idaho added a qualifying statement to the portion of the nurse practice act that prohibited nurses from diagnosing and treating patients to allow nurses to diagnose and treat as authorized jointly by the board of nursing and the board of medicine. Although this was a significant step, advanced practice nursing was still defined by both nursing and medicine.

In 1972, New York amended its nurse practice act to define registered nursing practice in broader terms, thereby accommodating the practice of diagnosing and treating by nurse practitioners. In 1974, Maine amended its nurse practice act to allow professional nurses with additional education to diagnose and treat if those responsibilities were delegated to them by physicians (Maine Revised Statutes, 1974).

In 1982, the NCSBN published a new model nursing practice act that defined the practice of nursing to include diagnosis, planning, implementation, and evaluation of care and treatment. Following publication of this definition, several states modified their nurse practice acts to define both advanced practice nursing as well as who holds regulatory responsibility for advanced practice nursing (nursing versus medicine, or a combination of both).

In 1992, the NCSBN recommended that the preferred method of regulation for advanced practice nursing be licensure rather than designation/recognition. That significant change hallmarked phase 4 of licensure. According to the position statement, advanced practice nursing should be based on graduate nursing education, and boards of nursing should regulate advanced nursing practice by licensure because the risk of harm from unsafe or incompetent clinicians at this complex level of care is quite high. The 1992 NCSBN model legislation was criticized for not addressing issues of clinical competency, mastery of skills, or validation of specific advanced practice knowledge (Hardy Havens, 1992).

The most recent NCSBN Model Nursing Practice Act of 2002 states that advanced practice registered nursing is based on knowledge and skills acquired in basic nursing education. Additionally, applicants for licensure as an advanced practice registered nurse must be licensed as a registered nurse, have graduated from a graduate-level APRN program that is nationally accredited, and hold current national certification in the appropriate APRN specialty (NCSBN, 2002, January 18). The intent of the 2002 Model Nursing Practice Act is to improve accountability of advanced practice registered nurses to clients, the nursing profession, and their respective board of nursing.

In August 2002 the NCSBN Delegate Assembly amended the Model Nursing Practice Act to address APRN applicants for whom there is no appropriate certifying exam available. The amendment allows states to develop alternative mechanisms to ensure initial competence of these applicants until January 1, 2005. After this date APRNs will not be issued a license without successful completion of an approved certification examination (NCSBN, 2002b).

In recent years several states have amended their nurse practice acts to expand their legal authority, APN reimbursement status, and prescriptive authority. As of 2001, at least 44 states have specific regulations in their nurse practice act that identify regulation of advance practice nursing as belonging to the state board of nursing. However, 19 of these 44 states require physician collaboration or supervision as part of the scope of practice definition for nurse practitioners. In another 6 states, advanced practice nursing was authorized by both the state board of nursing and the state board of medicine. Only 1 state (Tennessee) continues to define APN function under a broad nurse practice act. Several states are in the process of revising or refining their restrictive nurse practice acts to update the definition of advanced practice nursing and the regulatory mechanism of such practice (Pearson, 2002).

Advanced practice nurses have worked very hard in the past 10 years to obtain authority for autonomous practices in various states. Currently, nurse practitioners in 12 states (Alaska, Arizona, Iowa, Maine, Montana, New Hampshire, New Mexico, Oregon, Utah, Washington, Wisconsin, Wyoming, and the District of Columbia) have legal authority to prescribe independent of any required physician involvement in the prescription writing. Nurse practitioners in another 38 states (Alabama, Arkansas, California, Colorado, Connecticut, Delaware, Florida, Georgia, Hawaii, Idaho, Illinois, Indiana, Kansas, Kentucky, Louisiana, Massachusetts, Maryland, Michigan, Minnesota, Missouri, Mississippi, North Carolina, North Dakota, New Jersey, Nebraska, Nevada, New York, Ohio, Oklahoma, Pennsylvania, Rhode Island, South Carolina, South Dakota, Tennessee, Texas, Virginia, Vermont, West Virginia) can prescribe with "some" degree of physician involvement. Often this physician involvement refers to either a protocol or consultation and referral plan written that is agreed to by the nurse practitioner and consulting or supervising physician. All states now provide some degree of statutory or regulatory prescribing authority for nurse practitioners. Nurse practitioners in all states have authorized ability (via statutes or rules and regulations) to receive and/or dispense pharmaceutical samples (Pearson, 2002).

Slowly, unnecessary barriers are being removed and restraints lifted so that APNs can practice to the full scope of their ability, experience, and educational preparation. For more specific details, refer to the "Annual Legislative Update" published annually in the January issues of *The Nurse Practitioner* (Pearson, 2002).

The 1992 model identified an umbrella classification for advanced practice licensure for the purpose of regulation only. The classification is not intended to be used as a title, per se. Licensure at this level is designated as Advanced Practice Registered Nurse in one of the following four categories: nurse practitioner, certified registered nurse anesthetist, certified nurse-midwife, or clinical nurse specialist. The NCSBN believes that consistent titling and uniform use of terminology will improve public understanding of the roles, ensure safe advanced nursing practice, and provide a basis for regulating advanced practice.

Not all nurses support the concept of second licensure as a means to differentiate nurse generalists from nurse specialists. Not all nurses believe that differentiation is necessary. Rather, some critics believe the law should identify only the generic category of nurses and not specialists or advanced nurses. Some nurses believe that a rational, comprehensible system of credentialing needs to be established (Styles, 1990). For example, not all APNs are educationally prepared in the same manner. Although the majority of nurse practitioner programs in the United States are now master's-level programs (except the certificate programs that prepare women's health care nurse practitioners and certified critical care nurses), there is considerable concern about the recent proliferation of educational programs, particularly certificate-level and post-master's certificate programs. Graduates of all these programs are credentialed as nurse practitioners, yet clearly there is considerable variance among these educational programs in terms of length of coursework, curricula for nurse practitioner specialty areas of practice, number of required clinical hours, and faculty qualifications.

State boards of nursing are responsible for approval of their state's nursing education programs following review of curricula, faculty credentials, and teaching resources in an attempt to protect public health, safety, and welfare through safe and competent nursing practice. Criteria for program approval vary from state to state, which inhibits comparability of educational preparation of nurses. Variability in educational programs ultimately means variability in proficiency and skills of graduates. State boards of nursing have experienced major difficulties in credentialing and licensing nurse practitioners due to these variances. The difficulties and problems encountered in states' credentialing criteria and processes may significantly limit practice mobility and scope of practice, further underscoring the need for standardization of APN educational preparation. As discussed later in this chapter, it is doubtful that national certification by specialty organizations can serve to ensure a rational system of credentialing either.

In August 1997, the National Task Force on Quality Nurse Practitioner Education released a document entitled *Criteria for Evaluation of Nurse Practitioner Programs* in an attempt to provide a model for evaluating the quality of nurse practitioner education (National Task Force on Quality Nurse Practitioner Education, 1997). In 2002, the National Organization of Nurse Practitioner Faculty (NONPF) and the American Association of Colleges of Nursing (AACN) released a revised document entitled *Primary Care Nurse Practitioner Competencies: Adult, Family, Gerontological, Pediatric, and Women's Health* (National Organization of Nurse Practitioner Faculty, 2002). The revision was funded by the US Department of Health and Human Services, Health Resources and Services Administration, Bureau of Health Professions, Division of Nursing, and many national nursing organizations. The document identifies nationally recognized outcome competencies for each of the five primary care nurse practitioner specialties. The document is intended to be used in conjunction with existing documents and criteria such as *The Essentials of Master's Education for Advanced Practice Nursing* (American Association of Colleges of Nursing, 1996),

Philosophy, Conceptual Model, Terminal Competencies for the Education of Pediatric Nurse Practitioners (Association of Faculties of Pediatric Nurse Practitioner and Associate Programs, 1996), materials from national accrediting bodies (National League for Nursing, Commission on Collegiate Nursing Education), and other materials such as role delineation studies and practice standards developed by various specialty and certifying organizations. It is hoped that licensing (including definition of scope of practice) of APNs will become clearer as some of the titling and credentialing issues are addressed through evaluation and monitoring of advanced practice nurse education programs.

The ongoing debate about titling is directly related to licensure issues in that prescriptive authority had traditionally been afforded only to nurse practitioners. As the scope of practice for other APNs, such as clinical nurse specialists, expands, prescriptive authority becomes an increasingly more important necessity to the role. Nurse practice acts are beginning to change to reflect the need for all APNs, including clinical nurse specialists, to obtain prescriptive authority without having to meet licensure requirements as a nurse practitioner in addition to those for clinical nurse specialist.

There is continued interest among some nurse educators in merging the roles of clinical nurse specialist and nurse practitioner. Titles found in the literature addressing the combined clinical nurse specialist/nurse practitioner role include advanced nurse practitioner (Calkin, 1984), advanced registered nurse practitioner (Sparacino, Cooper, & Minarik, 1990), and advanced practice nurse (American Nurses Association, 1996; Safriet, 1992). Supporters of a merger claim that many similarities already exist in the educational preparation, clinical roles, and practice settings for both APNs, which are expanding and overlapping. Furthermore, supporters have suggested that professional unity would lead to greater power in activities with legislators, administrators, and consumers. Opponents of a merger assert that the scope of practice is quite different, graduate programs would need to be lengthened, and the legal entanglements outweigh the benefits of a merger (Soehren & Schumann, 1994). Full discussion of this issue is beyond the scope of this chapter.

Phase 4, second licensure for APNs, reflects the many internal and external forces acting on the nursing profession. The health care reform movement of the 1990s forced the nursing profession to increase professional accountability and set national practice standards, particularly at the advanced practice level. Changes in state nurse practice acts, including advanced practice licensure, represent responses by the profession to an increasing public demand for comprehensive, quality health care.

It seems that the fifth licensure phase, interstate licensure, has emerged reflecting the impact of technology on health care. The rapid growth of "telehealth" and "telenursing" stimulated the need to explore alternatives to the current licensing system for nurses. Telenursing is the practice of distance nursing using telecommunications technology including, but not limited to, telephones, interactive multimedia devices, computer monitoring systems, and the Internet (NCSBN, 1997). It is clear that nursing services are provided across state lines in a variety of ways.

In 1998, the NCSBN proposed a multistate licensure model entitled "Interstate Compact for Mutual Recognition of Nursing Regulation and Licensure" for registered nurses/practical nurses/vocational nurses, which ultimately was implemented January 1, 2000, by the states of Maryland, Texas, Utah, and Wisconsin. Implementation requires legislative activity by each state to address the development of an agreement or a compact with another state or states. In essence, this licensure model allows a nurse to maintain one license in his or her state of residency and to practice both electronically and physically in one or more other states. Involved nurses are subject to each state's practice laws, rules, and regulations. As of January 2002, 16 states have enacted the interstate nurse licensure compact, including Arizona, Alaska, Delaware, Idaho, Iowa, Maine, Maryland, Michigan, Nebraska, New Jersey, North Carolina, North Dakota, South Dakota, Texas, Utah, and Wisconsin. Georgia and Illinois have interstate compact legislation pending (NCSBN, 2003).

In August 2002, the NCSBN Delegate Assembly approved the adoption of model language for a Nurse Licensure Compact for Advanced Practice Registered Nurses (NCSBN, 2003). Only those states that have adopted the Nurse Licensure Compact for registered nurses, licensed vocational nurses, and visiting nurses, may implement a compact for APRNs. Many implementation issues need further discussion by stakeholders, including, but not limited to, variations across states relative to scope of practice, prescriptive authority, education, and certification. The concept of mutual recognition and interstate licensure remains controversial, as evidenced by the lack of support expressed by many professional nursing associations. Only two associations, the American Association of Occupational Health Nurses (AAOHN) and the Air and Surface Transport Nurses Association (ASTNA) have provided positive support. One association, the American Association of Poison Control Centers, Inc. (AAPCC) has provided endorsement. Two professional associations, the American Nurses Association (ANA) and the National Association of Pediatric Nurse Practitioners (NAPNP) have expressed numerous concerns regarding the multi-state licensure model for nursing practice (NCSBN, 2002, January 18).

CERTIFICATION

Certification is a credentialing process by which a nongovernmental agency or association attests that an individual licensed to practice a profession has met certain predetermined standards specified by that profession. In response to a proliferation of specialties in nursing and a growing emphasis on quality care in the health professions, the ANA initiated a national certification program in 1974 to recognize excellence in nursing practice. The certification process was voluntary, and initially 191 nurses were certified. In 1975, the National Certification Board of Pediatric Nurse Practitioners and Nurses (NCBPNP/Ns) began offering pediatric certification examinations, also on a voluntary basis.

In 1978, the purpose of the certification process had expanded to include assurance of quality beyond basic registered nurse licensure, identification of nurses who may be eligible for direct reimbursement for services, and recognition of professional achievement and quality of practice (Hawkins & Thibodeau, 1993). Ten generalist and specialty certification examinations were available from ANA in 1978. Three more specialty examinations were added in 1979. By 1996, more than 130,000 nurses had achieved ANA certification in 24 categories consisting of 21 clinical areas, 2 administrative areas, and 1 staff development area.

In 1980, the Nurses' Association of the American College of Obstetricians and Gynecologists assumed responsibility for certification of obstetric/gynecologic nurse practitioners, neonatal intensive care nurses, and inpatient obstetric nurses. In 1993, the name of the group was changed to National Certification Corporation for the Obstetric, Gynecologic, and Neonatal Nursing Specialties, and five other area-related certification examinations were added.

Although the ANA served as a leader in the development of national certification examinations for nurses, several professional organizations or associations offer APN certification processes. For example, the American College of Nurse Midwives certifies nurse-midwives, the American Association of Nurse Anesthetists certifies nurse anesthetists, and the National Certification Board of Pediatric Nurse Practitioners and Nurses (NCBPNP/N) certifies pediatric nurse practitioners. In 1991, the certification arm of ANA changed its name to American Nurses Credentialing Center (ANCC) and continues to offer certification examinations for generalist nurses in several specialty areas and for advanced practice nurses (CNS, NP, nurse administrators) in several advanced practice specialty areas. In 1993, the American Academy of Nurse Practitioners (AANP) began to offer national certification examinations for family and adult nurse practitioners.

Reflective of the rapid technological growth in the mid-1990s, the NCBPNP/Ns and ANCC exams became computer-based and are offered at specific technology centers throughout the United States. In fall 2001, ANCC offered its first certification examination for pediatric clinical nurse specialists.

In response to the growing need for appropriate credentialing of acute-care nurse practitioners, ANCC offered the first Acute-Care Nurse Practitioner Certification Examination in December 1995. A clear distinction between acute-care and primary care nurse practitioners was finally made within the nursing community.

Certification of APNs serves to protect the public by ensuring that an individual titled as an APN has mastered a certain body of knowledge and acquired a particular set of specialized skills. Specialists are expected to have expert competence, and certification serves as one means to verify the knowledge and skills of nurses who claim competence at a certain level. Certification of nursing specialists represents a judgment made by the nursing profession about an individual's credentials. Many nurses are certified in more than one area.

Because several specialty groups offer certification, much variability exists in certification processes. In the past, attempts to standardize certification processes have not been successful for several reasons, one being the intense concern of specialty organizations to maintain control of their specialty practice. For example, in the late 1970s, following 3 years of extensive study, an ANA committee on credentialing recommended that a separate national credentialing center be established (Hawkins & Thibodeau, 1993). The intent was to have one national credentialing center that would be responsible for certification for all nursing specialty groups. Although a national center was never established, the ANA did establish its own credentialing center, which now offers 24 certification exams for nurses. Another attempt to standardize certification processes in nursing was attempted recently in 1995–1996, perhaps in response to the concern about the proliferation of nurse practitioner programs and the quality of these programs and their graduates. The issue may also have been related to some accreditation process issues that were occurring with the National League for Nursing (NLN). This effort to standardize was unsuccessful as well because specialty organizations again fought to maintain control of their specialty practice.

Currently there are six national certifying agencies for APNs: the American Academy of Nurse Practitioners (AANP); the American Nurses Credentialing Center (ANCC); the National Certification Board for Pediatric Nurse Practitioners and Nurses (NCBPNP/N); the American College of

Nurse Midwives Certification Council; the National Certification Corporation (NCC) for Obstetric, Gynecologic, and Neonatal Nursing Specialities; and the Council of Certification of Nurse Anesthetists. Eligibility criteria to sit for a national APN certification examination vary by certifying agency, but all require RN licensure, a master's degree in nursing (since 1998) except for CNMs and CRNAs, graduation from a specialty program, and a minimum number of clinical experience hours.

Specialty designation and national certification also play a central role in both state licensure and reimbursement for specialty nursing services. Many states now require national specialty certification as a requirement for APN licensure. Medicaid reimburses only certified family and pediatric nurse practitioners for their services. These activities mandate that the professional organizations address the certification issue. What does certification mean in the 21st century? Should certification be linked to professional licensure or third-party reimbursement? Who should set the standards for certification?

Of special note is the requirement of state-specific certification for APN licensure by individual states. Currently, three states (California, Florida, New York) require state certification for APN licensure (Pearson, 2002). In addition to providing documentation of formal educational preparation as an APN, applicants must also meet other statutory requirements such as written protocols or supervisory agreements with a physician. The state certification may or may not be designated on the license. Some states recognize national certification in lieu of state certification.

CREDENTIALING

Credentialing refers to the validation of required education, licensure, and certification. Credentialing of APNs is necessary not only to ensure the public of safe health care provided by qualified individuals but also to ensure compliance with federal and state laws relating to nursing practice. Legal regulation provides clear authority for qualified APNs to provide advanced nursing care including certain aspects of health care such as diagnosing and prescribing. Credentialing acknowledges the APN's advanced scope of practice. Credentialing mandates accountability. Individual APNs must be held accountable for the quality of health care they provide as well as their continued professional growth. Credentialing systems must be accountable to the public by providing appropriate avenues for public or individual practice complaints. Credentialing allows the profession to be accountable to the public and its members by enforcing professional standards for practice.

The credentialing process for APNs usually involves validation or verification of educational preparation, state APN licensure, current certification, felony history, malpractice history, practice agreement with physician (if required), prescribing authority, and two or three professional references. Successful completion of the credentialing process is usually required to obtain hospital privileges and, most recently, to seek admission to managed care provider panels (Buppert, 1999).

A number of disturbing problems are evident in the nursing profession's current credentialing system for advanced practice nursing. Because the requirements for the various certification examinations vary widely, certification lacks uniform meaning (Hawkins & Thibodeau, 1993). In some states, the scope of advanced practice nursing is so severely restricted that the financial cost and time investment to become appropriately credentialed outweigh the benefits. This is particularly true if the employment situation also fails to recognize the significance of credentialing.

Currently, the issue of titling or name designation is also somewhat controversial. To most nurses, the particular advanced practice designation seems to signify certain professional accomplishments and some political advantages or disadvantages. In this era of health care reform, both legislators and the public are confused by nursing's many titles. What exactly is a "nurse practitioner," a "clinical nurse specialist," or a "certified nurse specialist"? Clarification through simplification of the APN title will foster professional unity and ultimately facilitate and cement the APN role in health care reform. To this end, the National Nurse Practitioner Marketing Campaign was instituted in 2000 with the expressed purpose of fostering the positive image of nurse practitioners. A national media campaign is being developed to educate the public and elevate the visibility of the nurse practitioner role. This unified effort by several national nurse practitioner organizations serves as an important step toward clarification of the role.

CONCLUSIONS

The health care reform movement of the 1990s has provided nursing with an opportunity to reevaluate the regulatory aspects of the APN role. At the state level, there is an increasing trend toward more physician involvement in regulation of advanced practice nursing. Many states require joint regulation of APNs by the board of nursing and the board of medicine. Many require restrictive controls, such as protocols or detailed written practice agreements between the APN and physician. Yet other states legally acknowledge the professional contribution of the APN to health care through regulation by the board of nursing only. There is also a trend to specify in state statutes that a master's degree in nursing be the mandatory minimum educational requirement for the APN role and that national certification serve as a requirement for APN licensure.

On the national level, the most significant trend is toward standardization and uniformity. APN licensure is being proposed as the most effective method of self-regulation. It is postulated that second licensure will facilitate mobility among states and increase professional accountability. The interstate compact legislation is an attempt to address some of the issues that have arisen due to the impact of technology on health care. It will be critical to monitor the development and likely implementation of the APRN interstate compact legislation. Current trends also include use of national certification as a credentialing mechanism rather than as a voluntary measure of competence. Nationally there is a growing need to set practice standards and monitor APN educational programs relative to these standards.

The legal authority for APNs to diagnose, prescribe, and receive reimbursement for services continues to expand. APNs continue to gain full practice autonomy, including deletion of requirements for physician supervision. There is sufficient research to support that APNs provide high-quality, cost-effective care. Patient satisfaction rates of health care provided by APNs are high. The collaborative relationship between APNs and physicians in providing quality health care is becoming more evident in several health care arenas despite organized medicine's attempts to maintain sole control of health care. It is definitely an exciting yet challenging time to be an advanced practice nurse.

REFERENCES

American Association of Colleges of Nursing. (1996). *The essentials of master's education for advanced practice nursing.* Washington, DC: Author.

American Nurses Association. (1996). *Scope and standards of advanced practice registered nursing.* Washington, DC: Author.

Association of Faculties of Pediatric Nurse Practitioner and Associate Programs. (1996). *Philosophy, conceptual model, terminal competencies for the education of pediatric nurse practitioners.* Cherry Hill, NJ: National Association of Pediatric Nurse Associates and Practitioners.

Bullough, B. (1976). Influence on role expansion. *American Journal of Nursing, 76,* 1476–1481.

Buppert, C. (1999). *Nurse practitioner's business practice and legal guide.* Gaithersburg, MD: Aspen.

Calkin, J. D. (1984). A model for advanced nursing practice. *Journal of Nursing Administration, 14*(1), 24–30.

Hardy Havens, D. (1992). Licensure for advanced practice: Be informed, be alert. *Pediatric Nursing, 18,* 540.

Hawkins, J. W., & Thibodeau, J. A. (1993). *The advanced practitioner: Current practice issues* (3rd ed.). New York: Tiresias Press.

Kelly, L. Y. (1974). Nursing practice acts. *American Journal of Nursing, 74,* 1310–1319.

Maine Revised Statutes. (1974). Title 32, Chapter 31, Section 2102.

National Council of State Boards of Nursing. (1982). *The model nursing practice act.* Chicago: Author.

National Council of State Boards of Nursing. (1992). *Position paper on the licensure of advanced nursing practice.* Chicago: Author.

National Council of State Boards of Nursing. (1993). *Advanced nursing practice* (fact sheet). Chicago: Author.

National Council of State Boards of Nursing. (1996). *Position paper on assuring competence.* Chicago: Author.

National Council of State Boards of Nursing. (1997). *Position paper on telenursing.* Chicago: Author.

National Council of State Boards of Nursing. (2002). Retrieved October 29, 2002, from http://www.ncsbn.org/publi

National Council of State Boards of Nursing. (2002, August 22). *Press release: NCSBN delegates vote on significant actions at delegate assembly, 2002.* Retrieved October 29, 2002, from http://www.ncsbn.org/

National Council of State Boards of Nursing. (2002, January 18). NCSBN model nursing practice act, ???? 2002. Retrieved February 11, 2002, from http://www.ncsbn.org/

National Council of State Boards of Nursing. (2003, April). *Nurse licensure compact map.* Retrieved May 5, 2003, from http://www.ncsbn.org/

National Council of State Boards of Nursing, APRN Compact Development Subcommittee. (2002). First draft of APRN compact prepared. *Council Connector, 2*(1), 4.

National Organization of Nurse Practitioner Faculty. (2002). *Primary care nurse practitioner competencies: Adult, family, gerontological, pediatric, and women's health.* Retrieved October 29, 2002, from http://www.nonpf.org

National Task Force on Quality Nurse Practitioner Education. (1997). *Criteria for evaluation of nurse practitioner programs.* Washington, DC: National Organization of Nurse Practitioner Faculty.

O'Neil, E. H., & the PEW Health Professions Commission. (1998). *Recreating health professional practice for a new century.* San Francisco: Pew Health Professions Commission.

Pearson, L. J. (2002). Fourteenth annual update of how each state stands on legislative issues affecting advanced nursing practice. *Nurse Practitioner, 27*(1), 10-52.

Safriet, B. J. (1992). Health care dollars and regulatory sense: The role of advanced practice nursing. *Yale Journal on Regulation, 9*(2), 417-487.

Soehren, P. M., & Schumann, L. L. (1994). Enhanced role opportunities available to the CNS/nurse practitioner. *Clinical Nurse Specialist, 8*(3), 123–127.

Sparacino, P. S. A., Cooper, D. M., & Minarik, P. A. (1990). *The clinical nurse specialist: Implementation and impact.* Norwalk, CT: Appleton-Lange.

Styles, M. M. (1990). Nurse practitioners creating new horizons for the 1990s. *Nurse Practitioner, 15*(2), 48–57.

Chapter 24

WORKFORCE POLICY PERSPECTIVES ON ADVANCE PRACTICE NURSING

Linda H. Aiken

S ubstantial growth in the number of advanced practice nurses over the past decade in a context of potential oversupply of physicians has fueled professional and policy debate about the optimal composition of the health care workforce and the future of advanced practice nursing (Cooper & Aiken, 2001; Cooper, Laud, & Dietrich, 1998). In 2000, almost 200,000 nurses, accounting for over 7% of all registered nurses, were prepared as nurse practitioners, clinical nurse specialists, nurse anesthetists, or nurse-midwives (Spratley, Johnson, Sochalsky, Fritz, & Spencer, 2002). Approximately 275,000 nurse practitioners, physician assistants, and nurse-midwives are projected to be in practice by 2015. In combination with other rapidly increasing nonphysician caregiver occupations such as chiropractors and acupuncturists, the total number of nonphysician caregivers could reach the equivalent of 65 primary care physicians per 100,000 population by 2015 (Cooper, Getzen, McKee, & Laud, 2002). There are currently 270 active physicians per 100,000 population, so by 2015 the total number of nonphysician caregivers would be the equivalent of increasing the supply of physicians by about 20%.

The supply of physicians has been growing faster than the population for decades and exceeds most estimates of need, although physicians are not distributed optimally by specialty or geography. Much of the increase in nonphysician caregiver supply has been in primary care, which, according

431

to past workforce projections, is where expansions in the health care workforce were needed. However, contrary to expectations, population demands for primary care have been relatively stable for some years, which casts some doubt over whether unabated increases in primary care providers, including advanced practice nurses, are desirable.

Debate about the rate of increase in advanced practice nurses (APNs) stems from the belief that APNs were a creation of public policy in the 1960s and 1970s for the express purpose of meeting a projected shortfall in primary care. If true, the policy warrant for continued subsidy of the training of nurse practitioners and other APNs is weakened if there is no longer a shortage of primary care physicians. Moreover, if there is an impending oversupply of primary care providers, future employment opportunities for APNs could be reduced. Finally, much has been written about the many barriers to APN practice that result from restrictive state practice acts and reimbursement policies. What does the future hold with regard to the practice climate for APNs? In this chapter, three myths that fuel debates about the future of advanced practice nursing are debunked: (1) the shortage of primary care physicians created the original demand for APNs, (2) an oversupply of physicians will reduce the demand for APNs, and (3) payment and practice restrictions are necessary to ensure APN participation in the care of underserved populations.

MYTH #1: ADVANCED PRACTICE NURSING EVOLVED PRIMARILY TO FILL A SHORTAGE OF PRIMARY CARE PHYSICIANS

Much of the early policy literature on the development of advanced practice roles for nurses refers to them as "physician extenders," in the sense that they could help ease perceived problems Americans were having obtaining access to generalist physician care. If this construction of the origins of APNs is accepted, the elimination of the shortage of primary care physicians should obviate the need for APNs in the future.

The first point in refuting this myth is the absence of evidence of an actual shortage of primary care physicians that could have been the major driver of consumer acceptance of nurses in expanded professional practice roles. The distribution of the physician supply in the United States in the latter two thirds of the 20th century shows a growing proportion of physicians electing to become specialists and a declining proportion of physicians selecting generalist practice. These trends were routinely interpreted to signal a shortage of primary care. However, the increase in the proportion of physicians electing specialty practice obscured the fact that the actual supply of generalist physicians per capita remained constant between 1950 and the late 1980s, when generalist physicians per capita started to increase to the historically high levels we see today (Cooper, 1994). Moreover, contrary to conventional wisdom, specialist physicians served as principal care providers for a substantial share of the American population during the period of presumed shortage of primary care physicians, blunting the effects of what was perceived to be a shortage of primary care (Aiken et al., 1979). Thus, there is little hard evidence that there was a shortage of primary care providers at the time advanced practice nursing began to become a mainstay in American health care.

Savvy nursing leaders exploited the opportunity presented by the perception of a shortage of primary care to advance their agenda to create expanded professional roles for nurses and to obtain public subsidies to support additional education. As Loretta Ford (1982, p. 232) noted, "The dearth of physician manpower *provided the opportunity* to test new roles [such as the nurse practitioner]; it was not, however, the *raison d'etre* for the initiation of the expanded role." Instead, the nurse practitioner concept developed as innovators recognized substantial unmet needs for a range of health care services among consumers with and without access to physicians, and saw the opportunity for nurses to fill that void. Thus, there is ample evidence that the successful integration of nurse practitioners into the medical division of labor had little to do with a shortage of primary care physicians and more to do with the perceived value of the services advanced practice nurse came to provide that had not routinely been provided by physicians, irrespective of their specialties. Thus, assuming that practice patterns of U.S. physicians remain as they were in the 20th century, growing numbers of physicians are not likely to obviate the "need" for APNs. Moreover, there is some indication that the predictions of a physician surplus made in the early 1990s have not materialized, and at least one prominent medical workforce expert predicts a growing shortage of physicians that could become severe by 2020 (Cooper, Getzen, et al., 2002).

MYTH #2: THE INCREASE IN ADVANCED PRACTICE NURSES WILL SATURATE DEMAND AND RESULT IN EMPLOYMENT DIFFICULTIES

The rapid increase in the number of nurses with educational preparation as advanced practice nurses in the decade of the 1990s has resulted in concern among health workforce analysts that the market for APNs will soon become saturated, thus leading to increased unemployment among advanced practice nurses (Cooper, 1994). These concerns are based on the assumption that the majority of advanced practice nurses will work in conventional patient care roles, with nurse practitioners working predominantly in primary care. However, the evidence suggests that APNs hold a wide range of positions, and that the large increase in nurses prepared as APNs over the decade of the 1990s has been absorbed without substantially affecting employment opportunities.

Employment patterns of nurse practitioners are of special interest to health workforce analysts because of the presumed connection between the employment opportunities for nurse practitioners and the supply of primary care physicians. The number of nurses educated as nurse practitioners grew from 70,993 in 1996 to 102,829 by 2000, an increase of 45% (Spratley et al., 2002). Over the same time, the supply of primary care physicians also increased. Nevertheless, there is no evidence of increased unemployment of nurse practitioners. An examination of the employment patterns of nurse practitioners shows that only slightly over half were employed in positions with the title "nurse practitioner." Of the approximately 55,000 nurses with educational preparation as clinical nurse specialists in 2000, only 12,000 worked in positions with that title. Most advanced practice nurses were employed in nursing or health care, but clearly not all were working in conventional advanced nursing practice roles.

These employment patterns suggest there is substantial demand for nurses with graduate preparation, which is being met, in part, by graduates from clinical master's degree programs in advanced practice. While we do not have published data on exactly what these nurses with advanced clinical practice degrees are doing, we can speculate on their possible types of employment by examining broad trends in health care and nursing education.

Nursing Education

Graduate nursing education has been shifting steadily over two to three decades from a focus on the functional specialties of teaching, administration, and practice to an increasingly dominant focus on clinical specialty practice. Moreover, during the 1990s many of the clinical master's programs shifted from clinical specialist to nurse practitioner programs. Other than programs in nursing administration, which have experienced declining enrollments in recent years, many nursing schools do not offer nonclinical or non-APN master's programs. Thus, it seems probable that a portion of those trained recently in nurse practitioner master's degree programs never intended to practice in conventional nurse practitioner roles but wanted or needed a master's degree to advance their career trajectories. The increase in the number of nurses pursuing graduate clinical education appears to represent, in part, a general trend toward higher average education for nurses, commensurate with a general increase in the education of all health professionals.

One potentially large source of employment for nurses with graduate preparation is in clinical faculty for the nation's large nursing education infrastructure. The National League for Nursing Accrediting Commission (NLNAC, 2002) lists a total of 1,396 nursing education programs in the country: 562 bachelor of science in nursing, 785 associate degree, and 89 diploma programs. The demand for faculty with graduate degrees and advanced clinical preparation to staff this large educational infrastructure is substantial and will increase in the future given the aging of the existing nursing school faculty and the estimates that a substantial portion of nursing school faculty will retire over the next decade (Sochalski, 2002).

Clinical Practice

Despite the long-standing animosity of organized medicine toward advanced practice nursing, a substantial proportion of physicians have, elected to work with nurse practitioners. During the period 1995–1999 approximately 25% of primary care office-based physicians worked with nurse practitioners and/or physician assistants. Almost 10% of all hospital outpatient visits between 1997 and 1999 involved nurse practitioners and/or physician assistants. During this time, nurse practitioners delivered 13 million hospital outpatient visits (Lin, Hooker, Lenz, & Hopkins, 2002). In addition, nurse practitioners provided 1.5 million hospital emergency department visits in 1999 (Hooker & McCaig, 2001).

Managed care organizations have shown substantially greater demand for advanced practice nurses than was the norm in fee-for-service indemnity insurance plans. The shift to managed care has been dramatic: 8 in 10 privately insured Americans nationwide are enrolled in some form of managed care (Draper, Hurley, Lesser, & Strunk, 2002). The expansion of managed care has altered in fundamental ways the medical division of labor, with physicians losing some of their control over other health professions, which has created new opportunities for APNs (Aiken, 2001; Hartley, 1999). Recently, the public backlash against health maintenance organizations' restrictions on choice of provider has resulted in a transition to less-restrictive managed care products, including the elimination of primary care gatekeepers in many plans. The primary care gatekeeper requirement often served in the past to limit consumers' access to nurse practitioners, and thus fewer restrictions on consumer provider choice should benefit nurse practitioners.

Demand for advanced practice nurses is also growing in specialty practice. The United States is unique among its peer countries in the large proportion of its physicians who elect specialty training and practice. Consumers in the United States have also shown, over time, a preference for specialty physicians. In a now classic study of physician practice, Aiken and colleagues (1979) documented that one in five Americans received their primary care from specialists in the mid-1970s. In a more recent study, Weiner (1994) found that in two well-known health maintenance organizations—Kaiser Permanente and Harvard Community Health Plan—nurse practitioners and physician assistants delivered 60% of dermatological care, between 38% and 56% of obstetric/gynecological care, 44% of orthopedic care, and between 28% and 47% of adult medicine care. Many U.S. patients with chronic illnesses prefer to obtain both specialty care for their chronic condition and primary care from the same physician. The development of less-restrictive products by managed care organizations could encourage this trend, which could be expected to increase the demand for nurse practitioners to work in specialty practices but concentrating on primary care for those with chronic illnesses. Such a trend toward greater utilization of advance practice nurses in specialty care may also be encouraged by shortages of specialty physicians that have been forecasted to occur possibly before the end of this decade.

Employment opportunities for clinically expert nurses are also increasing rapidly in a variety of roles outside of traditional health care organizations. Examples include case management, utilization review, quality assurance, health writing, occupational health, fitness training, consulting, and pharmaceutical research. Moreover, several trends affecting acute hospitals suggest a potential growing market for APN employment. The potential of a surplus of physicians led some teaching hospitals to reduce the number of medical residency positions. Advanced practice nurses provide an alternative to medical house staff. Also, the increasing acuity of inpatient hospital care is creating an increased demand for nurse practitioners and full-time hospital-based physicians known as "hospitalists" and "intensivists." Ever-expanding hospital quality assurance programs rely increasingly on advanced practice nurses. Finally, the needs of an aging population have created, and will continue to create, a host of roles for nurses in advanced practice.

In summary, the demand for APNs is strong and the increasing supply has been absorbed to the benefit of consumers and without problems of nurse practitioner unemployment. A number of trends in current health care arrangements suggest that demand for nurse practitioners will continue to remain strong. In addition, while overall growth in the number of nurse practitioners has been substantial, graduations peaked in 1998 and decreased each year through 2001. Thus, estimates of a large, possibly excess supply of nurse practitioners by 2010 need reconsideration. Fewer than anticipated nurse practitioners and a potential shortage of physician specialists lead some analysts to worry about a shortage of NPs rather than an surplus (Hooker & Berlin, 2002).

MYTH #3: PAYMENT AND PRACTICE RESTRICTIONS ARE NECESSARY TO ENSURE THE DISTRIBUTION OF APNS TO CARE FOR UNDERSERVED POPULATIONS

The policy rationale for public subsidies of the education of advanced practice nurses and the reimbursement of services provided by them is APNs' contribution to the provision of health care for populations with unmet needs for care. The idea of advanced practice nurses as physician extenders was thought to be a strategy to improve access to health care for the poor. Access-to-care problems for the poor were perceived to be associated with the geographic maldistribution of physicians, who were underrepresented in inner city and rural areas. Thus policy makers in the late 1960s and 1970s focused on how to use the reimbursement systems in Medicare and Medicaid to steer advanced practice nurses away from areas with physician surpluses and into physician shortage areas.

As is often the case in the highly decentralized American health care system, however, public policies regarding APNs often conflicted with one another. The national priority on improving access to care that accompanied President Johnson's Great Society Program of the 1960s was tempered in the 1970s and thereafter by the explosion of health expenditures and to the increasing costs to the federal government of Medicare and Medicaid. One strategy to contain costs favored by policy makers was to require physician supervision of APNs to promote their use as substitutes for physician visits and thereby limit new expenditures that would likely occur with the introduction of a new class of health care providers. Organized medicine supported the federal requirement for physician supervision of APNs because it was consistent with its agenda to exert control over the medical division of labor. Very quickly, organized medicine recast the purpose of the federal supervision requirement, which was originally intended as a cost-containment strategy, into a public issue of quality control that has persisted to this day (Cooper & Aiken, 2001). The point, however, is that public policies to steer nurses to underserved geographic areas conflicted with the requirement of physician supervision because, by definition, there were insufficient physicians to supervise APNs in physician shortage areas.

A consistent physician critique of APNs, from the inception of their expanded roles, is that APNs do not contribute to improving access to care because they desire to practice in locales where there are already sufficient numbers of physicians, the requirements for physician supervision notwithstanding (Kassirer, 1994).

Pennsylvania Survey Findings

The Center for Health Outcomes and Policy Research at the University of Pennsylvania undertook a survey of all nurse practitioners and nurse-mid-wives in Pennsylvania in the mid-1990s to obtain a better understanding of the distribution of their practices by specialty and location, and to shed new light on how implicit and explicit restrictions influenced their practice choices. The survey revealed that 40% of Pennsylvania's nurse practitioners practiced in underserved areas, and an additional 45% said that they would be willing to work in underserved areas if employment opportunities were available. Of those who were willing to work in underserved areas, 63% said that they would work in either rural or urban areas, 25% indicated that they would work in rural but not urban areas, and 12% said that they would work in urban but not rural areas.

In the case of certified nurse-midwives (CNMs), half reported already working in underserved areas, and an additional 39% said that they were willing to work in underserved areas. Of those CNMs who would work in an underserved area, 57% said they would work in a rural or urban area, 30% would work in a rural but not urban area, and 13% would work in an urban but not a rural area.

The data confirm that a significant percentage of APNs already work in underserved areas, and most would consider practicing there if employment opportunities existed. We did not find that APNs had a bias toward urban areas; in fact, the opposite was true. Significantly more nurse practitioners and nurse-midwives said they would be willing to work in underserved rural areas than in underserved urban areas. Hence, we concluded that the physician supervision requirement for nurse practitioners along with problems with prescriptive authority were primary impediments to advanced practice nurses locating in underserved areas. We predicted that lifting the physician supervision requirement would help achieve one of the original policy objectives of the federal government's subsidy of APN education—improving access to appropriate health services by those presently underserved. In recent years, the federal government has, for the most part, removed cumbersome direct physician supervision requirements for Medicare and Medicaid payment policies for APNs and now defers instead to state practice acts, the great majority of which have no requirements for direct physician supervision.

COMMENTARY

By all measures, the future for APNs looks very promising. Although organized medicine has not noticeably changed its negative stance toward advanced nursing practice, physicians, health care organizations, and public and private insurers have all exhibited growing openness to APNs. The landscape of health care has changed so dramatically since nurse practitioners were introduced that many of the original barriers to practice have fallen because of fundamental changes in the organization and financing of health care. Large multispecialty group practices and health maintenance organizations develop organizational solutions around outdated nurse practice act issues, such as lack of prescriptive authority for nurse practitioners (Jacobson, Parker, & Coulter, 1998). New organizational alignments have swept away many of the difficulties experienced by nurse-midwives and others in gaining hospital admission privileges. Innovators like Mundinger have challenged all the myths about nurse practitioners by demonstrating that nurse-managed primary care can compete head on with medicine in a highly competitive environment because consumers with a choice will elect care by advanced practice nurses (Mundinger, 2002; Mundinger et al., 2000).

One measure of the success of an innovation in health care is the extent to which it is replicated internationally. Within the past 5 years, an increasing number of countries have concluded that the evidence base amassed in the United States demonstrating safety, cost-savings potential, and consumer acceptance of nurse practitioners provides a rationale for the introduction of expanded roles for nurses elsewhere in the world. The United Kingdom (Horrocks, Anderson, Salisbury, 2002), Canada, and New Zealand (Hughes, 2002) are among the countries actively introducing nurse practitioners.

The APN movement in the United States can be proclaimed a success. The number of qualified practitioners has increased dramatically. Likewise, employer demand for APNs has more than kept pace with increasing supply. While concerns about the safety of APN care have not totally been put to rest (Sox, 2000), consumers', employers', and insurers' acceptance of

APNs has created a positive environment for practice. Escalating concerns about growing health care costs will no doubt result in continuing challenges for APNs and their practices, as occurred after the Balanced Budget Act of 1997 abruptly reduced reimbursement for many community-based nurse-managed programs, causing these programs to close. However, APNs have demonstrated considerable resourcefulness and tenacity over three decades to thrive in what has been, in years past, a hostile environment for growth. All the evidence suggests that APNs have become fully integrated into the mainstream of American health care and are likely to prosper in the future.

ACKNOWLEDGMENTS

Supported by grants from The Robert Wood Johnson Foundation Investigator Awards in Health Policy Research, and The Pew Charitable Trusts.

REFERENCES AND BIBLIOGRAPHY

Aiken, L. H. (1995). Health work force policy. In *For the public good: Highlights from the Institute of Medicine, 1970–1995* (pp. 70–83). Washington, DC: National Academy Press.

Aiken, L. H. (2001). Allied health professions. In N. J. Smelser & P. B. Baltes (Eds.), *International encyclopedia of the social and behavioral sciences* (Vol. 10, pp. 6591–6598). Oxford: Elsevier.

Aiken, L. H., Lewis, C. E., Craig, J. E., Mendenhall, R. C., Blendon, R., & Rogers, D. E. (1979). Contributions of specialists to primary care: A new perspective. *New England Journal of Medicine, 300,* 1363–1370.

Aiken, L. H., & Sage, W. M. (1993). Staffing national health care reform: A role for advanced practice nurses. *Akron Law Review, 26,* 187–211.

Cooper, R. A. (1994). Seeking a balanced physician workforce for the 21st century. *Journal of the American Medical Association, 272,* 680–687.

Cooper, R. A., & Aiken, L. H. (2001). Human inputs: The health care workforce and medical markets. *Journal of Health Politics, Policy and Law, 26,* 925–938.

Cooper, R. A., Getzen, T. E., McKee, H. J., & Laud, P. (2002). Economic and demographic trends signal an impending physician shortage. *Health Affairs, 21*(1), 140–154).

Cooper, R. A., Henderson, T., & Dietrich, C. L. (1998). Roles of nonphysician clinicians as autonomous providers of patient care. *Journal of the American Medical Association, 280,* 795–802.

Cooper, R. A., Laud, P., & Dietrich, C. L. (1998). Current and projected workforce of nonphysician clinicians. *Journal of the American Medical Association, 280,* 788–794.

Draper, D. A., Hurley, E., Lesser, C. S., & Strunk, B. C. (2002). The changing face of managed care. *Health Affairs, 21,* 11–23.

Ford, L. C. (1982). Nurse practitioners: History of a new idea and predictions for the future. In L. H. Aiken (Ed.), *Nursing in the 1980s: Crises, opportunities, and challenges* (pp. 231–242). Philadelphia: J. B. Lippincott.

Hartley, H. (1999). The influence of managed care on supply of certified nurse-midwives: An evaluation of the physician dominance thesis. *Journal of Health and Social Behavior, 40,* 87–101.

Hooker, R. S., & Berlin, L. E. (2002). Trends in the supply of physician assistants and nurse practitioners in the United States. *Health Affairs, 21,* 174–181.

Hooker, R. S., & McCaig, L. F. (2001). Use of physician assistants and nurse practitioners in primary care, 1995–1999. *Health Affairs, 20,* 231–238.

Horrocks, S., Anderson, E., & Salisbury, C. (2002). Systematic review of whether nurse practitioners working in primary care can provide equivalent care to doctors. *British Medical Journal, 324,* 819–823.

Hughes, F. A. (2002). Reflections from "down under" about NPs "up top." *Journal of Psychosocial Nursing and Mental Health Services, 40,* 6–8.

Jacobson, P. D., Parker, L. E., & Coulter, I. D. (1998). Nurse practitioners and physician assistants as primary care providers in institutional settings. *Inquiry, 35,* 432–446.

Kassirer, J. P. (1994). What role for nurse practitioners in primary care? *New England Journal of Medicine, 330,* 204–205.

Lin, S. X., Hooker, R. S., Lenz, E. R., & Hopkins, S. C. (2002). Nurse practitioners and physician assistants in hospital outpatient departments, 1997–1999. *Nursing Economics, 20,* 174–179.

Mundinger, M. O. (1994). Advanced-practice nursing—good medicine for physicians? *New England Journal of Medicine, 330,* 211–214.

Mundinger, M. O. (2002). Through a different looking glass. *Health Affairs, 21,* 163–164.

Mundinger, M. O., Kane, R. L., Lenz, E. R., Totten, A. M., Wei-Yann, T. Cleary, P. D., Friedewald, W. T., Siu, A. L., & Shelanksi, M. L. (2000). Primary care outcomes in patients treated by nurse practitioners or physicians: A randomized trial. *Journal of the American Medical Association, 283,* 59–68.

National League for Nursing Accrediting Commission (NLNAC). (2002). *Directory of accredited nursing programs 2002.* Retrieved September 16, 2002, from www.nlnac.org

Sage, W. M., & Aiken, L. H. (1997). Regulating interdisciplinary practice. In T. Jost (Ed.), *Regulation of the health professions* (pp. 71–101). Ann Arbor, MI: Health Administration Press.

Sochalski, J. (2002) Nursing shortage redux: Turning the corner on an enduring problem. *Health Affairs, 21,* 157–163.

Sox, H. C. (2000). Independent primary care practice by nurse practitioners. *Journal of the American Medical Association, 283,* 106–108.

Spratley, E., Johnson, A., Sochalski, J., Fritz, M., & Spencer, W. (2002). *The registered nurse population, March 2000: Findings from the National Sample Survey of Registered Nurses.* Rockville, MD: Division of Nursing, Bureau of Health Professions, Health Resources and Services Administration, U.S. Department of Health and Human Services.

Weiner, J. P. (1994). Forecasting the effects of health reform on U.S. physician workforce requirement: Evidence from HMO staffing patterns. *Journal of the American Medical Association, 272,* 222–230.

Chapter 25

ACADEMIC NURSING PRACTICE: IMPLICATIONS FOR POLICY

Lois K. Evans, Melinda Jenkins, and Karen Buhler-Wilkerson

REENVISIONING ACADEMIC PRACTICE IN SCHOOLS OF NURSING

For a practice discipline, the notion that those who generate and disseminate nursing knowledge should also be expert practitioners seems self-evident. However, the history of faculty practice in nursing academic circles has been anything but smooth. By the close of the 20th century, developments in health care organization and financing, in roles for advanced practice nurses, and in the struggle of academic nursing for greater equity with academic medicine had heightened the debate about faculty practice in academic nursing. Several ingredients critical for embracing practice as an equal arm of academic nursing's tripartite mission appeared finally to be in place: a richer mix of doctorally prepared faculty with research funding, widespread availability of practice reimbursement for advanced practice nurse faculty, and the potential for school of nursing control of community-based practice. As we enter fully into this new era, the challenge remains for academic nursing to amass, demonstrate, and disseminate the scientific evidence that nursing makes an essential difference in health care, both in quality and cost. If nursing as a discipline is to sustain

443

its renewed emphasis on the tripartite mission, then we must move beyond previous conceptions of faculty practice to institutionalize academic nursing practice, wherein research, education, and clinical care converge and are highly integrated. In continuing to map this course, we have considerably updated and expanded this chapter to discuss the parallels and disparities between historically community-based academic nursing and historically hospital-based academic medicine; to critique the current definition of faculty practice as it relates to academic nursing practice; to identify facilitators in the establishment and maintenance of academic nursing practice, including networks and collaborations; and to illustrate current challenges and opportunities for the future through use of a case example, the Penn Nursing Network.

ACADEMIC PRACTICE: AN HISTORICAL REVIEW

Academic Medicine

A comparison of the not-so-parallel development and trajectories of academic medicine and academic nursing is instructive in understanding the critical implications of the debate on faculty practice in nursing circles. Following a 150-year history of academically based training, early 20th-century reforms in American medical education established research as a significant expectation of the faculty and a crucial element in the educational milieu. Patient care was already incorporated into medical school activities through ownership of and/or strong affiliation arrangements with hospitals. Thus, the triad of teaching, research, and patient care came to be viewed as inextricably and vitally bound (Burondess, 1991). Federal training and biomedical research monies flowed into academic medicine after World War II, while medical faculty served as peer reviewers in the distribution of these research funds through the newly formed National Institutes of Health. Whereas income to schools of medicine had traditionally been derived from sources analogous to each of the three arms of the tripartite mission—state appropriations, endowment, and tuition; research grants and contracts, and patient care revenues—their relative proportions changed dramatically during the 1980s. Faculty practice plans that were initiated in schools of medicine in response to the introduction of Medicare and Medicaid in the mid-1960s provided an increasingly important supplemental funding source for medical education. Funds derived from teaching and research did not keep pace with inflation, while funds from patient care services continued to expand, both in absolute and relative terms (MacLeod & Schwarz, 1986; Turner, 1989). These shifts in funding likewise created shifts in time commitments of medical faculty, with increasing numbers of faculty appointed to teaching-practice tracks.

By the 1990s, however, the traditional faculty practice plan models were becoming less lucrative, primarily because of changes in reimbursement from fee-for-service to managed care. Academic medical centers acted quickly, building comprehensive health care systems to spread financial risk between and among system components and to increase positions of negotiating strength with managed care organizations while continuing to generate large revenues for their medical schools' education and research missions. At the same time, changes in the reimbursement stream forced schools of medicine to begin to shift their locus of teaching, practice, and research from the institution to the community (Krakower, Ganem & Beran, 1994). Today, academic medical centers still face unpredictable resources (including changes in Graduate Medical Education funding through Medicare [Nicholson, 2002]), changing institutional mandates, and growing demands for accountability (D'Alessandri et al., 2000; Karpf, Schultze, & Levey, 2000; Nonnemaker & Griner, 2001; Reinhardt, 2000; Rodgers, Zuckerman, & Goode, 2000). Within this increasingly competitive environment, medical faculty struggle to maintain a productive program of research and, at the same time, teach and care for patients. As academic physicians' careers become more and more dissimilar to those of faculty in the rest of the university, many medical schools are reexamining faculty titles and criteria for appointment, promotion, and tenure (Nonnemaker & Griner, 2001; Rubin, 1998; University of Pennsylvania School of Medicine, 2000). In addition, the uncertainties of reimbursement for patient care and medical school dependence upon extramural research funding have further heightened the tensions between academic medical centers and their parent universities. The most radical responses have resulted in corporate restructuring, including the selling of university teaching hospitals, while in other universities, centers have chosen simply to re-engineer their administrative systems in an effort to create a more responsive and flexible organizational model (Blumenthal & Weissman, 2000; Nonnemaker & Griner, 2001; Rodin, 2001).

Despite the volatility, complexity, and constraints of today's health care system, the teaching hospital is *not* an endangered species (Risse, 1999). Recent analyses of medical school finances (1998–1999) indicate continued expansion of both faculty size and revenues. Currently, practice plans still represent the largest single source of medical schools' revenues (average 34.5%), while hospital support accounts for an average 14.6%. Grants and contracts (primarily for federal research), which account for 30% of revenues, experienced the largest dollar increase in 1997–1998, and other sources (tuition, endowments, gifts, state appropriations, etc.) made up the final 21% (Blumenthal & Weissman, 2000; Krakower, Coble, Williams, & Jones, 2000; Krakower, Ganem, & Beran, 1994).

These recent shifts have posed additional challenges and conflicts, both within medical schools and between medical schools and their parent academic institutions. Nonetheless, a review of academic medicine's journey is instructive in understanding academic nursing's historical evolution and in charting its future course.

Academic Nursing

As is well known, nursing came late to academia, with little real presence until after World War II (Reverby, 1987). From the 1940s forward, nursing education shifted appreciably from a hospital-based apprenticeship model to a professional curriculum housed in institutions of higher education. Thus, nursing faculty and students became separated not only from direct practice responsibilities but also from reaping any direct benefits through (hospital) revenue generation.

Federal support for the education of nurses in academic settings dates from 1935 (for public health nursing), 1947 (for psychiatric nursing), and 1956 (for administration, teaching, and supervision in any nursing field). Changes in the educational preparation of the workforce were, however, slow; by 1954, only 1% of nurses had a master's degree and 7.2% a bachelor's degree (Kalisch & Kalisch, 1978). Despite increasing federal aid, by 1962 only 14% of nurses had graduated from a baccalaureate program. After 1964, federal investment in nursing education became even more generous. By 1970, $15.4 million had been given to schools of nursing, 30,000 nurses had received tuition support, $73 million in construction grants had been awarded, and an additional $103 million was dedicated to training nurse administrators and supervisors (Lynaugh & Brush, 1996). Doctoral education for nursing faculty was the most delayed: Only 4% of nursing faculty had earned doctoral degrees in 1962, and even today only 4% of all nurses are doctorally prepared (American Nurses Association, 2003). The first comprehensive doctoral program in nursing was not initiated until 1964, at the University of California, San Francisco. Thus, at a time when schools of medicine were benefiting from the influx of federal research dollars, few nursing faculty were eligible to apply. Further, from the first $500,000 allocated in 1956 until the late 1970s, federal dollars for research projects in nursing focused on educational issues and studies of nurses and nursing practice roles rather than on clinical nursing problems.

While a few schools of nursing (notably the University of Florida, Case Western Reserve, Rush-Presbyterian University, and the University of Rochester) made valiant attempts to structurally reunite practice and education through such models as "academic leadership" and "unification," these were not important sources of revenue for their schools and have not been widely adopted (Fagin, 2000). Finally, while medical schools' practice incomes soared in the 1960s, direct reimbursement for much of nursing practice remained essentially unavailable until the late 1990s. Even now, for most nursing schools, revenue from practice activities remains insubstantial, scarcely (if at all) covering associated costs.

Reuniting Education and Practice

Concern over the widening split between education and practice reached a high pitch with the advent of advanced practice roles in the 1960s and 1970s (Walker, 1995). Like academic medicine, academic nursing developed model teaching centers for students where the best of nursing practice could be observed, learned, and examined. Unlike medicine, nursing's academic origins were community based. Nursing's first forays into academia in the early 1920s were postgraduate study for public health nurses (Kalish & Kalish, 1978). O. Marie Henry, Director of the Division of Nursing during the 1970s and 1980s, challenged nurse educators to take control of practice by creating centers for the integration of practice, education, and research where new methods of nursing care and delivery could be developed, tested, and demonstrated. She proposed that such centers should be in a variety of settings that are dependent on high-quality nursing care and that nursing could readily influence, such as nursing homes, rehabilitation centers, and the community (Henry, 1986). While there was consensus regarding the necessity to create centers where nursing would be the primary focus, debate over these centers' practice agendas mirrored that of nursing in the aggregate (Fehring, Schulte, & Reisch, 1986). Like public health nurses who preceded them and created the first nursing centers (Thwing, 1919; Walsh, 1920), contemporary nurses' early "insider" debates reflected the profession's continued struggle to achieve professional autonomy in practice, to legitimize claims for direct reimbursement for practice, to control practice environments, and to define requirements for entry into advanced practice nursing.

The 1970s saw a renewed effort among nursing school faculties to establish their own practices, related at least in part to the requirement for nurse practitioner program faculty to be current in clinical care. The 1979 American Academy of Nursing resolution in support of faculty practice, followed by a series of symposia cosponsored by the Academy and the Robert Wood Johnson Foundation, served to further escalate the debate on the role of practice in academia and to stimulate the evolution of a variety of models, including partnerships, faculty practice plans, and nursing centers. By the early 1980s, 63 schools of nursing were affiliated with or were sponsoring nurse-managed centers, the National League for Nursing had established a Council for Nursing Centers, and the first national conference on nursing centers had been held. Consensus was building that nursing faculty must increase control of practice environments in order to influence education, conduct research, and facilitate research-based care. Many of these practice initiatives were directed to low-income and vulnerable populations, and adequate attention was not given to post-grant financial sustainability. The revenue-generating, business aspects of the integrated mission, thus, lagged far behind (Aiken, 1992). Finally, these practice models often espoused an emphasis on independent or nurse-managed practice, in part reflecting nursing's difficulty in attaining a "place at the table" to plan and provide such services within organized health care. In addition, there was an identified need for nursing to demonstrate its value to society.

Context of Sociopolitical Forces

As the 1990s drew to a close, an unprecedented window of opportunity existed for academic nursing, especially in research-intensive environments, to achieve a more powerful position by finally integrating its tripartite mission. For the first time, many schools of nursing had a critical mass of faculty, prepared at the doctoral level and successfully engaged in programs of funded research, to compete for research dollars. The National Institute for Nursing Research, together with other institutes and sources, was providing important support for the development of the science ($120 million was allocated to nursing by NIH in fiscal year 2002 (National Institute of Nursing Research, n.d.) as well as opportunities for nurse faculty to define the national nursing research agenda and to participate in peer review.

Further, there was a critical mass of advanced practice nurse (APN) faculty for whom there now existed greater opportunities for practice reimbursement (Jenkins & Torrisi, 1995). APNs in most states had prescriptive privileges (Pearson, 2002), and other constraints on the advanced practice of nursing were gradually lifting. Interdisciplinary resistance to the APN role, while still prevalent, had lessened as the data consistently demonstrated quality and cost-effectiveness as well as public acceptance, trust, satisfaction, and demand (Brown & Grimes, 1995; Brush & Capezuti, 1996; Kerekes, Jenkins, & Torrisi, 1996; Mundinger et al., 2000; "Split decision," 2001). The passage by Congress in 1989 and 1997 of legislation that opened direct reimbursement to APNs under Medicare and Medicaid began to pave the way for other insurers to follow suit (Sullivan-Marx, Happ, Bradley, & Maislin, 2000). Simultaneously, the rapid escalation of managed care continued to have important positive implications for the practice of APNs.

Thus, in the dawn of the new century, academic nursing remains at one of those rare moments in history when all the forces are right—research dollars, practice dollars, and educational and societal demand—to permit successful integration of the tripartite mission, enabling nursing to gain equity with the other academic health professions and to make a visible difference in the health of the nation. Yet in no sphere of resources—federal support for education, federal research opportunities, or practice income—is there comparability with schools of medicine. Thus, embracing this new paradigm will not be for the faint of heart. There still remain the formidable tasks of retaining control of nursing's community practice environments, creating acceptance in academic circles for integrating the practice component of the tripartite mission (Rudy, Anderson, Dudjak, Robert, & Miler, 1995), and finding fresh ways of partnering that will capitalize on earned power and equity. Working from this new power position, nursing will no longer need to emphasize the nurse-managed or independent focus of its work that dominated the 1990s, but can again recognize the collaborative models that it has always espoused (Hegyvary, 2001). Given increasing interest from both the community and schools of medicine in working with nursing to achieve mutual goals, such collaboration is most likely to evolve within the context of interdisciplinary practice, education, and research that is community based, focused, or partnered (Gersten-Rothenberg, 1998; Rubin, 1998; Schwartz, 2001; Taylor & Marion, 2000).

DEFINITIONS AND MODELS OF ACADEMIC NURSING PRACTICE

A critique of the current definitions and models of academic nursing practice is important if we are to move toward a new paradigm. Until recently, the literature has utilized primarily the term *faculty practice* rather than *academic practice* when referring to the role of practice in schools of nursing. In our view, this term is limiting in regard to the integration of the tripartite mission, as can be seen in a critique of the following definition:

Faculty practice includes all aspects of the delivery of health care through the roles of clinician, educator, researcher, consultant and administrator. Faculty practice activities within this framework encompass direct nursing services to individuals and groups, as well as technical assistance and consultation to individuals, families, groups, and communities. In addition to the provision of service, the practice provides opportunities for promotion, tenure, merit, and revenue generation. *A distinguishing characteristic of faculty practice within the School of Nursing is the belief that teaching, research, practice, and service must be closely integrated to achieve excellence. Faculty practice provides the vehicle through which faculty implement these missions.* There is an assumption that student practica and residencies as well as *research opportunities for faculty and students are an established component of faculty practice.* (Taylor & Marion, 2000, p. 800; italics added)

The notion of integrating the tripartite mission does not frame this definition of faculty practice, but rather is added near the end, either as an afterthought or in acknowledgment of its "presumed" existence. The scant research literature (Brown, 2001; Jones & VanOrt, 2001; Macnee, 1999; Sawyer et al., 2000; Walker, 1995; Zachariah & Lundeen, 1997), and our own experience, however, dictate that the latter is hardly the case. At the University of Pennsylvania, we have defined academic nursing practice as "the intentional integration of education, research and clinical care in an academic setting for the purpose of advancing the science and shaping the structure and quality of health care" (University of Pennsylvania School of Nursing, 2002, p. 6). This broader vision of academic nursing practice clearly articulates the deliberate integration of the three arms of the tripartite mission, placing emphasis on the generation and dissemination of nursing practice knowledge through health service provision. Such a view also allows for the possibility that faculty may move between and among the three arms of the mission, at any one point in time concentrating more heavily on one or two roles rather than being master of all three simultaneously (Norbeck, 1998). Academic medicine recognized this necessity long ago and created a range of roles and tracks for faculty, including those for clinical practice and research. In academic nursing, however, the problem of "role overload" when faculty attempt to do everything has been acknowledged in survey after survey as a contributing factor in nurse faculty burnout (Rudy 2001; Walker, 1995).

Models

Historically, nursing has experimented with a variety of practice models (see Broussard, Delahoussaye, & Poirrier, 1996; Hutelmyer & Donnelly,

1996; Potash & Taylor, 1993; Taylor & Marion, 2000). Academic practice models may vary by structural type (e.g., school-owned nursing centers or other equity enterprises, joint appointments or contracts, partnerships or joint ventures), by faculty roles (e.g., practitioner, consultant, teacher, researcher), by specialty practice (e.g., community health, elder care, primary care, school health, midwifery, and so on), or by administrative aspects of practice (e.g., volunteer, joint practice collaborative arrangements, revenue-generating, contractual) (Taylor & Marion, 2000). While any school may simultaneously operate examples of several of these types, the entrepreneurial model appears to afford the most flexibility for strength and growth of academic practices within a rapidly changing market. Vanderbilt University School of Nursing's ability to advance its practice mission by taking advantage of a statewide conversion to Medicaid managed care is an example (Conway-Welsh, 1995; Spitzer et al., 1996). The entrepreneurial model allows for a variety of revenue-generating practice designs that may be wholly or partially owned by a school or its affiliates. Other prominent examples include the University of Texas-Houston Health Science Center School of Nursing (Mackey & McNiel, 1997), the University of Rochester (Coggiola & Walker, 1995), and Columbia University School of Nursing (Auerhahn, 1997; Boccuzzi, 1998). Some schools have a faculty practice plan that delineates how faculty-generated practice is governed and revenues shared (Taylor, 1996). For faculties considering academic practice, resource guidelines are available (Marion, 1997; Potash & Taylor, 1993).

Facilitators

A distinguishing feature of academic nursing practice is the opportunity for *all* faculty, regardless of the degree of intensity of their clinical practice activity, to participate in practice-related research within school-owned or -affiliated practices. Thus, academic practice becomes the medium for testing innovative models, developing a common language to measure nursing outcomes, and generating new knowledge and evidence-based practice (Lang, Jenkins, Evans, & Matthews, 1996; Zachariah & Lundeen, 1997) rather than just another opportunity for faculty to maintain clinical skills, gain personal satisfaction, teach students by serving as a role model, and so on. As in academic medicine, academic nursing practice spawns increased research funding and educational program development resources, and holds the potential to generate much-needed revenues for schools' educational programs.

For this to happen, however, faculty governance and an infrastructure tuned to the business of practice are essential. Patient care responsibilities that feed the teaching and research missions are constant and demanding and have a rhythm very different from that of the usual academic calendar. Discontinuity and tragic consequences can result unless the business of the practice is well managed. Faculty governance and business infrastructure facilitate stability of practices and development of community trust in their ongoing presence (Lang & Evans, 1999; Swan & Evans, 2001). Other facilitators of the practice mission include flexible faculty scheduling and workload, administrative recognition and support for practice, and a valuing of practice in tenure and promotion criteria (Burns, 1997; Norbeck & Taylor, 1999; Nugent, Barger, & Bridges, 1993; Potash & Taylor, 1993; Taylor, 1996; Walker, 1995). In addition, practices that fit third-party reimbursement streams and contracts are most likely to achieve fiscal viability. This has remained a challenge for many community nursing centers (Frenn, Lundeen, Martin, Riesch, & Wilson, 1996; Mackey, Adams, & McNiel, 1994; Vincent, Oakley, Pohl, & Walker, 2000), especially those serving primarily the economically disadvantaged. Facilitators in achieving the teaching mission associated with academic practice are faculty confidence in their own skills and expertise and willingness to reach beyond the traditional academic role. The practice-associated research mission is facilitated by the establishment of common databases through collaboration among several schools of nursing to monitor client data, assess costs, and investigate faculty effectiveness in practice (Anderko & Kinion, 2001; Frenn, et al., 1996; Iowa Intervention Project, 1997; Lang, Jenkins, et al., 1996; Marek, Jenkins, Westra, & McGinley, 1998; Pohl, Bostrom, Talarczyk, & Cavanagh, 2001). Role integration is enhanced when faculty are able to generate research from within their practice (Brown, 2001; Macnee, 1999).

Institutional support from the university and the dean is essential. In fact, administrative support is perceived to be the greatest overall facilitator of faculty practice (Barger & Bridges, 1987; Norbeck & Taylor, 1999). In schools where administrative policies support practice as a promotion criterion, the mean number of reported practice hours is nearly twice as high. Schools with doctoral programs and those that are public institutions reported higher levels of faculty practice time. Practice, however, is not a criterion for promotion and tenure in most schools, and many schools do not have formalized faculty practice plans (Barger, Nugent, & Bridges, 1993; Norbeck & Taylor, 1999). For individual faculty members, workload and time demands must be balanced with financial and academic promotion incentives. As mentioned previously, individual faculty members pay a high price in role strain and work overload unless roles are well integrated. Institutional commitment to policies supporting implementation of an integrated tripartite mission is critical (Walker, 1995).

Several nursing schools have formal criteria for clinical scholarship within the tenure track or on a separate, parallel clinician-educator track (Burns, 1997; Fagin, 2000). Oregon's criteria, for example, mesh with Boyer's (1990) proposal that scholarship include the four domains: discovery, integration, application, and teaching. Currently, higher education emphasizes research and the scholarship of discovery. Universities that also house medical schools, however, are likely familiar with promotion criteria that honor practice. Valuing the scholarship of research application, including the development of evidence-based care, through inclusion in nursing promotion and tenure criteria enhances excellence in practice, education, and scholarship for individual faculty members and for the school (Burgener, 2001; Jones & Van Ort, 2001).

Finally, schools of nursing are forming collaborative arrangements to enhance both sustainability and research opportunities. The Regional Nursing Centers Consortium is a Philadelphia-based organization that was initiated in the mid-1990s to enhance potential for sustainability and growth of neighborhood-based nursing centers (Hansen-Turton & Kinsey, 2001; Regional Nursing Centers Consortium, 2000). Recently renamed the National Nursing Centers Consortium (NNCC), it now has membership from over 30 nursing centers, many owned by schools of nursing, from across the country. NNCC has developed guidelines for quality management in member centers, including structure, process, and outcome criteria. With support from the Philadelphia-based Independence Foundation, a primary emphasis of the NNCC is to collect common data elements across centers to derive information that can be used in educating policy makers and shaping public policy in order to mainstream nursing centers' access to reimbursement (National Nursing Centers Consortium, 2002). Currently, installation and implementation of electronic office management and patient record software is in process. The Midwest Regional Nursing Centers Consortium (MRNCC) was recently formalized with similar goals (University of Wisconsin—Milwaukee and School of Nursing, 2002), and funding from the Agency for Healthcare Research & Quality (AHRQ) in support of a practice-based research network among member centers has been obtained. Similarly, the Michigan Consortium contains four schools of nursing in a project supported by the Kellogg Foundation to enhance education in, and evaluation of, academic community nursing centers (Pohl et al., 2001). In addition to benefiting from shared educational materials, joint policy efforts, and "business of practice" advice, the

Consortium has also agreed to a shared database that is facilitating evaluation and research efforts. The National Organization of Nurse Practitioner Faculty (NONPF) has recently created a targeted action group to promote networking among academic nursing centers (see http://www.nonpf.com). One action being explored is the promotion of collaborative collection and storage of common data from faculty practices. The Penn Macy Fellows is a loosely bound group comprising faculty teams from 21 schools of nursing in research-intensive environments that participated in the Penn Macy Initiative (1999–2001). This University of Pennsylvania project, supported by the Josiah Macy, Jr., Foundation, assisted such schools to successfully advance their academic practice agendas (Lang, Evans, & Swan, 2002). Because the small size of each practice limits research, fellows have expressed strong interest in creating a Penn Macy Research Alliance that would facilitate greater research access to populations served by academic nursing practices nationally. Currently, the Knowledge Center on the Penn Macy Web site (http://www.pennmacy.com) facilitates access to sets of common data elements being used by several entities. Finally, a network of nurse clinicians (APRNET) has been formed with support from AHRQ to facilitate practice-based research (Grey & Walker, 1998). These examples indicate recognition of need for, and the synergistic empowerment that can derive from, partnerships rather than competition. A rarity in the past, such partnerships across nursing educational institutions likely represent important new realities for growth of the academic practice agenda.

THE UNIVERSITY OF PENNSYLVANIA: A CASE EXAMPLE

An examination of the evolution of academic practice at the University of Pennsylvania School of Nursing may be instructive in helping to understand the forces that have influenced, and continue to shape, development of advanced practice nursing. Academic medicine and nursing at Penn will first be compared, then the school's evolving academic practice will be described to demonstrate Penn Nursing's unique window of opportunity to fully integrate its tripartite mission.

School of Medicine

The School of Medicine (SOM) at the University of Pennsylvania is ranked second among the top U.S. academic medical centers, with over $325 million in annual federal research and training dollars. Opening in 1765 as the first medical school in America, Penn Med early on gained control of its practice environment through developing in 1874 the first American university teaching hospital built expressly for that purpose (Baltzell, 1996). The Hospital of the University of Pennsylvania (HUP), together with several large nearby teaching hospitals with close medical school affiliations, enabled faculty to educate students, practice, and conduct research relatively unencumbered. The School's 22 faculty practice plans (Clinical Practices of the University of Pennsylvania) grew rapidly after the influx of Medicare and Medicaid dollars in the 1960s. Responding to a more recent challenge posed by health care financing changes in Philadelphia, the Medical Center embarked on a bold strategic plan in 1993 to develop the nation's first fully integrated academic health system, the University of Pennsylvania Health System (UPHS). This initiative enabled UPHS to expand its influence and strengthen its position in a budding managed care market by acquiring, through purchase, merger, or affiliation, multiple community-based sites, including primary care practices, community hospitals, nursing homes, home care and hospice agencies, and rehabilitation centers. Access to a clinically diverse patient population and a range of health care delivery settings was believed necessary to ensure continued achievement of its educational and research goals and to maintain its financial resource base (Iglehart, 1995). The experience and maturity required to bring this strategic plan to fruition proved overwhelming for an immature system in what turned out to be a very volatile environment. Facing huge deficits and operating losses, the trustees and University administration considered a number of options, but settled on a new structure within the University with a single executive vice president and dean of medicine and a single umbrella organization—Penn Medicine. A unified board provides for integration, nimbleness, efficiencies, and economies of scale and "references every decision about health service delivery through its impact on and its benefit for the School of Medicine, which is why we are running health services in the first place" (Rodin, 2001, p. 3). Continued support for the SOM's initiatives is thus secured.

School of Nursing

The University of Pennsylvania remains the only Ivy League University that prepares nurses at the baccalaureate, master's, doctoral, and postdoctoral levels. Its School of Nursing has maintained top rankings in the level of federal research funding, totaling nearly $6 million in total federal dollars in fiscal year 2001 (N.I.H. Awards, n.d.). Like the School of Medicine, Penn Nursing also has a distinctive history. By 1950, an autonomous

School of Nursing had evolved at Penn from programs initiated earlier at the Hospital of the University of Pennsylvania Training School (1886), the School of Education (1935), and the Division of Medical Affairs (1945). Master's study was begun first in nursing education (1937) and psychiatric-mental health nursing (1961), then in other clinical areas. Penn's first nurse practitioner program was opened in 1972. Doctoral study (DNSc in 1978, then PhD in 1984) soon followed. While the University's research emphasis and the academic practice histories of the School of Medicine and the other health science schools (dentistry, veterinary medicine) lent precedent for developing the tripartite mission in the autonomous but younger School of Nursing, there was from the beginning disparity between nursing and these other schools in size, educational preparation, research funding, access to practice incomes, and control over practice environments.

Building the Base for the Tripartite Mission

The numbers of doctorally prepared faculty in the School of Nursing grew through the 1970s; yet even by the end of the decade, the level of funded research was modest at best. The recruitment of Dean Claire Fagin and faculty with expertise in clinical research, as well as the securing of external funding for a Center for Nursing Research, helped ensure the growth of the research mission and development of a doctoral program. Doctorally prepared advanced practice faculty were also recruited during this period, thus enhancing the focus on advanced practice within the educational and research domains.

Under Dean Fagin's leadership, a number of collaborative medicine and nursing faculty practice and research initiatives were implemented during the 1980s, and a partnership plan between the School of Nursing and the HUP evolved to relink the two entities (Fagin, 1986). Independent of structural change, the partnership focused on ways that the related but separate goals of the School of Nursing and the hospital—for clinical excellence, development of a research and scholarly base, and provision of excellent educational programs—could be best achieved. In 1984, the extension by the University Faculty Senate to nursing faculty of a track for clinician-educator standing faculty that was parallel to the tenure track facilitated the engagement of faculty in scholarly practice initiatives (Fagin, 2000). Doctorally prepared nurse practitioner and clinical nurse specialist faculty practiced within a variety of models, including joint appointment, contractual, and entrepreneurial private practices.

Other initiatives that helped create an environment to embrace the tripartite mission included directing the national Robert Wood Johnson

Teaching Nursing Home Project that emphasized the critical linkage of schools of nursing and clinical facilities to achieve high-quality care (Mezey, Lynaugh, & Cartier, 1988); serving as a training site for the Robert Wood Johnson Clinical Scholars program, which demonstrated faculty practice-research role integration; cultivating a faculty research agenda that was primarily clinically focused (Lang, Sullivan-Marx, & Jenkins, 1996); developing several intradisciplinary research centers that helped to successfully target the faculty's research efforts (Lang, 1996); and building strong affiliations with community partners such as with the Philadelphia Visiting Nurses Association (Buhler-Wilkerson, Naylor, Holt, & Rinke, 1998) and the Philadelphia Department of Recreation (Reed, 1997). Institutionally, the entrepreneurial model already existing within the University, strong advanced clinical practice educational programs, and clinical research programs, together with existing effective partnerships with health care entities and a formalized standing faculty clinician educator role, supported the continued development of academic practice in Penn Nursing. Thus, the stage was set for truly integrating the tripartite mission, a primary emphasis of Dean Norma Lang (Lang, 1996; Lang, Jenkins, et al., 1996; Lang, Sullivan-Marx, & Jenkins, 1996). Lang viewed the intentional integration of the tripartite mission as essential to facilitate the evolution of the science, the implementation of evidence-based practice, and the shaping of health care structure and quality. Under her leadership, several new clinically focused research centers were established, the school-owned Penn Nursing Network was formalized to complement existing practice affiliations and partnerships, and the Penn Macy Initiative to Advance Academic Nursing Practice was launched to provide other schools in research-intensive environments with a framework for establishing or strengthening academic practices. This phase of the evolution is described below.

Academic Nursing Practice at Penn

Over an 8-year period, the concept of academic practice at Penn Nursing evolved to encompass several dimensions. These include the practices of the faculty (both clinician educator and tenure track); the practices of the school-owned Penn Nursing Network; the partnerships and alliances with nursing at the University of Pennsylvania Health System, Children's Hospital of Philadelphia, the Visiting Nurse Association of Greater Philadelphia, and others; and interdisciplinary collaborative practices afforded through partnerships and alliances ("About our academic nursing practice," 2002–2003) (see Figure 25.1). Major teaching partner/affiliate institutions

Academic Practice Components

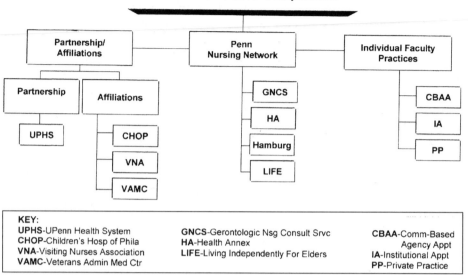

FIGURE 25.1   Penn Nursing academic nursing practice components.

are formally linked through clinician educator faculty appointments. Currently, 37.5% of the faculty are clinician educators (CEs) whose practice responsibilities range from administrative leadership (n =3), to advanced nursing practice and research with special populations (n = 14) to private practice (n = 1). The models for the CE and affiliated practices have not changed dramatically since they were conceived (Fagin, 2000), but the Penn Nursing Network, still a relatively young and innovative model, will be briefly described to illustrate challenges and opportunities for the future.

The school-owned component of its academic practices, the community-based Penn Nursing Network (PNN), was formalized in 1994 to help facilitate full integration of the school's tripartite mission (see Table 25.1).

Formal consultation provided assistance with developing the strategic plan for PNN, laying out an aggressive projected growth, from just under $0.5 million in gross revenues in fiscal year 1993 to $10 million in fiscal year 2001. (In actuality, for fiscal year 2001, the practices generated some $5.4 million in total gross revenues; in fiscal year 2002, PNN was conservatively projected to generate $7.4 million.) Building on a history of successful nurse-midwifery and geriatric services, clinician educator appointments,

TABLE 25.1   Penn Nursing Network Mission
and Vision Statements

Mission

Penn Nursing Network (PNN), a multipractice health care delivery network spanning the life cycle, is committed to community-based health care of the highest standard. PNN embraces health as a cornerstone for quality of life as defined by the person and supported by PNN staff. PNN promotes proactive health care, fostering active participation and personal responsibility in health care decisions.

PNN adheres to the belief that quality health care is defined as the degree to which health services for individuals and populations increase the likelihood of desired health outcomes and are consistent with current professional knowledge. Such outcomes are achieved through partnership with individuals, families, and the community and the integration of research-based practice, education of professionals and community members, and scientific inquiry.

PNN is committed to quality health care that is cost-effective, utilizing the most advanced and appropriate health care models and interventions.

Vision

PNN seeks to provide individuals, families, and the community with respectful and confidential quality care while educating health care professionals, developing research-based guidelines, and maintaining economic stability. PNN strives to improve health services to the community and is committed to affirm this vision with the care of each individual.

and the partnership with HUP, several practices for which the school was financially at risk were clustered together under the PNN umbrella. The model was designed to be flexible and responsive to market forces while meeting community need, research agendas, and educational mission. Thus, over the years, practices have been added (e.g., Living Independently For Elders, Hamburg) or closed (e.g., Collaborative Assessment and Rehabilitation for Elders Program [Evans & Yurkow, 1999], Neighborhood Midwifery, Community Midwifery Services, Perinatal Newborn Service, Continence Program) as appropriate, that is, in response to dramatic changes in reimbursement, population shifts, managed care emphases, and/or local competition. Currently the school operates practices that provide services primarily to underserved and vulnerable populations, including primary care, family planning and women's health, men's health, mental health, a Program of All-Inclusive Care for the Elderly (PACE) named Living Independently For Elders [LIFE], and consultation services (see Table 25.2). These practices are based on the school's strengths in research and advanced practice education as well as community preferences, needs, and service gaps.

While the practices of the PNN carry out Henry's (1986) agenda in that they are community based and focus on populations that are dependent on high-quality nursing, their development within the autonomous School of Nursing, as opposed to the Health System, has not been without challenges in a research-intensive university (Evans, 1994; Iglehart, 1995). Perceiving that its successful implementation would be important to long-term achievement of mutual goals, however, the faculty and administration persevered in their efforts to build the PNN.

Governance and Operations Management

Faculty governance, including review of new practice proposals, business plans, and quality management plans and outcomes, is accomplished through a standing committee of the school's faculty senate; this practice committee also has responsibility for the school's overall practice mission. Every practice is directly linked to the standing faculty through faculty academic directors, each of whom sits on the practice committee. The faculty academic director has responsibility for designing and maintaining the practice model and closely ties the practice to the academic enterprise of the school by facilitating educational and research opportunities and setting the research agenda. Day-to-day operations of each practice are accomplished by a professional manager and/or master clinician who serves as practice and/or clinical director. A director for academic nursing practices position, with a direct reporting line to the dean, was created to facilitate achievement of operating, fiscal, and quality outcomes within the tripartite mission over the entire network of practices. Recently vacated, the position is currently unfilled and its functions are being shared by the faculty academic directors and the associate dean for practice while the faculty is engaged in reexamining mission, organization, and leadership for practice, including the PNN, as a part of its strategic planning.

Business Infrastructure and Revenues

Infrastructure in support of practice is dynamic and constantly evolving, commensurate with overall practice growth and needs. Within a "make," "use," or "buy" framework, PNN has focused its central resources on strategic planning, monitoring, analysis, system and new service development, and quality management. Functions essential to effective management at the practice level, including facilities management, managed care credentialing,

**TABLE 25.2   University of Pennsylvania School of Nursing
Penn Nursing Network**

Overview

Penn Nursing Network (PNN) provides best practice models of community-based, family-focused health care services to people of all ages in a variety of settings. Advanced practice nursing services include well-child care, preteen and adolescent care, family planning, women's health, primary care for children and adults, consultation, mental health, and integrated acute and long-term care services for frail older adults. As an academic practice of a major research school of nursing, the PNN serves uniquely to demonstrate community-based practice fully integrated with education and research.

Brief Descriptions of Each Practice

Gerontologic Nursing Consultation Service (GNCS)/PNN Consulting provides education and consultation focusing on research-based care of older adults and a range of other fields, including academic nursing practice.

Hamburg. The PNN also provides women's health services to residents of the Hamburg Center in Hamburg, Pennsylvania, under contract with the Pennsylvania Department of Public Welfare.

The Health Annex at the Francis J. Myers Recreation Center is a result of a unique cooperative effort between the School of Nursing, the City of Philadelphia Department of Recreation, and community partners. The practice promotes health and wellness, identifies and treats illness, and delivers integrated primary and mental health services to a culturally diverse community. The **Health Corner at West Philadelphia Community Center**, a satellite of the Health Annex, provides primary care, gynecologic, family planning, teen, and women's health services.

Living Independently For Elders (LIFE) is a risk-based program providing integrated acute and long-term care services for frail older adults who are nursing home certifiable and prefer to live in the community. A comprehensive range of health and social services, provided by an interdisciplinary team, is available on a 24-hour basis, with adult day health centers serving as the focal point. The practice is a Medicare-certified PACE provider.

www.nursing.upenn.edu/clinicalpractice

Clinical Practice—Penn Nursing Network (2003).

clinical billing and collections, practice-specific contract negotiations and management, marketing, and so on, have gradually been moved to the individual practice level. School of Nursing and University resources are used/purchased for payroll management, human resources, legal, insurance and risk management, finance and accounting, development, public relations, and clinical/management information systems (Lang & Evans, 1999; Swan & Evans, 2001). Members of the school's board of overseers with health care interest and expertise have, since inception, voluntarily served in various capacities to advise and assist the practices. Revenue sources include, primarily, patient revenues (Medicare and Medicaid [fee for service and capitation], commercial insurance, managed care capitation, out of pocket, and service contracts), and, secondarily, public and private grants and gifts. Most practices are dependent on these latter sources during start-up, and thereafter to support new innovations in programming. After establishing appropriate levels of risk reserve, excess revenues over expenses generated by any one practice have been placed in a practice loan pool to be borrowed by other practices during their developmental phases. In addition, a line of credit was established within the University to permit planned operating shortfalls during start-up of new practices.

With University and foundation support, the Office for Research in Academic Practice (ORAP) was opened in 1997 to facilitate practice-based research (Lang, Jenkins, Evans, & Matthews, 1996). Clinical, financial, and administrative data from PNN practices were housed there for quality management and research purposes. Faculty and students could access databases on other populations of interest, tables of evidence on current clinical problem areas, and relevant electronic clinical research and quality management programs. The ORAP also centralized funded work on evidence-based reviews and guidelines, clinical information system development and refinement, collection of common data elements by primary care students and faculty, and Web-based, practice-oriented research projects.

Early Outcomes and the Challenge for the Future

As "living laboratories," Penn's academic practices have fostered and stimulated new developments in health care research, practice, and education. Development of new research methods suitable for evaluating practice outcomes in small, unique practice settings (Lang, Jenkins, Evans, & Matthews, 1996; Sochalski, 2001), comparing impacts on health-related quality of life in a range of living environments and services for frail elders (Naylor & Buhler-Wilkerson, 1999), scholarly leadership in database development within the National Nursing Centers Consortium, graduate-level courses in the business of nursing and health care informatics, and federal and state policy changes (Jenkins, 2002; Jenkins & Torrisi, 1995; Sullivan-Marx et al., 2000) have all evolved from the academic practices at the University of Pennsylvania School of Nursing.

Penn is the only school of nursing in the country to have operated a comprehensive outpatient rehabilitation facility (Evans, Yurkow, & Siegler,

1995) or a Program of All-Inclusive Care for the Elderly (Naylor & Buhler-Wilkerson, 1999). New models for community-based and interdisciplinary education are evolving (Salmon et al., 2000; University of Pennsylvania School of Nursing, 2002). In its short history, the PNN alone has yielded more than 60 scholarly publications, 11 research studies, and 10 national, regional, and local awards. The school's early leadership in clinical information system development for nursing practices (Marek et al., 1998), synergistic networking through the RNCC/NNCC and Penn Macy Fellows Initiative, and development of settings that facilitate research-based practice and policy change (Barnsteiner, 1996; Barnsteiner & Prevost, 2002; Lang, Sullivan-Marx, Jenkins, 1996; Sochalski, 2001) reflect a culture increasingly ready to embrace fully the practice arm of its mission.

The clinician educators have played a vital role in developing the practice mission at Penn, and the school's research centers are increasingly engaged in developing clinical research proposals that will employ the resources of the academic practices. The school provides national leadership in developing integrated academic practice models through the Penn Macy Initiative (PMI). Consisting initially of an intensive week-long conference, together with ongoing consultation and electronic networking, the PMI continues to offer an annual Penn Macy Institute: Academic Nursing Practice: Building the Evidence Base.

At this decisive moment in history, Penn School of Nursing remains uniquely poised to help move forward the discipline through academic nursing practice. A critical mass of seasoned and funded nurse scholars at Penn are producing clinically relevant research findings that are influencing practice on national and international levels. Nearly 150 advanced practice nurses are graduated each year, along with substantial numbers earning bachelor's and doctoral degrees. Faculty members have been instrumental in expanding scope of practice and reimbursement opportunities on a national and state level. And the school controls a small portfolio of innovative community-based and community-focused clinical settings, demonstrating economic and operational success. The academic practices of the school will increasingly serve as important vehicles for testing the implementation of clinical findings from nursing faculty research, seeking cost-effective ways to bring innovative programs to market, testing best practices, developing evidence-based care, and preparing students to practice in a new era in health care. Thus, albeit on a much different scale from that of the School of Medicine, the academic practices of the School of Nursing do feed its research and educational missions and provide limited financial resources for the school.

As academic medicine at the University of Pennsylvania launches more community-based initiatives, there exist opportunities for the School of

Nursing to partner and collaborate in new ways in reaching mutual service, education, and research goals. LIFE (PACE), certified to provide fully integrated primary, acute, and long term care services to a very frail group of elders in the community (see Table 25.2), is enabling the development and enhancement of such partnerships through the appointments of faculty from geriatric medicine to interdisciplinary practice and leadership teams and negotiation of service agreements for acute and specialty services with the UPHS. New opportunities for interdisciplinary research and education will follow. Now that the School of Nursing has moved toward maturity in its own tripartite mission, it brings a new level of parity to the table. That the value-added strengths of the school's academic practices can complement those in the health system, and vice versa, is increasingly recognized. Like academic medicine, nursing at Penn is at a critical juncture for review and recommitment. In recognition of the opportunities presented by major changes in national and regional health care structure and finance, the recent appointment of new deans in the Schools of Nursing and Medicine, changes in academic nursing practice leadership, and the presence of a more equal position "at the table" with our medical colleagues, the faculty are taking stock of where we have been and where we need to go, and developing new strategies for how to get there.

We believe that academic nursing practice, in its ability to integrate the tripartite mission, clearly represents a unique and powerful resource for nursing in the 21st century. Indeed, the discovery, demonstration and dissemination of scientific evidence that nursing makes an essential difference is dependent on academic practice. Schools of nursing must continue to develop and evolve their practice missions if nursing is to survive and thrive as a discipline and a profession.

REFERENCES

About Our Academic Nursing Practice. (2002–2003). Retrieved April 25, 3003 from http://www.pennmacy.com/practice/index.cfm

Aiken, L. H. (1992). Charting nursing's future. In L. H. Aiken & C. M. Fagin (Eds.), *Charting nursing's future: Agenda for the 1990s* (pp. 3–12). Philadelphia: Lippincott.

American Nurses Association. (2003). *NursingFacts*. Retrieved April 25, 3003 from http://www.nursingworld.org/readroom/fsdemogrpt.htm#summ

Anderko, L., & Kinion, E. (2001). Speaking with a unified voice: Recommendations for the collection of aggregated outcome data in nurse-managed centers. *Policy, Politics & Nursing Practice, 2*, 295–303.

Auerhahn, C. (1997). Columbia University School of Nursing faculty practice: A cross-site model. In L. N. Marion (Ed.), *Faculty practice: Applying the models* (pp. 65–72). Washington, DC: National Organization of Nurse Practitioner Faculties.

Baltzell, E. D. (1996). *Puritan Boston & Quaker Philadelphia*. New Brunswick: Transaction Publishers.

Barger, S. E., & Bridges, W. C. (1987). An assessment of academic nursing centers. *Nurse Educator, 15*(2), 31–36.

Barger, S. E., Nugent, K. E., & Bridges, W. C. (1993). Schools with nursing centers: A 5-year follow-up study. *Journal of Professional Nursing, 9,* 7–13.

Barnsteiner, J. H. (1996). Research-based practice. *Nursing Administration Quarterly, 20*(4), 52–58.

Barnsteiner, J., & Prevost, S. (2002). How to implement evidence-based practice. *Reflections on Nursing Leadership, 28*(2), 18–21.

Blumenthal, D., & Weissman, J. S. (2000). Selling teaching hospitals to investor-owned hospital chains: Three case studies. *Health Affairs, 19,* 158–166.

Boccuzzi, N. K. (1998). CAPNA: A new development to increase quality in primary care. *Nursing Administration Quarterly, 22*(4), 11–19.

Boyer, E. (1990). *Scholarship reconsidered: Priorities for the professoriate*. Princeton, NJ: The Carnegie Foundation for the Advancement of Teaching.

Broussard, A. B., Delahoussaye, C. P., & Poirrier, G. P. (1996). The practice role in the academic nursing community. *Journal of Nursing Education, 35*(2), 82–87.

Brown, M. A. (2001). Academic faculty practice: Enrichment through synergism. *Applied Nursing Research, 14*(1), 56–61.

Brown, S. A., & Grimes, D. E. (1995). A meta-analysis of nurse practitioners and nurse midwives in primary care. *Nursing Research, 44*(6), 332–339.

Brush, B. L., & Capezuti, E. A. (1996). Revisiting 'A nurse for all settings': The nurse practitioner movement, 1965–1995. *Journal of American Academy of Nurse Practitioners, 8*(1), 5–11.

Buhler-Wilkerson, K., Naylor, M., Holt, S., & Rinke, L. (1998). An alliance for academic home care. *Nursing Outlook, 46*(2), 77–90.

Burgener, S. C. (2001). Scholarship of practice for a practice profession. *Journal of Professional Nursing, 17*(10), 46–54.

Burns, C. E. (1997). Faculty clinical practice as a tenurable activity. In L. N. Marion (Ed.), *Faculty practice: Applying the models* (pp. 41–48). Washington, DC: National Organization of Nurse Practitioner Faculties.

Burondess, J. (1991). The academic health center and the public agenda: Whose three-legged stool? *Annals of Internal Medicine, 115,* 962.

Clinical Practice—Penn Nursing Network. (2003). Retrieved April 25, 2003 from http://www.nursing.upenn.edu/clinical_practices/

Coggiola, P., & Walker, P. H. (1995). Building an entrepreneurial multi-site autonomous practice in a rural community. In B. Murphy (Ed.), *Nursing centers: The time is now*. Pub. No. 41-2629. New York: National League for Nursing.

Conway-Welsh, C. (1995). At the table: Nursing in managed care. *Nursing Policy Forum, 1*(5), 10–16.

D'Alessandri, R. M., Albertsen, P., Atkinson, B. F., Dickler, R. M., Jones, R. F., Kirch, D. G., Longnecker, D. E., McArnarney, E. R., Parisi, V. M., Selby, S., Stapcznski, J. S., Thompson, J. W., Wasserman, A. G., & Zuza, K. L. (2000). Measuring contributions to the clinical mission of medical schools and teaching hospitals. *Academic Medicine, 75*(12), 1232–1237.

Evans, L. K. (1994). Overcoming intra-institutional challenges to collaborative practice. In E. Siegler & F. Whitney (Eds.), *Overcoming barriers to nurse-physician collaboration* (pp. 33–42). New York: Springer Publishing.

Evans, L. K., & Yurkow, J. (1999). Balanced Budget Act of 1997: Impact on a nurse-managed academic nursing practice for frail elders. *Nursing Economics, 17,* 280–282, 297.

Evans, L. K., Yurkow, J., & Siegler, E. (1995). The CARE Program: A nurse-managed collaborative outpatient program to improve function of frail elders. *Journal of the American Geriatrics Society, 43,* 1155–1160.

Fagin, C. M. (1986). Institutionalizing faculty practice. *Nursing Outlook, 34*(3), 140–144.

Fagin, C. (2000). *Essays on Nursing Leadership.* New York: Springer Publishing.

Fehring, R. J., Schulte, J., & Reisch, S. K. (1986). Toward a definition of nurse-managed centers. *Journal of Community Health Nursing, 3,* 59–67.

Frenn, M., Lundeen, S. P., Martin, K. S., Riesch, S. K., & Wilson, S. A. (1996). Symposium on nursing centers: Past, present and future. *Journal of Nursing Education, 35*(2), 54–62.

Gersten-Rothenberg, K. (1998). Should schools of nursing develop nursing centers? *Clinical Nurse Specialist, 12*(2), 59–63.

Grey, M., & Walker, P. H. (1998). Practice-based research networks for nursing. *Nursing Outlook, 46,* 125–129.

Hansen-Turton, T., & Kinsey, K. (2001). The quest for self-sustainability: Nurse-managed health centers meeting the policy challenge. *Policy, Politics & Nursing Practice, 2,* 304–309.

Hegyvary, S. T. (2001). Join the forum. *Journal of Nursing Scholarship, 33,* 304.

Henry, O. M. (1986). Demonstration centers for nursing practice, education and research. In M. D. Mezey & D. O. McGivern (Eds.), *Nurses, nurse practitioners: The evolution of primary care* (pp. 239–241). Boston: Little, Brown.

Hutelmyer, C. M., & Donnelly, G. F. (1996). Joint appointments in practice positions. *Nursing Administration Quarterly, 20*(4), 71–79.

Iglehart, J. K. (1995). Academic medical centers enter the market: The case of Philadelphia. *New England Journal of Medicine, 333,* 1019–1023.

Iowa Intervention Project. (1997). Proposal to bring nursing into the information age. *Image: Journal of Nursing Scholarship, 29*(3), 275–281.

Jenkins, M. (2002). Policy case study: Nurse-managed health centers. In D. J. Mason & J. K. Leavitt (Eds.), *Policy and politics in nursing and health care* (4th ed., pp. 87–91). Philadelphia: Saunders.

Jenkins, M., & Torrisi, D. (1995). Nurse practitioners, community nursing centers and contracting for managed care. *Journal of the American Academy of Nurse Practitioners, 7,* 1–6.

Jones, E. G., & VanOrt, S. (2001). Facilitating scholarship among clinical faculty. *Journal of Professional Nursing, 17*(3), 141–146.

Kalisch, P. A., & Kalisch, B. J. (1978). *The advances of American nursing.* Boston: Little, Brown & Co.

Karpf, M., Schultze, R. G., & Levey, G. (2000). The decade of the nineties at the UCLA Medical Center: Responses to dramatic marketplace changes. *Academic Medicine, 75*(8), 781–792.

Kerekes, J. J., Jenkins, M. L., & Torrisi, D. (1996). Nurse-managed primary care: Abbottsford Community Health Center. *Nursing Management, 27*(2), 44–47.

Krakower, J. Y., Coble, T. Y., Williams, D. J., & Jones, R. F. (2000). Review of US medical school finances, 1998–1999. *Journal of the American Medical Association, 284,* 1127–1129.

Krakower, J., Ganem, J., & Beran, R. L. (1994). Medical school financing: Comparing seven different types of schools. *Academic Medicine, 69,* 72–81.

Lang, N. (1996). Academic nursing practice: A case study of the University of Pennsylvania School of Nursing. *Penn Nursing: The Publication of the University of Pennsylvania School of Nursing, 1*(1), 17–19, 36.

Lang, N. M., & Evans, L. (1999). Case study: Forging new partnerships for financial development. In J. A. Ryan (Ed.), *Market-driven nursing* (pp. 115–124). Chicago: Health Forum.

Lang, N. M., Evans, L. K., & Swan, B. A. (2002). Penn Macy Initiative to Advance Academic Nursing Practice. *Journal of Professional Nursing, 18*(2), 63–69.

Lang, N. M., Jenkins, M., Evans, L. K., & Matthews, D. (1996). Administrative, financial, and clinical data for an academic nursing practice: A case study of the University of Pennsylvania School of Nursing. *The power of faculty practice* (pp. 79–100). Washington, DC: American Association of Colleges of Nursing.

Lang, N. M., Sullivan-Marx, E. M., & Jenkins, M. (1996). Advanced practice nurses and success of organized delivery systems. *American Journal of Managed Care, 11*(2), 129–135.

Lockhart, C. A. (1995). Community nursing centers: An analysis of status and needs. In B. Murphy (Ed.), *Nursing centers: The time is now* (pp. 1–88). Pub. No. 41-2629. New York: National League for Nursing Press.

Lynaugh, J., & Brush, B. (1996). *American nursing: From hospital to health system.* Cambridge: Blackwell Publishing.

Mackey, T. A., Adams, J., & McNiel, N. O. (1994). Nursing centers: Service as a business. *Nursing Economics, 12,* 276–279, 282.

Mackey, T. A., & McNiel, N. O. (1997). Negotiating private sector partnerships with academic nursing centers. *Nursing Economics, 15*(1), 52–55.

MacLeod, G. K., & Schwarz, M. R. (1986). Faculty practice plans. *Journal of the American Medical Association, 256,* 58–62.

Macnee, C. L. (1999). Integrating teaching, research, and practice in a nurse-managed clinic. *Nurse Educator, 24*(3), 25–28.

Marek, K. D., Jenkins, M., Westra, B. L., & McGinley, A. (1998). Implementation of a clinical information system in nurse-managed care. *Canadian Journal of Nursing Research, 30*(1), 37–44.

Marion, L. N. (Ed.). (1997). *Faculty practice: Applying the models.* Washington, DC: National Organization of Nurse Practitioner Faculties.

Mezey, M., Lynaugh, J., & Cartier, M. (1988). A report card on faculty practice: The Robert Wood Johnson Teaching Nursing Home Program, 1982–87. *Nursing Outlook, 36,* 285–288.

Mundinger, M. O., Kane, R. L., Lenz, E. R., Totten, A. M., Tsai, W., Cleary, P. D., Friedewald, W. T., Siu, A. L., & Shelandski, M. L. (2000). Primary care outcomes in patients treated by nurse practitioners or physicians: A randomized trial. *Journal of the American Medical Association, 283,* 59–68.

National Institute of Nursing Research. (n.d.). *NINR Congressional Justification 2004* (p. 12). Retrieved April 25, 2003 from http://www.nih.gov/ninr/about/legislation/CJ2004.pdf

National Nursing Centers consortium. (2002). About vision, mission, goals. Retrieved April 25, 2003 from http://www.nationalnursingcenters.org/NNCC_About/VMG/VisionMissionGoals.htm

Naylor, M. D., & Buhler-Wilkerson, K. (1999). Creating community-based care for the new millennium. *Nursing Outlook, 47*(3), 120–127.

Nicholson, S. (2002). The effects of Medicare payment subsidies to teaching hospitals. *LDI Issue Brief, 7*(4), 1–4.

NIH Awards to Health professional Components FY 2001: Nursing. (n.d.). Retrieved April 25, 2003 from http://grants1.nih.gov/grants/award/trends/dhenrsg01.htm

Nonnemaker, L., & Griner, P. F. (2001). The effects of a changing environment on relationships between medical schools and their parent universities. *Academic Medicine, 76*(1), 9–18.

Norbeck, J. S. (1998). Teaching, research, and service: Striking the balance in doctoral education. *Journal of Professional Nursing, 14,* 197–205.

Norbeck, J. S., & Taylor, D. L. (1999). Faculty practice. In E. J. Sullivan (Ed), *Creating nursing's future* (pp. 125–136). St Louis: Mosby.

Nugent, K. E., Barger, S. E., & Bridges, W. C. (1993). Facilitators and inhibitors of practice: A faculty perspective. *Journal of Nursing Education, 32,* 293–300.

Pearson, L. J. (2002). Annual update of how each state stands on legislative issues affecting advanced nursing practice. *Nurse Practitioner, 27*(1), 10–22.

Pohl, J. M., Bostrom, A. C., Talarczyk, G., & Cavanagh, S. (2001). Development of an academic consortium for nurse-managed primary care. *Nursing and Health Care Perspectives, 22,* 308–313.

Potash, M., & Taylor, D. (1993). *Nursing faculty practice: Models and methods.* Washington, DC: National Organization of Nurse Practitioner Faculties.

Reed, D. (1997). The development of a community-based, nurse managed practice network by the University of Pennsylvania School of Nursing. In *The Third*

National Primary Care Conference Case Studies (pp. 229–140). Washington, DC: HRSA.

Regional Nursing Centers Consortium. (2000). *Nurse-managed health centers: Leaders for healthy neighborhoods*. Philadelphia: Author.

Reinhardt, U. E. (2000). Academic medicine's financial accountability and responsibility. *Journal of the American Medical Association, 284*(9), 1136–1138.

Reverby, S. M. (1987). *Ordered to care: The dilemma of American nursing, 1850–1945*. Cambridge, MA: Cambridge University Press.

Risse, G. B. (1999). *Mending bodies, saving souls: A history of hospitals*. New York: Oxford University Press.

Rodgers, K. W., Zuckerman, L., & Goode, T. (2000, December 4). An overview of academic medical centers. *Standard & Poor's Credit Week Municipal* (pp. 9–15).

Rodin, J. (2001). Proposal to create Penn Medicine. *University of Pennsylvania Almanac, 48*(12), 1–3.

Rubin, E. R. (1998). Making sense of the tenure debate. In E. R. Rubin (Ed.), *Mission management: A new synthesis* (pp. 187–216). Washington, DC: Association of Academic Health Centers.

Rudy, E. B. (2001). Supportive work environments for nursing faculty. *AACN Clinical Issues, 12,* 401–410.

Rudy, E. B., Anderson, N. A., Dudjak, L., Robert, S. N., & Miler, R. A. (1995). Faculty practice: Creating a new culture. *Journal of Professional Nursing, 11,* 78–83.

Salmon, M., Cotroneo, M., Couch-Jones, M. A., Mark, H., Hennrich, M. L., & Mood, L. (2000). Community-based nursing leadership curriculum: Planning for the future health of communities (Abstract #2939). *American Public Health Association 128th Annual Meeting*, Boston.

Sawyer, M. J., Alexander, I. M., Gordon, L., Juszczak, L. J., & Gilliss, C. (2000). A critical review of current nursing faculty practice. *Journal of American Academy of Nurse Practitioners, 12,* 511–516.

Schwartz, A. (2001). Collaborative practice and research: Making the link to patient care. *UCSF Science of Caring, 13*(2), 110–119.

Sochalski, J. A. (2001). Outcomes of a nurse-managed geriatric day hospital (Special Issue I). *Gerontologist, 41,* 51.

Spitzer, R., Bandy, C., Bumbalough, M., Frederiksen, D., Gibson, G., Howard, E., McIntosh, E., Pitts, V. N. & Reeves, G. (1996). Marketing and reimbursement of faculty-based practice. *Nursing & Health Care, 17,* 309–311.

Split decision. (2001). *NurseWeek*, April 16. Retrieved April 25, 2003 from http://www.nurseweek.com/news/features/01-04/splitdecision.asp

Sullivan-Marx, E. .M., Happ, M. B., Bradley, K. J., & Maislin, G. (2000). Nurse practitioner services: Content and relative work value. *Nursing Outlook, 48,* 269–275.

Swan, B. A., & Evans, L. K. (2001). Infrastructure to support academic nursing practice. *Nursing Economics, 19*(2), 68–71.

Taylor, D. (1996). Faculty practice: Uniting advanced nursing practice and education. In A. B. Hamric, J. A. Spross, & C. M. Hanson (Eds.), *Advanced nursing practice: An integrative approach*. Philadelphia: Saunders.

Taylor, D., & Marion, L. (2000). Innovative practice models: Uniting advanced nursing practice and education. In A. Hamric, J. Spross, & C. Hanson (Eds.), *Advanced nursing practice: An integrative approach* (2nd ed., pp. 795–831). Philadelphia: Saunders.

Thwing, M. D. (1919). The university public health nursing district in Cleveland. *The Public Health Nurse, 11,* 362–365.

Turner, B. (1989). Future role of academic centers. *Health Care Management Review, 14,* 73–77.

University of Pennsylvania School of Medicine (2000). *The Faculty-2000 Project: Final report.* Philadelphia: Author.

University of Pennsylvania School of Nursing (2002). Practice. *Penn Nursing, 5*(1), 6.

University of Wisconsin—Milwaukee School of Nursing. (2002). *Welcome from Sally Lundeen.* Retrieved April 25, 2003 from http://www.uwm.edu/Dept/Nursing/deanwelc.htm

Vincent, D., Oakley, D., Pohl, J., & Walker, D. S. (2000). Survival of nurse-managed centers: The importance of cost analysis. *Outcomes Management for Nursing Practice, 4*(3), 124–128.

Walker, P. H. (1995). Faculty practice: Interest, issues, and impact. In J. Fitzpatrick & J. Stevenson (Eds.), *Annual review of nursing research* (pp. 217–235). New York: Springer Publishing.

Walsh, M. S. (1920). A teaching district in St. Louis. *Public Health Nurse, 13,* 994–996.

Zachariah, R., & Lundeen, S. P. (1997). Research and practice in an academic community nursing center. *Image: The Journal of Nursing Scholarship, 29,* 255–260.

INDEX

Abbottsford Community Health
    Center, 324–326
Abuse, 409–411
Academic discipline
    historical perspective, 74–76
    primary care, 65–82
Academic medicine
    historical review, 444–446
Academic nursing practice, 443–464
    defined, 449–454
    historical review, 444–449
    models, 450–454
    reenvisioning, 443–444
    sociopolitical forces, 448–449
Acceptance of nurse practitioners,
    see Recognition
Accountability, 44–47; *see also*
    Recognition; Standardization
Accreditation; *see also* Credentialing;
    Licensure
    National League for Nursing, 76–77
    program for modern nurse
        anesthesia education, 272–273
Acupuncture, 236
Acute care, 97–98, 135–147
Acute care of the elderly (ACE) units,
    203
Acute care nurse practitioners
    (ACNP), 135–147
    allied health, 145
    educational preparation, 136–138
    interdisciplinary health care team,
        141–143
    medical colleagues, 143–144

other acute care nurse practitioners
    (ACNP), 145
patient care, 141–143
physician consultants, 144
practice privileges, 140–141
role, 138–141
scope of practice and standards,
    135–136
service-based, 140
unit-based, 139
Veterans Administration, 290–291
Adolescent family practice, 376–388
    characteristics and components,
        377–379
    collaborative practice issues,
        381–383
    consultation and referral,
        379–380
    primary care practice perception,
        384–386
    research findings, 383–384
    teaching program, 380–381
Advanced practice acts, 43, 305,
    417–418
Advanced practice holistic nursing,
    238–247
Advanced practice nurses (APN)
    acute care services, 135–147
    defined, 305
    discharge planning, 112–113
    home care, 160
    long-term care
        need, 160–162
    long-term outcomes, 108–128

Advanced practice nurses (APN)
   (*continued*)
  managed care, 150–163
    ambulatory care, 158–159
    settings, 156–160
  preparation and clinical practice,
    3–36
  projections, 156
  school-based health care, 166–188
  statistics, 156
  vs. physicians
  benchmarking, 96–97
Advanced practice nursing
  defined, 3–5
  financial and professional
    recognition, 11
  future, 25–29
  history, 3–5
  internalization extension, 27
  philosophical and historical role
    bases, 37–62
  preparation and clinical practice,
    3–29
  vs. clinical nurse specialists
    curriculum, 17
  workforce realities and projections,
    5–9
Advocacy, 67
Air and Surface Transport Nurses
    Association (ASTNA), 423
Alabama, 311
Alaska, 311, 423
Alcoholic client
  care of, 114, 197, 225–228
Ambulatory setting for APNs, 93,
    158–159, 357–361
American Academy of Nurse
    Practitioners (AANP), 309, 425
  certification, 307
American Association of Colleges of
    Nursing (AACN), 421
American Association of Critical Care
    Nurses (AACCN), 136
American Association of Nurse
    Anesthetists (AANA), 272

American Association of Occupational
    Health Nurses (AAOHN), 423
American Association of Poison
    Control Centers (AAPCC), 423
American College of Nurse Midwifery
    (ACNM), 23
  certification council, 254
American College of Nurse Midwives
    Certification Council, 425
American College of Nurse
    Practitioners (ACNP), 408
American Holistic Nurses' Association
    (AHNA), 249
  Standards of Advanced Holistic
    Nursing Practice for Graduate
    Prepared Nurses, 238, 240–241
American Holistic Nurses Certification
    Corporation (AHNCC), 249
American Nurses Association (ANA),
    51, 136, 316, 400, 408, 423
  Code of Ethics for Nurses, 325
  Scope and Standards of Advanced
    Practice Nursing, 325
  Scope and Standards of Psychiatric-
    Mental Health Nursing Practice,
    223–224
American Nurses' Credentialing
    Center (ANCC), 218, 309, 425
Anesthesia practice arena, 278–281
Arizona, 311, 423
Arkansas, 307
Assembly for School-Based Health
    Centers, 187
Association of Faculties of Pediatric
    Nurse Practitioner and
    Associate Programs, 421–422
Asthma
  research, 110
ASTNA, 423
Atherosclerosis, 114
AUDIT, 226
Authority of nurse practitioners, 39,
    41–47, 52; *see also* Licensure;
    Recognition; Reimbursement
Autonomy, 39, 41–47

Balanced Budget Act of 1997, 314–316, 335
Beliefs, 244
Benchmarking
    advanced practice nurses *vs.* physicians, 96–97
Billing challenges to APNs, 374, 402; *see also* Reimbursement
Biological science
    mental health, 217–218
Botulinum injections
    research, 111
Bureau of Primary Health Care (BPHC), 329

CAGE questionnaire, 226
Cardiovascular disease risk factors, 114–115
Carlisle, George W., 272
Case management, 291–292
Case managers, 145, 223
Center for Health Outcomes and Policy Research
    University of Pennsylvania, 438–439
Center for Medicare and Medicaid Services, 408
Central Florida Health Care Coalition, 152
Certification, 305–311, 424–426
    Council on Certification of Nurse Anesthetists, 310
Certified nurse-midwives (CNM), 70, 254–265, 307, 402–403
Certified registered nurse anesthetists (CRNA), 70, 272, 279–281, 307, 402–403
CHAMPUS, 316, 406
Chronic obstructive pulmonary disease (COPD), 111
Cigna, 152
Civilian Health and Medical Program of the Uniformed Services (CHAMPUS), 316, 406
Clinical nurse specialists (CNS), 17, 218

Clinical practice, 435
    advanced practice nursing, 3–29
    holistic nursing, 250
Clinical practicum, 137
Clinical preceptors, 137
Clinical rotations, 138
Clinical scholarship
    criteria, 453
Clinical staff
    development, 146
Clinical success, 93
Clinical thinking, 58
Clinton Administration, 178
Collaboration; *see also* Recognition; Reimbursement
    of APN and physician, 26–27
    future, 26–27
    practice agreements, 312, 336–339
    practice of, 376–388
    school outcomes, 184–185
Collaborative Assessment and Rehabilitation for Elders (CARE), 200
Columbia Advanced Practice Nurse Associates (CAPNA), 159
Commission on Collegiate Nursing Education (CCNE), 23
Communication
    holistic, 243
Community-based practice
    alcohol abuse, 227–228
    health care agencies, 6
    interventions for, 114–117
    outpatient clinics (CBOC), 289
    primary care of elderly, 192–207
    support of school-based student health centers, 246–247
Community Health Accreditation Program (CHAP), 23
Community Nursing Organization (CNO), 200
Compensation, *see* Payment
Competency, 86, *169t–170t*

Competition, 86–89, 91–92; *see also*
    Managed Care; Recognition;
    Reimbursement
Complementary and alternative
    medicine, 294–295; *see also*
    Holistic nursing
Complementary/integrative health
    care, 235–237
Comprehensive geriatric assessment,
    196–198
Consultation by nurse practitioners,
    379–380
Consultations, 223–224, 340
Consumer health education, 176
Continuing education
    modern nurse anesthesia education,
    277–278
Controlled substances
    prescribing, 311–312
Conventional/allopathic and holistic
    perspectives of care, *240t*
Coordination of care, 93
Coronary artery bypass graft (CABG),
    110, 115
Corporatization in health care, 13–14;
    see also Managed care
Cost, 90–91, 93, 121, 193–194, 236
Cost-effectiveness of nurse
    practitioners, 89–94, 122–124;
    see also Effectiveness of nurse
    practitioners
Cost-utility analysis, 124
Council on Certification of Nurse
    Anesthetists, 310
Credentialing, 22–24, 51, 308–311,
    426–427; *see also* Licensure;
    Recognition
*Criteria for Evaluation of Nurse
    Practitioner Programs,* 421
Culturally based care, 18,
    243–244
Current Procedure Terminology
    (CPT), 55–56, 398
Curriculum of APN programs, 16–20,
    258; *see also* Education

Decision-making process, 382
Delaware, 423
Department of Defense, 288
Depression, 110–111, 328
Developmental assessments, 175
Developmental progress, 176
Diabetes mellitus, 110, 158
*Diagnostic and Statistical Manual
    of Mental Disorders,* 220
Disaster response, 28–29
Discharge planning effectiveness,
    112–113; *see also* Effectiveness
    of nurse practitioners
Disease prevention, 196–198
Disease-specific model, 203
Distance learning, 168, 288
District of Columbia, 311
Diversity, 8
Drug Enforcement Administration
    (DEA), 311–312

Early nurse anesthesia education
    program, 272
Economics in health care
    environment, 8–10
Education, 56–58, 168, 288, 434–435;
    see also Recognition;
    Reimbursement
    of certified nurse-midwives,
    257–258
    health, *see* Health education
    higher, 14–24
    holistic, 240–242
    for holistic nursing, 248–249
    medical, 74–76
    of nurse anesthetists, 272–278
    nursing, 434–435
    practice, 24–25
    for primary care, 65–82
    professional, 14, 16–22
    of psychiatric-mental health APNs,
    220, 224–225
    reunited with practice, 447–448
    self-care, 260
    standards for, 52

Effectiveness of nurse practitioners
  in geriatric care, 192–214
  impetus to enhance, 10–11
  in managed care settings, 156–160
  research in support of, 84–107
  in school-based health care,
    166–188
E-health, 28
Eisenberg, D. M., 236–237
Elderly, 192–214
  assessment of, 114, 196–198
  cost of care, 193–194
  demographics of, 193–194
  health promotion to, 196–198
  health services for, 193–194
  hospital-based primary care, 201–204
  nursing home care, 204–205
  palliative care, 205–206
  primary care models, 199–206
Elementary schools, 178
Emergency departments
  acutely ill children
    research, 111
  emergency nurse practitioners
    vs. physicians, 143
Emergency managed care systems, 195
Emotional and behavioral disorders,
    173
Employee Incentive Scholarship
    Program (EISP), 288
Employee support programs, 295
Employment
  contracts, 318–319
  difficulties, 433–437
Equal Rights Amendment
  lack of nursing support, 49
Essentials of Master's Education for
    Advanced Practice Nursing, 421
Ethics
  holistic, 238–240
EverCare Program, 205
Expenditures, see Cost

Facilitators in academic nursing
    practice, 451–454

Faculty in advanced nursing practice
    programs, 20–21, 449
Fagin, Claire, 456
False Claims Act, 410
Family Educational Rights and Privacy
    Act (FERPA), 172
Family nurse practitioners, 321–330
Federal Bureau of Primary Care, 178
Federal Employees Health Benefit Plan
    (FEHBP), 406
Federally qualified health centers,
    324, 329, 405
Fee-for service plans, 317
Financial and professional recognition
    of APNs, 11
Florida, 311
Fraud, 280, 409–411
Frontier Nursing Service, 84–85
Funding for nursing education, 21–22

General practitioners, 74–75
Geriatric care, 158, 192–214
Geriatric evaluation and management
    units, 201
Geriatric nurse practitioners (GNP),
    160, 355–357
Gerontologic advanced practice nurses
    (GAP), 203
Gerontologic nursing, 198–199
Gerontology/extended care centers,
    295–296
Globalization, 27
Graduate Medical Education, Nursing,
    and Allied Professions
    Commission (GMENAC), 90
Graduate prepared holistic nurse, 238
Graham, Dinah, 271
Graham, Edith, 271
Gross domestic product (GDP), 152
Guide to Clinical Preventive Services,
    197

Handicapped Children's Act, 173
Harvard Pilgrim Health Care, 153
Healers in operating rooms, 236

Health care, 8–14, 100, 151–152, 166–188
Health Care Common Procedural Coding System (HCPCS), 399
Health Care Professional Advisory Committee (HCPAC), 400
Health centers
 nurse-managed, 321–330
Health education, 176–177, 258–259
Health insurance, 317, 373–374, 405–406
Health Insurance Portability and Privacy Act (HIPPA), 172, 316, 409–410
Health maintenance organizations (HMO), 151
HealthPACT, 176
Health promotion, 196–198
Health Resources and Services Administration (HRSA), 178, 329
Health screening, 261–262
Healthy People, 196, 256
Healthy People 2010, 166
Healthy Rewards, 152
HeartCare, 128
Heart Failure Program, 157–158
HEDIS, 159
Heide, Wilma S., 50
HELP, 201–202
Henderson, Virginia, 51
Henry Street Settlement, 50, 76
Hill-Burton Act, 75
HIPPA, 172, 316, 409–410
HIV, 116
HMO, 151
Hodgins, Agatha, 272
Holistic nursing, 233–252
 advanced practice, 238–247
 clinical practice, 250
 education, 248–249
 issues, 247–251
 policy, 250–251
 research, 249–250
Home care, 296–297, 333–346
 advanced practice nurses, 160

 case vignettes, 342–346
 physician–nurse practitioner relationships, 362–364
 replacing hospitalization, 111
Hospital Elder Life Program (HELP), 201, 202
Hospitals
 advanced practice nurses and managed care, 156–158
 financing growth, 75
 home support replacing, 111
 managed care, 154–155
 primary care for older adults, 201–204
 traditional nursing role, 95–96
House calls, 334–335
Human immunodeficiency virus (HIV), 116

Idaho, 418, 423
IDEA, 166
Imagery, 236
Indemnity plans, 317, 406–407
Independent activities of daily living (IADL), 114
Independent practice association (IPA), 393
Individuals with Disabilities Education Act (IDEA), 166
Infants, 112–113, 115
Innovations, quality and cost, 89–94
Insurance, 317, 405–406
Integrated Health Care Consortium, 247
Interdisciplinary practice, 26–27, 141–143, 224
International Classification of Diseases (ICD), 399
Internet, 28, 127–128, 423
Iowa, 311, 423

Jackson, Charles T., 270
Joint Commission on Accreditation of Healthcare Organizations (JCAHO), 23, 146

Journal of Alternative Medicine, 235
*Journal of the American Medical
    Association,* 236

Kaiser-Permanente, 159
Kentucky, 311
Kissick, William, 89
Knowledge, 41–47, 57

Learning, *see* Education
Legal issues and advance practice
    nursing, 42, 55–56, 361, 420
Licensure, 306–311, 417–423; *see also*
    Credentialing; Recognition
    interstate, 423
    interstate nurse, 423
    second, 305–307
LIFE, 404
Living Independently for Elders
    (LIFE), 404
Long, Crawford W., 270
Long-term care need for advanced
    practice nurses, 160–162
Long-term outcomes for advanced
    practice nurses, 108–128

Magaw, Alice, 271
Maine, 311, 423
Malpractice claims, 361
Managed care, 10, 150–163, 317, 324,
    393–395, 435
    and advanced practice nursing,
        150–163
    background, 151
    challenges presented by, 162–163
    defined, 150–151
    future, 153, 163
    impact on employers, 154
    impact on health care providers,
        154–155
    impact on hospitals, 154–155
    present, 152–153
Maraldo, Pam, 50
Maryland, 423
Masters, 7

Maternal Child Health (MCH), 178
Mayo, Charles H., 271
Mayo, William W., 271
Medicaid, 158, 314, 324, 404–405
Medical education
    historical perspective, 74–76
Medicare, 314–316, 396–403,
    407–411
    fee schedule, 398
    fraud, 280
    part B, 401–403, 408–409
Medicare and Medicaid Patient
    Protection Act, 410
Medicare+Choice organizations, 403
Medicare Professional Advisory
    Committee, 408
Medicine's Dilemmas, 89
Meditation, 236
Mental health–psychiatric advanced
    practice nursing, 215–229
Michigan, 423
Midwest Regional Nursing Centers
    Consortium (MRNCC), 453
Military health insurance, 405–406
Mississippi, 311
Missouri, 311
Mobile health and wellness program,
    297–298
Montana, 311
Moral authority, 55
Morton, William T., 270
Mount Sinai Hospital-New York City
    Visiting Doctors Program, 160

National Association of Pediatric
    Nurse Practitioners (NAPNP),
    423
National Center for Complementary
    and Alternative Medicine
    (NCCAM), 235
National Center for Quality Assurance
    (NCQA), 186
National Certification Board of
    Pediatric Nurse Practitioners,
    309, 424–425

National Certification Corporation (NCC), 310
National Commission for Certifying Agencies (NCAA), 307
National Council of State Boards of Nursing (NCSBN), 5, 306, 416, 419
National League for Nursing Accreditation Commission (NLNAC), 23
National League for Nursing (NLN), 76–77
National Nurse Executive Council (NNEC), 287
National Nurses Response Team, 29
National Nursing Centers Consortium (NNCC), 329
National Organization for Women (NOW), 50
National Organization of Nurse Practitioner Faculty (NONPF), 421, 454
National Provider Identifier (NPI), 316
National Task Force on Quality Nurse Practitioner Education, 421
Nebraska, 423
Neighborhood-based nursing centers, 453
New England Journal of Medicine, 92
New Hampshire, 311
New Jersey, 423
New Mexico, 311
New York, 307, 418
Nightingale, Florence, 42–43, 51
North Carolina, 423
North Dakota, 423
Nurse anesthetists, 269–275
  certification of, 310
  education of, 272–278
  future of, 282
  historical context, 270–275
  professionalism organization, 272–273
  research arena for, 281

Nurse Education Act, 22
Nurse executive, 299
Nurse Improving Care to Health Systems Elders (NICHE), 203
Nurse-midwives, 84–85, 254–265
  curriculum for, 258
  defined, 256
  future of, 265
  and health education, 258–259
  and primary health care, 254–265
Nurse practitioners
  acceptance of, 4, 88, 360–361
  case load of, 357–361
  in emergency care, 143
  in family care, 324–325
  in geriatric care, 160, 355–357
  in pediatric care, 168
  preparatory programs for, 4–5
  relationships with physicians, 355–365
  research supporting, 84–102
  role in acute care, 97–98
  scheduling visits, 359
  in school based environments, 178–184
  status of, 305–319
  in surgical intensive care unit, 347–354
  unique contributions of, 93
Nurse Reinvestment Act, 9
Nurses' Association of the American College of Obstetricians and Gynecologists, 424
Nursing
  academic, 446–447
  definition of, 51
  development, 76–77
  discipline, 46–47
  and knowledge, 41–47
  nature of, 78–81
  shortage of, 8, 95
Nursing homes, 160–161, 204–205, 362
Nursing Systems Toward Effective Parenting-Preterm (NSTEP-P), 116

Occupational category, 39
Older adults, *see* Elderly
Oregon, 311
Outcomes research, 96–99
Outpatient services, 289, 299–300

Payment, 292–294, 391–411
Pediatrician–pediatric nurse practitioner
    relationships, 367–375
Pediatric nurse practitioner (PNP), 168
Pension from Veterans Administration,
    292–294
PEW Memorial Trust, 378
Philosophy, Conceptual Model, Terminal
    Competencies for the Education
    of Pediatric Nurse Practitioners,
    421–422
Physician extenders, 432, 435
Physician Payment Review
    Commission (PPRC), 397
Physicians
    compared to advanced practice
        nurses, 96–97, 143
    as consultants for acute care nurse
        practitioners, 144
    in entrepreneurial practice
        relationships with nurse
        practitioners, 60
    and managed care, 154
    nurse practitioner perceptions of, 95
    and oversupply of specialist, 81
    relationships with nurse
        practitioners, 355–365
        ambulatory practice, 357–361
        geriatricians *vs.* geriatric nurse
            practitioners, 355–357
        home care, 362–364
        nursing home care, 362
        pediatrician-pediatric nurse
            practitioner, 367–375
Planned Parenthood, 50
Power, 47–49, 58–61
Practice
    acute care, 97–98, 135–147
    education, 24–25

family practice, 324–325
future opportunities, 26
gerontologic, 158, 192–214, 355–357
health maintenance organizations,
    151
home care, 333–346
long-term care facilities, 160–162
managed care, 393–395
neighborhood health clinics, 454
nursing homes, 204–205
outpatient clinics, 289, 299–300
privileges for acute care nurse
    practitioners, 140–141
protocols for, 312–313
psychiatric-mental health, 215–229
public health agencies, 76
schools, 166–188
selecting, 318
Prescriptive privileges, 66, 287,
    311–312, 420; *see also*
    Licensure; Recognition
Primary care
    as an academic discipline, 65–82
    defined, 40–41
    as an emergency managed care
        system, 195
    future of, 386–387
    home-based, 296–297
    hospital-based for older adults,
        201–204
    model for mental health care, 216,
        218
    models for older adults, 199–206
    and nurse-managed delivery clinics,
        289
    and nurse-midwifery, 254–265
    and nursing education, 79–80
    for older adults, 192–207
    perception of, 384–386
    and research, 113–114
    shortage of physicians for, 432–433
    for women, 264
        model, 259–264
Primary Care Nurse Practitioner
    Competencies, 421

Professionalism, 45–49
Program of All-Inclusive Care for the
    Elderly (PACE), 158–159, 200,
    403–404, 463
Protest, 47–49
Psychiatric–mental health advanced
    practice nursing, 215–229
Public health nursing, 76
Public housing residents, 322–323

Quality Cost Model of Clinical
    Specialist Transitional Care,
    112–113
Quality improvement, 18, 90–91;
    see also Accountability

Recertification
    modern nurse anesthesia education,
        277–278
Recognition, 68
    by international community, 72
Recognition of advanced practice
    nursing; see also Managed care;
    Reimbursement
    financial and professional, 11
    historical acceptance, 37–64
    by managed care, 150–163
    of nurse-midwives, 84–85, 254–265
    practice privileges, 140–144
    prescriptive privileges, 66, 287,
        311–312, 420
    of psychiatric mental health, 219–221
    by state nurse practice acts, 43, 305,
        417–418
Regional Nursing Centers Consortium,
    see National Nursing Centers
    Consortium (NNCC)
Regulation, 416–417
Reiki, 236
Reimbursement, 313–317, 391–414;
    see also CHAMPUS; Cost;
    Managed Care; Medicaid;
    Medicare; Payment; Salaries
    for care of elderly, 193–194
    for CNMs and CRNAs, 402–403

coding and classification systems,
    399
of commercial health insurance,
    317, 373–374, 405–406
direct, 66, 71
nurses, 66
of psychiatric mental health, 219–221
Relative Value Update Committee
    (RUC), 400
Research, 84–107
    acceptability of, 95
    condition/symptom interventions,
        109–110
    examples of long-term outcomes,
        109–117
    future of, 100–101
    historical context of, 99–100
    holistic, 240–242, 249–250
    innovations, quality and cost, 89–94
    and nurse anesthetists, 281
    role of psychiatric–mental health
        advanced practice nursing,
        224–225
    roles advanced practice psychiatric-
        mental health nursing, 224–225
    supporting nurse practitioners,
        84–102
Resource-based relative value scale
    (RBRVS), 397, 399–401
Roles
    of acute care nurse practitioners,
        37–64, 138–141
    philosophical and historical bases
        for, 37–62

Safety net providers, 329–331
Salaries, 392–393
Sanger, Margaret, 50
School-based health care, 166–188
School-based student health centers
    (SBHC), 178–184
    access to care, 180–181
    collaboration, 184–185
    community support, 179–180
    financing, 185–186

future, 186–187
outcomes evaluation, 182–184
student usage patterns, 181–182
School nurse practitioner
competency guidelines, *169t–170t*
conceptual framework, 174–176,
175f
educational preparation, 167–171
educational preparation guidelines,
171t
future, 177
health education, 176–177
role, functions, and effectiveness,
172–174
*Scope and Standards of Advanced
Practice Nursing (ANA)*, 325
*Scope and Standards of Psychiatric-
Mental Health Nursing Practice
(ANA)*, 223–224
Second licensure, 305–307
Self-care, 255, 260
Self-referral, 411
Sexism, 49
Skilled nursing facility (SNF), 160–161
South Dakota, 423
Standardization; *see also*
Credentialing; Licensure
demands of credentialing, 9, 22–24
of education for nurse practitioners,
52
of nurse-midwives curriculum,
257–258
*Standards and Scope of Gerontologic
Nursing Practice*
American Nurses Association
(ANA), 198
*Standards and Scope of Gerontologic
Nursing Practice*, 198
*Standards of Advanced Holistic Nursing
Practice for Graduate Prepared
Nurses*, 238, 240–241
Stark laws, 411
State boards of nursing, 421
State Child Health Insurance Program
(SCHIP), 185–186

State nurse practice acts, 43, 305,
417–418; *see also* individual
states
Statistical methods in nursing
outcomes research, 125–126
Status, *see* Recognition
Surgical intensive care unit nurse
practitioner, 347–354
characteristics and components of,
351–352
current clinical practice of, 352–353
role of, 348–351

Tax Equity and Fiscal Responsibility
Act (TEFRA), 280
Teaching hospital, 445–446
Telehealth, 19, 423
Telenursing, 423
Tennessee, 419
Texas, 311, 423
Therapeutic touch, 236
Thompson Women's Primary Health
Care Model, 262–264
Torrisi, Donna, 324
Traditional authority, 42
Transitional care model, 202
Tricare, 405–406

Uniformed Services University of the
Health Sciences (USUHS), 288
Uninsured, 12, 181
University of Colorado Health
Sciences Center school nurse
practitioner program, 167–168
University of Pennsylvania academic
practice development, 438–464
U.S. Department of Veterans Affairs
acute care nurse practitioners
(ACNP), 290–291
case management, 291–292
complementary and alternative
medicine, 294–295
nurse practitioner roles, 289–299
U.S. Preventive Services Taskforce, 197
Utah, 311, 423

Values, 244
Vanderbilt Medical Center Heart
    Failure Program, 157–158
Veterans, 114
Veterans Integrated Service Network
    (VISN), 201, 289
Visiting Doctors Program of Mount
    Sinai Hospital-New York City,
    160
Visiting Nurse Association (VNA) of
    Greater Philadelphia, 335–340
  clinician perspectives, 339–340
  collaborative practice agreements,
    336–339
  consultations, 340
  day-to-day operations, 337–340
  patient perspectives, 337–340
Visiting Nurse Service, 76
Visiting Nurse Service of New York
    (VNSNY), 200

Wald, Lillian, 50, 76
Washington, 311
Wattleton, Fay, 50
Wells, Horace, 270
White House Commission on
    Complementary and Alternative
    Medicine Policy (WCHHAMP),
    237, 247
Wisconsin, 311, 423
Women
  primary health care for, 254–267
Women's Health, Obstetric and
    Neonatal Nurses, 109
Workforce
  policy perspectives, 431–440
  realities and projections for
    advanced practice nursing, 5–9
Worth
  research proving, 84–89
Wyoming, 311